PHYSIOLOGY OF THE HEART AND CIRCULATION

Fourth Edition

Physiology of the Heart and Circulation

Fourth Edition

Robert C. Little, M.D.

Professor, Department of Physiology and Endocrinology
Professor, Department of Medicine
School of Medicine
Medical College of Georgia
Augusta, Georgia

William C. Little, M.D.

Associate Professor
Division of Cardiology
Department of Medicine
Bowman Gray School of Medicine
Wake Forest University
Winston-Salem, North Carolina

YEAR BOOK MEDICAL PUBLISHERS, INC.
CHICAGO • LONDON • BOCA RATON

2   3   4   5   6   7   8   9   0   MR   93   92   91   90   89

LIBRARY OF CONGRESS
Library of Congress Cataloging-in-Publication Data

Little, Robert C.
  Physiology of the heart and circulation/Robert C. Little,
William C. Little.—4th ed.
    p.   cm.
  Includes bibliographies and index.
  ISBN 0-8151-5478-X
  1. Cardiovascular system—Physiology.   I. Little, Robert C.
II. Title.
  [DNLM: 1. Blood Circulation.   2. Cardiovascular System-
-physiology.   3. Heart-physiology.   WG 202 L778p]
QP102.L57 1989
612'.1—dc19
DNLM/DLC   88-20673
for Library of Congress   CIP

Sponsoring Editor: Kevin M. Kelly
Assistant Director, Manuscript Services: Frances M. Perveiler
Copyeditor: Sally J. Jansen
Production Project Manager: Gayle Paprocki
Proofroom Manager: Shirley E. Taylor

PREFACE TO THE FIRST EDITION

This book is based on the material I have used in presenting cardiovascular physiology to medical and beginning graduate students. The organization and depth of coverage of each topic are designed to outline the essentials of the subject in a form that will be useful for individuals at that level. Physicians, more advanced graduate students and others may find it useful as a concise review of the field. In the compilation of this material, it has been assumed that the reader has some knowledge of anatomy, biochemistry and elementary physics. Basic biophysical and structural aspects of cardiovascular function are discussed in Part I. Students without a background in these areas and who wish a less rigorous discussion of the heart and circulation may elect to skip parts of this first section and concentrate on the more descriptive coverage in the remaining chapters that deal with the function of the heart and the circulation.

In the interest of brevity, a moderately dogmatic approach has been used, and extensive documentation or presentation of research results has been avoided. If a fuller discussion of the data base that underlies these explanations is desired, larger encyclopedic texts and research monographs should be consulted. In adopting this method I have not meant to suggest that the explanations discussed are always settled or that there are not other viewpoints. Nevertheless, when the data appeared to justify such an approach and the explanation utilized appeared to be generally accepted, only one opinion is given. Discussion of alternate explanations is left for the course instructor or outside reading by the student. A few pertinent references that I have found to be helpful are listed at the end of each chapter. The serious student may find them, along with the credits listed for some of the illustrations, an access point to the literature.

Our knowledge of cardiovascular physiology stems from the work of many investigators. The names of a few individuals who have made significant contributions to the development of the field have been included in this discussion to provide historical relevance. I regret that space has not permitted the listing of many others who perhaps have made even greater contributions to our understanding of cardiovascular physiology.

Since this book is directed largely to medical students and others in the health care field, reference, where appropriate, is made to disease conditions as part of the discussion of normal cardiovascular physiology. In addition, a somewhat more detailed discussion of such clinical matters as heart sounds, the electrocardiogram and cardiac arrhythmias is included than is usual for a basic science text. These areas are discussed to provide an understanding of the underlying physiologic principles and how they are modified by disease conditions. No attempt, however, has been made to cover these areas in a comprehensive clinical fashion.

Many individuals have helped in the preparation of this book. My thanks go to many colleagues and students who have encouraged me in this venture and have given valuable help and criticism during the preparation of the manuscript. Special thanks go to Drs. Gene L. Colborn, Jack M. Ginsburg, Mary Ella Logan and Vernon T. Wiedmeier of the Medical College of Georgia and to Dr. Carleton H. Baker and the members of the Department of Physiology of the School of Medicine, University of South Florida, who reviewed sections of the manuscript and made helpful suggestions. Final responsibility must, however, remain with the author. I am indebted to Shirl Melton for preparation of the finished typescript and to Jim Wilson and his staff of the Department of Medical Illustration at the Medical College of Georgia for original drawings and illustrations.

Robert C. Little, M.D.

PREFACE TO THE FOURTH EDITION

The organization and depth of coverage of this book is designed to present the essentials of cardiovascular physiology in a form that will be useful to students approaching the subject for the first time. In addition, we hope that physicians, advanced students, and health professionals will continue to find it helpful as a concise review of the field.

The rapid expansion of basic cardiovascular knowledge during the past decade and the newer insights it has provided into the operation of the heart and circulation have dictated an extensive revision for this edition. In undertaking this task, we have emphasized basic principles and areas of immediate importance for students entering their clinical studies. Extensive documentation and presentation of research data have been avoided, and the moderately dogmatic approach utilized in earlier editions has been continued. A few pertinent references that we have found helpful are, however, provided at the end of each chapter as an access point to the literature.

Each chapter has been revised or extensively rewritten to incorporate newer material; illustrations have been added as needed. Some chapters have been rearranged for greater clarity. Information on the microcirculation has been grouped into a separate chapter, and the section on special circulations has been expanded. In order to conserve space, some discussions have been abbreviated and outdated explanations have been deleted.

Because this book is directed to first year medical students and other health professionals, reference is made, where appropriate, to the pathophysiology of clinical conditions as part of the discussion of normal cardiovascular physiology. These clinical notes are presented only to provide an understanding of the underlying physiologic principles, and no attempt has been made to cover them in a comprehensive clinical fashion.

Many individuals have helped in the preparation of this book. We are indebted to students and colleagues who have provided valuable comments and suggestions. It is our hope that readers will continue to provide such input. Special thanks are due to Dr. Carl F. Rothe of Indiana University and Dr. Carleton H. Baker of the University of South Florida, who reviewed the previous edition and made many helpful suggestions; and to Drs. W. F. Jackson, T. M. Nosek, and V. T. Weidmeier of the Medical College of Georgia, who reviewed portions of the manuscript. The Department of Medical Illustration of the Medical College of Georgia and of the Bowman Gray School of Medicine, Wake Forest University, supplied a number of new drawings and illustrations. It is a pleasure to acknowledge the excellent secretarial assistance provided by Valerie E. Smith and Joye Zafuto. During the preparation of this book, Dr. William C. Little was the recipient of an Established Investigatorship from the American Heart Association.

Robert C. Little, M.D.
William C. Little, M.D.

CONTENTS

Chapter 1

Introduction to Cardiovascular Physiology

The cardiovascular system is the material transport network of the body. It interfaces with diffusion sites throughout the body and exchanges fluids, oxygen, carbon dioxide, hormones, electrolytes, nutrients, and other substances with the interstitial compartment. Because of the importance of this activity, a discussion of the forces that govern movement between body compartments is a logical starting point for a text on cardiovascular physiology. Accordingly, these factors, along with a brief discussion of cellular transport mechanisms and a listing of some of the characteristics of blood important to the function of the vascular system, will be summarized in this chapter.

MOVEMENT OF FLUID AND DISSOLVED SOLUTE IN THE BODY

Body water is usually subdivided into three general compartments: *intracellular*, *interstitial* (outside both the cell and vascular system), and *vascular*. Other classifications can be used (Fig 1–1). Water and its dissolved solute move more or less independently within and between these compartments by the processes of diffusion, osmosis (a special case of diffusion), ultrafiltration, and carrier-mediated transport, which can be either active or facilitative in nature. In addition, the fluid inside the vascular system

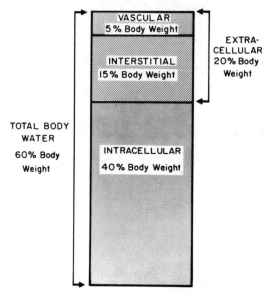

FIG 1–1.
Body water compartments showing approximate distribution of total body water for an adult male. The vascular volume does not include cellular elements of the blood.

(blood) is circulated by the pumping action of the heart. This hydraulic movement of fluid (bulk flow) will be discussed in subsequent chapters.

Diffusion

The process of diffusion is important for the function of the vascular system. For example, most of the interchange in the capillary bed between blood plasma and body cells takes place by diffusion through the bounding membranes of each compartment and the intervening interstitial fluid. Diffusion can be simply defined as the spontaneous movement of particles as a consequence of thermal agitation from areas of high concentration to areas of low concentration. This movement is specific for each species of particles and is independent of the movement of other particles in the medium.

In the macroscopic sense, the basic molecular energy of a substance (assuming there are no chemical bonds or other forms of extraneous energy) exists primarily as the kinetic energy of its component molecules due to their motion and the electrostatic forces (van der Waal forces) among adjacent particles. The intermolecular distances in a gas are normally so great that significant internal force fields do not develop in that medium, and the molecules are relatively free to move. In contrast, the molecules of a liquid are close together and are more likely to form intermolecular combinations. As a result, their motion is restrained. Some molecules (the number varies with the temperature) have sufficient energy to break away from these restraining forces and are able to move about in a random, straight-line manner until they hit another particle. When this happens, kinetic energy is transferred to the less active member. The consequence of many such collisions is a relatively uniform distribution of kinetic energy among all the particles in the bulk phase of a homogeneous solution.

The kinetic energy (KE) of a moving particle can be determined by the following equation:

$$KE = \frac{mV^2}{2} \tag{1-1}$$

where m is the mass of the particle and V is the linear velocity. The temperature and the average kinetic energy of a system are directly related. It follows, therefore, that at a given temperature (i.e., level of kinetic energy), particle velocity is inversely related to the square root of the mass (Graham's law). The water molecules in an aqueous solution of glucose will, for example, move three times as fast as the glucose molecules, which are approximately ten times heavier. In addition, the greater the density of the medium, the greater the probability that a moving particle will strike another particle and thereby shorten the length of its free path of movement. For this reason, other things being equal, the net linear velocity of a particle is inversely related to the density of the medium.

These factors have physiologic significance. With the exception of the pulmonary system, diffusion in the body takes place primarily in solutions. Even apparently solid structures such as membranes act as if they were liquids. As a result, lipid-soluble particles that are too large to travel through the aqueous channels that apparently penetrate the membrane are able to move from one side to the other. This is accomplished by their dissolving in the lipoid center of the membrane and diffusing to the opposite side before reentering the aqueous phase. Because of the greater density of the lipid interior compared to body fluids, the diffusion velocity through the membrane will be considerably slower than in the bulk aqueous phase on either side (Fig 1–2). As a consequence, significant concentration gradients in the body occur primarily across cell or epithelial membranes. Appreciable concentration differences within a local fluid compartment are observed only in conjunction with unique vascular arrangements such as the countercurrent system of the kidney, which supports a solute concentration gradient within the renal extracellular fluid.

The diffusion process can be illustrated (Fig 1–3) by separating sucrose

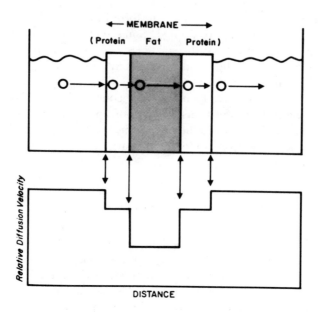

FIG 1–2.

Top, schematic diagram showing movement of a diffusing particle in the aqueous phase on each side of a membrane and in each of the three layers of the membrane. For purposes of illustration, the random walk of the diffusing particles is shown as a net forward movement through the membrane. *Bottom,* graph showing the relative velocity of movement of the particle in each membrane phase.

solutions by means of a freely permeable divider. There is a greater probability that a sucrose molecule during its random movement will move from solution A (high concentration) to solution B (low concentration) than the reverse. Although some sucrose molecules will move through the divider in both directions, the net movement will be from the area of high concentration to the area of low concentration. It should be noted that, due to the random motion of the water molecules, there will also be a net diffusion of water (osmosis) in the direction opposite to the movement of sucrose as water moves from an area of high water concentration to one of lower water concentration.

The rate of diffusion for a single species of particles was described in 1855 by the German biophysicist Adolph Fick and formulated into what is known as Fick's law.* In a simplified form this law states

$$\dot{Q} = -AD\left(\frac{dc}{dx}\right) \tag{1–2}$$

*This should be distinguished from the Fick principle, discussed in Chapter 7.

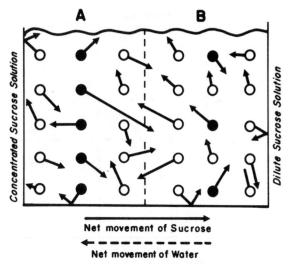

FIG 1–3.
Schematic diagram showing a concentrated sucrose solution **(A)** separated from a dilute sucrose solution **(B)** by a freely permeable divider. *Open circles* represent water molecules; *closed circles* represent sucrose molecules. See text for further discussion.

where $\dot{Q}$ is the rate of flow of solute at right angles to the interface (milligrams per second), dc/dx is the concentration gradient (i.e., the change in the concentration [milligrams per cubic centimeter] across the interface [centimeters] separating the two solutions), A is the area of the interface (square centimeters), and D is the diffusion coefficient (square centimeters per second). The magnitude of D is dependent on the temperature and the properties of the diffusing substance and the medium through which diffusion occurs. The negative sign is used because diffusion is downhill, i.e., from areas of high concentration to areas of low concentration.

Physiologists are interested in the diffusion of substances across a wide variety of membranes. The width of the membrane (analogous to dx in equation 1–2) can be included as part of the diffusion coefficient to form a permeability constant (P) as follows:

$$P = \frac{D}{d} \tag{1–3}$$

where d is the width of the membrane. An average value of 75 A is frequently assumed for cell membranes. The permeability constant for a species of particles has the units of velocity (centimeters per second) and gives

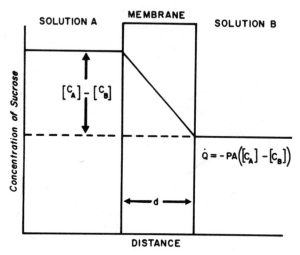

FIG 1–4.

Diagrammatic representation of the diffusion of sucrose through a membrane that separates a more concentrated sucrose solution from a dilute sucrose solution. The concentration of sucrose in each solution is indicated by $[C_A]$ and $[C_B]$, respectively. See text for description of other terms.

the diffusion rate per unit membrane area when the membrane is exposed to a unit concentration difference.* This value will be utilized in Chapter 3 as part of the discussion of the electric activity of the heart.

When the permeability constant is substituted in equation 1–2 and the assumption is made that there is a linear drop in concentration of the diffusing substance as it travels through the membrane (Fig 1–4), Fick's law becomes

$$\dot{Q} = -PA([c_1] - [c_2]) \qquad (1\text{–}4)$$

where $[c_1]$ and $[c_2]$ are the concentrations of the solute on each side of the membrane. (Technically, activities should be used instead of concentrations, but for dilute solutions the two values are almost identical.)

This relationship between the concentration of dissolved particles on each side of a membrane and their rate of diffusion is particularly important in the microcirculation where it underlies much of the movement of nutrients and metabolites in and out of the capillary bed. This aspect of dif-

---

*Diffusion and permeability constants are temperature dependent. As body temperature is normally closely regulated, this factor will not be considered in the discussion presented here.

fusion will be covered in Chapter 12 as part of the discussion of capillary function. Diffusion is only practical for the transport of biologic substances over short distances as its effectiveness decreases with the square of the diffusion path. As a result, the time required for equilibrium to occur over a distance of a few microns is usually measured in milliseconds, while this interval may become hours when the diffusion distance is increased to millimeters.

Osmosis

As indicated earlier, *osmosis* is the special case of diffusion where movement of solvent is studied. It usually is defined in terms of the solute concentration. Therefore, osmosis is the movement of water from solutions of *low solute* concentration of those of *high solute* concentration. Most students are aware of the importance of osmosis, along with other factors such as capillarity (the tendency of fluids to rise in a narrow tube), for the movement of sap to the top of a tree. These same osmotic forces are equally important in the body for the movement of fluid among body compartments.

Osmosis can be illustrated by separating two solutions containing different concentrations of sucrose by means of a membrane that will freely permit solvent (water) but *not* solute (sucrose) to pass (Fig 1–5). In such a system, water will move from solution B that contains a low concentration of sucrose to solution A, which has a higher concentration of sucrose and, therefore, less water per unit of volume. This movement of water will con-

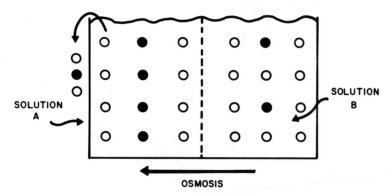

FIG 1–5.
Diagram showing diffusion of water through a semipermeable membrane from an area of higher water concentration to one of lower water concentration. Note that because of osmosis, solution A overfills its container. (The volume of solution B is considered to be infinite so that its level does not fall due to movement of water into solution A.)

tinue until the concentration of sucrose becomes equal on both sides of the membrane, assuming there is no change in hydrostatic level. If the experiment is modified so that solution A (at body temperature) has the same composition as intracellular fluid and is enclosed in an osmometer with a vertical manometer tube and pure water is substituted for solution B, water will move into the osmometer and rise approximately 227 ft in the manometer (Fig 1–6). This hydrostatic pressure is equivalent to a pressure of 6.7 atm. At this point the backflow of water from solution A to solution B, due to the hydrostatic pressure of the fluid column in the manometer tube, will exactly counter the diffusional flow from solution B to solution A, and the net flux of water (osmosis) will stop. This equilibrium (bucking) pressure is called the osmotic pressure (π). It is equal, but oppositely directed, to the diffusional force available for the migration of water molecules. The pressure is usually expressed in millimeters of mercury or atmospheres (1 atm = 760 mm Hg).

As illustrated by the above experiment, intracellular fluid has an amazingly high osmotic pressure. Because the fluid in each body unit has its

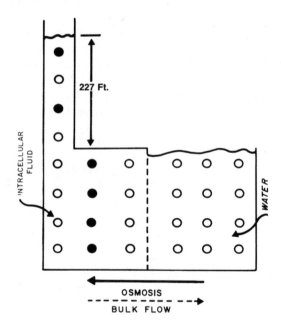

FIG 1–6.
Diagram showing an osmometer with a manometer tube filled with intracellular fluid. Water diffuses *(solid arrow)* through the semipermeable membrane into the osmometer until hydrostatic pressure of the fluid in the manometer produces an equal flow *(dashed arrow)* out of the osmometer.

own osmotic activity, osmotic forces of this magnitude are not encountered between compartments. Rather, the resultant osmotic force for the movement of solvent between body fluid compartments becomes the difference between their individual osmotic pressures. The use of the term "pressure" in expressing the osmotic force can lead to conceptual difficulties unless it is recognized that it is not a pressure in the usual sense but rather a way of expressing the *potential chemical energy* of a solution. For example, an erythrocyte has an internal osmotic pressure of over 5,000 mm Hg. This is the force available to move fluid into the cell *if it were suspended in pure water*. However, it should be clear that the real internal pressure of an isolated red blood cell is essentially atmospheric, and the transmembrane pressure (i.e., difference in pressure between inside and outside) is zero.

Osmotic pressure, as one of the colligative properties of a solution, varies directly with the number of solute particles* as follows:

$$\pi = \Sigma cRT \tag{1–5}$$

where Σc is the sum of the osmotically active solute particles expressed as a concentration per unit volume, R is the universal gas constant, and T is the absolute temperature. This equation was proposed in the 1880s by the Dutch physicist J. H. van't Hoff, and is known as van't Hoff's rule. Because of practical difficulties in the use of this equation to calculate osmotic pressure of biologic solutions due to ionization and the formation of osmotically active subgroups of particles, it is customary to express osmotic pressure in terms of osmoles (Osm). A solution containing 1 mole of a nonionizable solute in 1 L of water will have an osmotic pressure of 22.4 atm. As a result, any solution, regardless of its chemical composition, that has an osmotic pressure of this value is said to have an effective osmotic concentration of 1 Osm/L. This unit is much too large for most physiologic applications so the milliosmole (mOsm) usually is used (1 Osm = 1,000 mOsm).

In an ideal solution, each milliequivalent of dissolved monovalent substance (i.e., the amount of material that will react with or displace 0.001 gm atomic weight of hydrogen) will produce 1 mOsm of osmotic activity per liter of solvent. However, as mentioned above, the constituents of body fluids have a tendency to interact with each other to form units that then act as osmotic particles. In addition, 2 mEq of a divalent ion, such as SO_4^{2-}, produce only one osmotically active particle. As a result, the osmolar concentration of body fluid is somewhat less than the sum of the dissolved materials, and it must be specifically measured, usually by determination of its freezing point.†

---

*The number of osmotically active particles and not the type of particle is important.
†Also one of the colligative properties.

As body membranes are freely permeable to water, an osmotic gradient will not normally be maintained between compartments, and except as noted below, the osmotic concentration of intracellular and extracellular fluid will be approximately equal. The average osmotic pressure of body fluid (6.72 atm) is nearly 30% of the value of 1 Osm (22.4 atm); therefore, the osmolarity of body water is about 0.3 Osm or 300 mOsm (290 to 310 mOsm).

In spite of an overall osmotic equilibrium between body fluids, several local mechanisms operate to produce small but important regional differences in the concentration of osmotically active particles. The most important of these mechanisms are (1) the uneven distribution of charged particles across a semipermeable membrane due to the presence of nondiffusible polar molecules (Gibbs-Donnan equilibrium), (2) the activity of metabolic "pumps" that are able to move solute through membranes against its concentration gradient (active transport), and (3) the effect of blood pressure on the movement of fluid through capillary epithelium against an osmotic gradient (ultrafiltration).

Gibbs-Donnan Relationship

The presence of the negatively charged protein moiety inside the cell changes the distribution of the diffusible charged particles on each side of the cell membrane.

The nondiffusible protein attracts positive diffusible ions and repels other negatively charged particles. As a result, electric and concentration gradients are established so that the product of the diffusible anions and cations on each side of the membrane is equal* (Fig 1–7). The total concentration of particles is unequal on each side of the membrane and an osmotic gradient is produced toward the compartment that contains the nondiffusible molecules. At the same time, an electric potential difference is produced across the membrane. (See Chapter 3 for a further discussion of the electric potentials produced by the unequal distribution of charged particles.) This equilibrium was suggested on theoretical grounds by the American biophysicist J. Willard Gibbs from 1874 to 1878 and was experimentally demonstrated by the British chemist Frederick R. Donnan in 1911.

Because of the semipermeable nature of the capillary epithelium, plasma proteins are retained in the vascular compartment, and their osmotic activity becomes of pivotal importance to the movement of fluid between the capillary and interstitial fluid compartments (see Chapter 12).

*This equilibrium can only be achieved if volume is controlled by a balance of opposing osmotic and hydrostatic pressures.

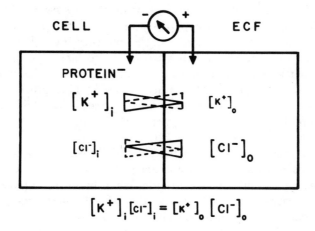

$$[K^+]_i [Cl^-]_i = [K^+]_o [Cl^-]_o$$

FIG 1-7.

Illustration of a Gibbs-Donnan equilibrium for a theoretical cell that contains only protein$^-$, K$^+$, and Cl$^-$. The intracellular protein$^-$ attracts the K$^+$ and repels the Cl$^-$. This electrostatic gradient is shown by the *dashed line*. The concentration gradients for the diffusion of K$^+$ and Cl$^-$ are shown by the *solid line*. At equilibrium, both gradients are equal but oppositely directed. The distribution of diffusible ions across the cell membrane is shown. Relative concentrations are indicated by the size of the brackets. *ECF* = extracellular fluid.

The Gibbs-Donnan equilibrium established across the capillary epithelium by the nondiffusible plasma proteins adds a small but important increment to this osmotic activity. Plasma proteins provide an osmotic pressure of approximately 20 mm Hg. The extra diffusible particles held in the vascular system by the nondiffusible protein molecules add an additional osmotic pressure of 6 or 7 mm Hg. The total oncotic pressure developed as a result of the plasma proteins is 26 to 27 mm Hg. This is discussed further in Chapter 12.

Active Transport

As indicated earlier, the movement of particles against their concentration gradient requires a pump mechanism. This process can be illustrated by the movement of sodium out of the cell into the extracellular fluid where it is already in high concentration. Active transport of this type permits a large sodium gradient to be maintained across the cell wall in spite of an inward diffusional force. Metabolic pumps are complex. A discussion of their properties is in the province of cell physiology, and specific texts should be consulted for detailed information. It is only necessary here to briefly summarize a few of the characteristics of these pumps.

Active transport makes use of a *membrane carrier system*. This mechanism, in its simplest form, is apparently utilized in the passive absorption of such substances as amino acids from the intestinal tract. The transported particles (Fig 1–8,A) are bound to a carrier at one surface of the cell membrane. The particle-carrier complex then diffuses through the membrane to the other side where the particles are released. This process, variously called *facilitated* or *mediated transport*, must operate "downhill" in that the concentration of particles must be greater on the entering side of the membrane than on the side where they exist. With active transport, the carrier mechanism is able to move the particles "uphill" against their concentration gradient. This is achieved by supplying sufficient energy (the breakdown of adenosine triphosphate [ATP] to adenosine diphosphate [ADP]) to uncouple the carrier-particle complex at the far side of the membrane and deliver the particle with sufficient chemical potential for it to diffuse into the fluid, where it is already in high concentration (Fig 1–8,B).

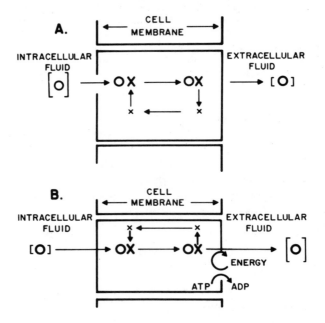

FIG 1–8.
Diagrammatic representation of transport of particles *(O)* from intracellular fluid to extracellular fluid by combination with a carrier *(X)*. **A,** passive carrier-mediated diffusion from a high intracellular concentration to a low extracellular concentration. **B,** active transport from a low intracellular concentration to a high extracellular concentration. Uncoupling of particle and carrier at outer edge of membrane by energy liberated from adenosine triphosphate *(ATP)* is indicated. (This carrier mechanism may be coupled with transport of a second particle in the opposite direction.) *ADP* = adenosine diphosphate.

In these systems the number of carrier sites is limited, and each carrier is highly selective and will bind only specific particles. For this reason these mechanisms show saturation kinetics and can be inhibited by substances that compete for binding sites. In addition, the energy source for active transport is vulnerable to the action of metabolic poisons or to the withdrawal of oxygen.

Active transport is important to a number of cellular activities. Its role in the electric activity of the heart will be discussed in Chapter 3. The sodium pump is also important for osmotic regulation of the cell. For example, the osmotic gradient produced across the cell membrane by the intracellular protein and the Gibbs-Donnan forces (see above) is directed so that fluid will enter the cell. This inward osmotic gradient results largely from the intracellular accumulation of diffusible potassium. This osmotic effect of potassium is opposed by the active transport of sodium out of the cell where sodium can act to maintain the effective osmolar concentration of the extracellular fluid. This factor explains the tendency for cells to swell if their active transport mechanisms are disturbed and has led to the clinical dictum, "a sick cell swells."

Ultrafiltration

The concentration of particles and the osmotic pressure of a fluid represent potential energy that can be used to do work. Osmotic work is carried out, for example, when fluid diffuses down its concentration gradient as it moves from one compartment to another. In conformity with thermodynamic principles, systems move from states of higher potential energy to those of lower potential energy. To reverse this process, it is necessary to add energy. This fact underlies the active transport of solute against its concentration gradient described above. In the microcirculation, a similar situation exists in that fluid and its dissolved particles are forced out of the arterial end of the capillaries against an osmotic gradient by the energy of the blood pressure. This process is called *ultrafiltration*. It can be illustrated using two sucrose solutions separated by a semipermeable membrane (Fig 1–9). If solution A, which has the larger concentration of sucrose, is subjected to a hydrostatic pressure that is greater than the difference between the osmotic pressures of the two solutions, the net movement will be against the osmotic gradient, and the water will move from solution A to solution B.

As already indicated, ultrafiltration is an important physiologic process that is involved both in the movement of fluid out of the capillaries and in the formation of urine. In each case, the energy required to move fluid against its gradient is supplied by the arterial blood pressure. This mechanism is also discussed in Chapter 12.

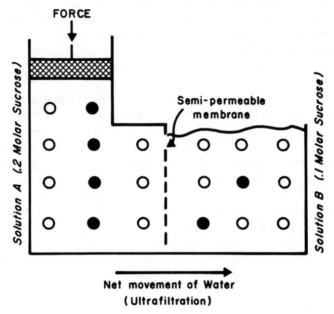

FIG 1–9.
Diagram showing net movement of water from solution A into solution B against the gradient for water when solution A is subjected to a pressure that exceeds its osmotic pressure.

COMPOSITION OF BLOOD

A discussion of cardiovascular function would not be complete without mentioning the fluid that fills the vascular system and plays such an important role in the activities of the body. This aqueous slurry of blood cells, electrolytes, foodstuffs, dissolved gas, and other substances serves a variety of functions. For example, blood transports metabolic fuels and respiratory gases to the tissues along with the building elements for growth and repair of body structures. It carries away the waste products of cellular metabolism and distributes the heat generated by these activities. It coordinates cellular function by its carriage of chemicals, hormones, and other messengers and plays an important role in the defense of the body. Because of these and the many other functions of blood, an adequate discussion of this organ system would require more space than available here. Nevertheless, a brief listing of some of its characteristics is appropriate for an understanding of cardiovascular function.

Composition

Blood, which constitutes about 7% to 9% of body weight, is a suspension of cellular elements in an aqueous solution. Approximately 45% of this volume is made up of cellular elements (the hematocrit) and the remainder is plasma. Because of the constant motion of blood, the cellular elements are relatively evenly distributed within the larger vessels, although sludging and rouleau formation (adherence of erythrocytes into cylindrical aggregates) may occur when blood flow is reduced. In the smaller vessels, the relative percentage of formed elements to the plasma fraction may be altered by the process of axial streaming. This aspect will be covered as part of the discussion of hemodynamics in Chapter 9. The average cellular composition of human blood is shown in Table 1–1.

Plasma is a complex fluid that contains a variety of proteins, lipids, and carbohydrates as well as both inorganic and organic chemicals. Approximately 8% of the plasma volume is solute, and the remainder is water. Because of its ability to absorb a considerable amount of heat with only a relatively small change in temperature (high specific heat), the large water content permits blood to serve as an efficient transport system for the heat generated by metabolic activity. The concentration of significant plasma electrolytes is summarized in Table 1–2. The major plasma proteins, albumin and globulin, have important physiologic functions in maintaining the osmotic relationships of blood. Their role in the establishment of a Gibbs-Donnan equilibrium in the microcirculation has been described earlier. The action of the plasma proteins in the microcirculation is discussed in Chapter 12.

Blood Clotting

An important feature of blood is its ability to clot. This hemostatic mechanism and the ability of local vessels to undergo significant vasocon-

TABLE 1–1.

Cellular Composition of Human Blood

Erythrocytes (RBCs)	4,500,000–5,000,000/cu mm
Platelets	200,000–400,000/cu mm
Leukocytes (WBCs)	5,000–10,000/cu mm
Neutrophils	63.5%
Lymphocytes	30.0%
Monocytes	4.0%
Eosinophils	2.0%
Basophils	0.5%

TABLE 1–2.

Concentration of Significant Plasma
Electrolytes*

	Range	Mean Value
Sodium	136–145	143.0
Chloride	98–106	103.0
Bicarbonate	25–28	27.0
Potassium	3.6–5.0	4.0
Phosphate	2.0–2.2	2.0
Calcium	4.5–6.0	5.0
Magnesium	2.0–2.2	2.0

*All values are expressed as milliequivalents per liter.

striction when injured serve to limit the loss of blood when breaks occur in the vascular system. Under normal conditions, blood in the vascular system remains fluid; however, if the delicate endothelial lining of the vascular system is injured, blood platelets collect in the injured area and tend to occlude small openings. At the same time, the clotting activity of the blood is locally activated by a cascade of coagulation factors triggered by contact with the damaged vessel wall and the platelet aggregations. These activities take place rapidly and usually are effective in preventing a major loss of blood.

In addition to an ability to clot, the blood has a complicated clot removal system containing a special proteolytic enzyme, *plasmin*. This material is able to split fibrin, the major component of the clot. Plasma also contains a number of inactive polypeptides called *kinins*, which are converted to their active form by the same stimulus that leads to blood clotting. These polypeptides lead to local vasodilation of neighboring small blood vessels and may produce a local inflammatory reaction in the tissue of the area.

SUMMARY

The cardiovascular system is the major transport system of the body. Material moves between it and the body compartments largely by diffusion or one of various transport mechanisms. (The hydraulic bulk flow of fluid and dissolved materials is discussed in Chapter 12). Diffusion and osmosis utilize the energy of thermal agitation to move particles or fluid from areas of higher concentration to areas of lower concentration, while the transport mechanism combines this force with a more complex carrier system and the use of metabolic energy. An understanding of these forces is important for the discussion of cardiovascular function that follows in subsequent chapters.

BIBLIOGRAPHY

Andreoli T, Hoffman JF, Franestil DD (eds): *Membrane Physiology*. New York, Plenum Medical Book Co, 1980.

Brown AC: Passive and active transport, in Ruch TC, Fulton JF (eds): *Medical Physiology and Biophysics*, ed 19. Philadelphia, WB Saunders Co, 1965.

Curran PF, Schultz SG: Transport across membranes: General principles, in Fenn WO, Rahan H (eds): *Handbook of Physiology, Section 6: Alimentary Canal*, vol 3. Washington, DC, American Physiological Society, 1965.

Dick DAT: *Cell Water*. Washington, DC, Butterworth, 1966.

Dyson RD: *Cell Biology: A Molecular Approach*, ed 2. Boston, Allyn and Bacon, Inc, 1978.

Florey E: *An Introduction to General and Comparative Animal Physiology*. Philadelphia, WB Saunders Co, 1966.

Hoppe W, Lohmann W, Markl H, et al. (eds): *Biophysics*. Berlin, Springer-Verlag, 1983.

Keynes RD, Aidley DS: *Nerve and Muscle*. Cambridge, Cambridge University Press, 1981.

Kyte J: Molecular considerations relevant to the mechanism of active transport. *Nature* 1981; 292:201.

Mathews GC: *Cellular Physiology of Nerve and Muscle*. Palo Alto, Blackwell Scientific Publications, 1986.

Randall JE: *Elements of Biophysics*, ed 2. Chicago, Year Book Medical Publishers, 1962.

Schultz SG: *Basic Principles of Membrane Transport*. New York, Cambridge University Press, 1980.

Wilbrandt W, Rosenberg T: The concept of carrier transport and its corollaries in pharmacology. *Pharmacol Rev* 1961; 13:109.

Chapter 2 _____

Physical Characteristics and Functional Significance of Cardiovascular Structure

_____

The function of the heart is to transfer sufficient blood from the low-pressure venous system to the arterial side of the circulation under the proper pressure to maintain the circulatory needs of the body. Arterial vessels distribute this blood to the tissues. Here the capillary microcirculation permits the exchange of fluid, dissolved gases, foodstuffs, hormones, metabolic waste products, and other small solute molecules between blood and interstitial fluid. The veins then serve to return blood to the heart. The architectural features and physical characteristics that permit the circulatory system to meet these requirements are summarized in this chapter. The physiologic mechanisms that underlie this circulatory function will be developed in more detail in the chapters that follow.

STRUCTURE OF THE HEART

The heart is an efficient force pump that few, if any, mechanical pumps can equal. In an engineering sense, the heart is made up of two separate pump systems. The right atrium and ventricle act as a single unit (the right heart) to move venous blood from the great veins to the pulmonary circulation. The left atrium and ventricle (the left heart) act together in a similar manner to pump blood from the pulmonary system to the high-pressure systemic circulation. This directional flow of blood, as well as some of the important structural features of the heart, are shown in Figure 2–1. The terms "right heart" and "left heart," although physiologically correct, are not descriptive of their position in the body. Due to the normal rotation of the heart on its longitudinal axis, the right ventricle is in front of the left and occupies a position immediately behind the sternum, whereas the left ventricle is rotated so that it faces toward the left side and the back of the thorax.

The heart is suspended in the pericardial cavity by its attachments to the great vessels and is oriented so that its base is directed upward, slightly backward, and tipped to the right. As a result, the apex of the heart is directed downward, forward, and to the left. The anatomical position of the base is relatively fixed due to its attachments, whereas the apex is free to move. During ventricular contraction, dimensional changes that take place within the ventricle cause the apex to move forward and to strike

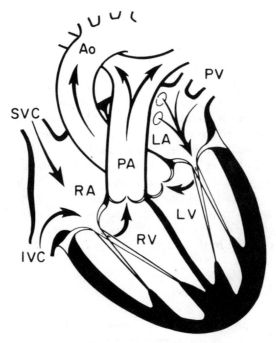

FIG 2–1.
Blood flow through the heart. *SVC* = superior vena cava; *IVC* = inferior vena cava; *RA* = right atrium; *LA* = left atrium; *PA* = pulmonary artery; *PV* = pulmonary veins; *RV* = right ventricle; *LV* = left ventricle; *Ao* = aorta.

against the left chest wall in the area of the fifth intercostal space; this characteristic systolic thrust is felt as the apical impulse.

Cardiac Skeleton

In relating the anatomical features of the heart to its function as a pump, it is helpful to focus first on the fibrous zone of fixation for the cardiac musculature, the *cardiac skeleton*. During early embryologic life, the endocardial cushions push in from the sides of the primitive cardiac tube in the area of the future atrioventricular (AV) valves. Tough fibrous rings are formed in this area that ultimately encircle the orifices of the two AV valves. Two additional *fibrous annuli* develop in relation to the bases of the aorta and pulmonary trunk. The aortic fibrous annulus is connected to the pulmonary annulus by a fibrous band, the *tendon of the conus*. Moreover, it is joined to the AV annuli by the small, *left fibrous trigone* and the larger, *right fibrous trigone* (or central fibrous body). The right fibrous trigone is the strongest point of fixation of the cardiac skeleton and attaches the mitral annulus, the tricuspid annulus, and the aortic annulus (Fig 2–2). It is further extended as the membranous *septum* of the interventricular septum. The right trigone merges inferiorly with the developing interventricular septum and superiorly with the atrial septum. The four valve annuli and their interconnections constitute a resistive connective tissue framework, the *cardiac skeleton*, or fibrous base of the heart. The cardiac skeleton serves as the attachment for the heart valves and is the origin and, in some instances, the insertion of muscle fibers from both the atria and ventricles. Interposition of this fibrous skeleton between the atria and ventricles of the heart prevents myocardial continuity between these areas. This separation permits the bundle of His, which penetrates the central fibrous body, to be the only bridge of excitable tissue between the atrial and ventricular myocardium. As will be discussed in Chapter 4, this anatomical feature is of considerable physiologic importance as it provides the only normal pathway for the excitation process associated with each heartbeat to reach the ventricles.

Heart Valves

The dynamic effect of cardiac contraction is surprisingly effective in moving blood through the heart even in the absence of competent valves. Nevertheless, these thin, delicate valves that guard the entrance and exit of each ventricle greatly enhance the efficiency of the cardiac pump by preventing backflow. In spite of their fragile appearance, the cusps of these valves are deceptively strong and resilient. Their movements are essentially

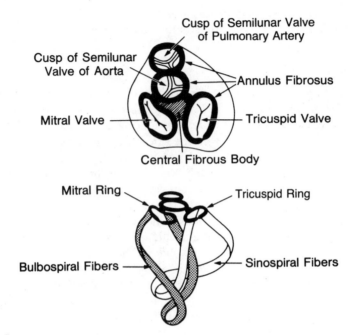

FIG 2–2.
Top, fibrous skeleton of the heart and cardiac valves viewed from above. *Bottom,* schematic diagram showing spiral arrangement of ventricular muscles with their origin and insertion on the fibrous skeleton. (Modified from Truex RC, in *Encyclopaedia Britannica,* vol 2, Chicago, Encyclopaedia Britannica, 1967.)

passive even though some of the leaflets have been shown to contain muscle fibers.

The crescent-shaped (semilunar) cusps of the pulmonic and aortic valves permit these structures to open maximally during ventricular ejection and still provide a perfect seal when closed during diastole. Eversion or bulging of the closed cusps into the ventricle due to the pressure of blood in the pulmonary artery or aorta does not normally interfere with closure of the valve because of the stout attachments of the valve leaflets to the annulus fibrosus.

A slight enlargement of the aorta and to a lesser extent of the pulmonary artery in the area of the semilunar valves (the sinus of Valsalva) serves two physiologic functions: (1) it provides space behind the open aortic valve cusps so that the leaflets do not occlude the orifices of the coronary arteries, and (2) this space favors the development of eddy currents behind the open valve cusps (Fig 2–3). This latter mechanism holds the open valve leaflets away from the vessel wall in a position where they will be promptly caught

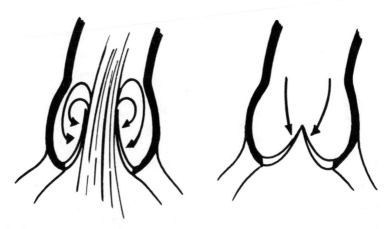

FIG 2–3.
Left, flow pattern through aortic valve during ejection. The rapid axial stream of blood through the open valve results in eddy currents behind the valve cusps that hold them away from the wall of the aorta. *Right,* closed position of valve cusps during diastole. When the flow through the open valve tends to reverse at the end of systole, the semi-open valves are promptly closed. (Modified from Rushmer RF: *Cardiovascular Dynamics,* ed 4. Philadelphia, WB Saunders Co, 1975. Used by permission.)

and closed by blood as it attempts to regurgitate back into the ventricle at the end of systole (see Chapter 4).

The structure of the *mitral* and *tricuspid* valves, which guard the entrance into the ventricles, is more complicated than that of the semilunar valves. The annulus that surrounds each of these AV valves is also quite compliant. As a result, contraction of the ventricular muscle fibers that insert on these elastic rings distorts their shape and reduces the diameter of the valve opening. For this reason, the valve cusps are larger than the area to be covered. This disparity in size ensures complete closure of the valve orifice during systole. If this disproportion is too great, the valve leaflets may, however, prolapse into the atrium during systole. This abnormal movement may then produce a midsystolic click and allow late systolic regurgitation.

The mitral valve, in contrast to the tricuspid valve on the right side of the heart, has only two cusps. These are slightly fused near their origin and form a funnel-like structure that points into the left ventricle. Attached to the free edge of both the mitral and tricuspid valves are fibrous strands (the *chordae tendineae*) that connect to papillary muscles deep in the ventricle. Fibers from similar areas on each of the valve cusps insert on the same or adjacent papillary muscles. This crossing arrangement (Fig 2–4) is functionally significant, as it causes the valve to move toward a position of closure

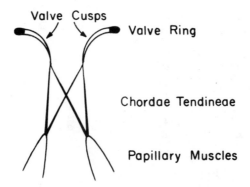

Valve Cusps

Valve Ring

Chordae Tendineae

Papillary Muscles

FIG 2–4.
Schematic diagram showing crossing arrangement of chordae tendineae from each papillary muscle to insert on the similar areas of each mitral valve cusp. (Modified from Rushmer RF: *Structure and Function of the Cardiovascular System,* ed 2. Philadelphia, WB Saunders Co, 1976.)

when tension is exerted on the cusps by contraction of the papillary muscles. These support structures also prevent eversion of the valve edge or bulging of the cusps into the atria during ventricular systole.

The Atria

The cardiac atria occupy the most anterior dorsal part of the heart. The right atrium is divided internally by a ridge, the *terminal crest,* into the right *atrial appendage* and the *sinus of the venae cavae.* The latter contains the openings of the cavae, the *coronary sinus,* and several small *thebesian veins.* Surrounding the openings of the inferior vena cava and the coronary sinus are several rudimentary folds of endocardium that resemble crescentic valve cusps. These folds are remnants of the right valve of the sinus venosus. The physiologic function, if any, of these folds is not clear. They are frequently fenestrated and undoubtedly do not act as true valves; however, it has been suggested that they may serve to deflect the flow of blood within the atrium. The left atrium, which is smaller than the right, is divided into a venous sinus containing the openings of the four pulmonary veins, and the left atrial appendage.

The wall of the atria contains three anatomically distinct layers: (1) the outer epicardium, (2) the muscular myocardium, and (3) the inner endocardium. The epicardium is continuous with the outer covering of the ventricles and is composed of mesothelium, connective tissue, and some fat. It also contains small nerve branches and the coronary blood vessels that send smaller branches into the atrial wall. The endocardium consists of endothelium and a layer of fibroelastic connective tissue that is somewhat thicker in the atria than in the rest of the heart.

The inner myocardial layer contains many nerve fibers and sensory endings. These are particularly abundant in the areas of the sinus node, the AV node, and the junction of both the venae cavae and right atrium and the pulmonary veins and the left atrium (see Chapter 10). In general, the atria have a richer supply of sensory endings than the ventricles. Small ganglion cells occur in the atrial myocardium, and nerve trunks accompany the main branches of the coronary arteries.

The muscular layer of the atrial myocardium may be divided into two groups: (1) a superficial layer that encircles both atria and (2) a deep layer that is independent for each chamber. These fibers form two muscular loops that encircle the venous inlet into each atrium (Fig 2–5). A number of distinct muscle bundles have been identified in each layer. The superficial muscle fibers fan out over the surface from their origin in the anterior part of the septum and the base of the superior vena cava. Most of these fibers insert into the annulus fibrosus. A prominent group of superficial fibers, the *interatrial band,* arises near the base of the superior vena cava and passes on the anterior surface of the atria to the left atrium, where it divides and encircles the left atrial appendage. This band has been suggested as a direct path for conduction of the excitatory process to the left atrium. Other fibers extend to the right from the base of the superior vena cava and encircle the right atrial appendage.

In general, the deep muscle fibers run at right angles to the superficial fibers and make up the major muscular elements of the atria. Annular fibers surround the orifice of the superior vena cava, the coronary sinus, and the

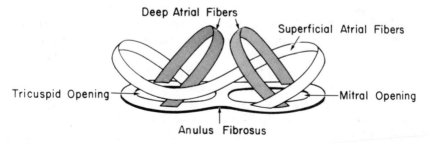

Deep Atrial Fibers   Superficial Atrial Fibers

Tricuspid Opening   Mitral Opening

Anulus Fibrosus

FIG 2–5.
Highly schematic representation of atrial muscle fibers. The superficial fibers encircle both atria; the deep fibers are independent for each chamber. Contraction of these muscle bands tends to propel the atrial contents toward the tricuspid opening on the right side and the mitral opening on the left.

pulmonary veins. In addition, muscle bundles extend across the atrial septum to form the musculature of the atrial septum.

Atrial-Venous Junction

High-speed angiocardiographic studies show that both the orifice of the superior and inferior vena cava and the entrance of the pulmonary veins into the left atrium narrow and become elliptical during atrial systole due to contraction of the annular muscle fibers that surround these openings. As a consequence of this dimensional change, the resistance offered to the movement of blood through the caval openings is increased. This increase is usually sufficient to prevent regurgitation from the atria during the brief reversal of the caval-atrial pressure gradient produced by atrial contraction. However, as these vessels remain patent, they will permit blood to reflux into the veins if atrial pressure becomes unduly elevated.

On the left side of the heart, the pulmonary vein-left atrial junction tends to collapse if atrial pressure is low. Under these circumstances, the elliptical cross section is maintained throughout diastole. As a result, a *vascular waterfall* is produced in that backflow of blood is prevented but forward flow is only minimally restricted. This occurs because interference with the normal flow will lead to an elevation in venous pressure and dilation of the atrial-venous junction. However, a modest increase in left atrial pressure will not have much effect on the collapsed segment of pulmonary vein. Thus, backflow from the atrium under these circumstances will be inhibited by the high resistance at the atrial-venous junction.

Physical Characteristics of the Atria

The cardiac atria serve as storage reservoirs for blood returning to the heart. This function is particularly significant during ventricular systole when the forward movement of blood is stopped by the closed AV valves and blood collects in the atria. The volume-distensibility characteristics of the atria, therefore, become an important determinant of both systemic and pulmonary venous pressure.

The atria are similar to the venous system in that they are collapsible when partially filled but function as an elastic structure when overfilled (Fig 2–6). In the dog the transition between these two states occurs in the right atrium at a filling volume that is about twice that of the left atrium. In man the capacity of the normal adult atria when filled but not distended is approximately 160 ml for the right atrium and 140 ml for the left atrium. The left atrium, in addition to being smaller, is also less distensible. Volume elasticity curves of the distended right and left atria plotted for the dog but probably representative of most hearts are shown in Figure 2–7.

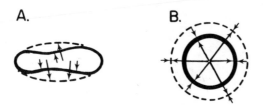

FIG 2–6.
Schematic drawing of the cross-sectional area of **A,** a collapsible system (vein) and **B,** a distensible system (artery). An increase in the volume inside each vessel causes a change in its shape *(dashed lines)*. The change in internal pressure *(arrows)* produced by this volume change represents essentially the change in hydrostatic pressure in the collapsible system, whereas in the elastic system the pressure is the internally directed force produced by stretched elastic elements in the wall.

The Ventricles

The thick-walled ventricles are the major force pumps of the heart. The more circular left ventricle is designed to support the systemic blood pressure and is quite effective in developing a high intracardiac pressure. The bellows-shaped right ventricle is designed to move blood through the pulmonary circuit under a low pressure (Fig 2–8). In cross section the ventricular wall shows the same three major subdivisions (endocardium, myocardium, and epicardium) as described earlier for the atria. The myocardium is much thicker than in the atria and is arranged in a complicated

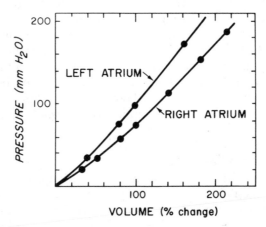

FIG 2–7.
Pressure-volume plot for right and left atrium of the dog. Volume is shown as the percentage change of the filling volume of each atrium. (From Little RC: *Am J Physiol* 1949; 158:237. Used by permission.)

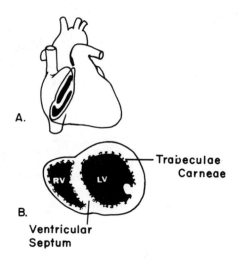

FIG 2–8.
Schematic drawing of the heart illustrating the difference in shape of the right and left ventricle. **A,** approximate anatomical position of the AV ring and tapered, bellows-like shape of the right ventricle. **B,** circular cross section of the left ventricle. *RV* = right ventricle; *LV* = left ventricle. (Modified from Schlant RC, in Hurst JW, Logue RB: *The Heart,* ed 2. New York, McGraw-Hill Book Co, 1970. Used by permission.)

sequence of layers and bundles. On its inner border it shows a trabeculated zone, the *trabeculae carneae,* where the muscle bundles are undercut by open spaces. It has been suggested that this highly irregular inner border eliminates the need for wrinkling of the endocardium and prevents possible damage as the heart becomes smaller during systole. The dense myocardial layer is quite thick in the left ventricle, whereas the trabeculated layer is relatively thicker in the right ventricle. The ventricular septum is the thickest part of the ventricular wall and has trabeculations on both sides. It is made up of muscular groups from both ventricles; however, a predominance of the muscle fibers in the septum comes from the left side of the heart.

Anatomy of the Ventricles
The traditional description of the muscle groups of the ventricle has recently been questioned. Two main groups were previously recognized: (1) a superficial layer that followed a predominantly clockwise helical course from base to apex where it then turned inward and spiraled upward toward the base in the opposite direction, and (2) a deep muscle layer that followed a similar but counterclockwise path. This formalized arrangement of muscle bundles may represent an oversimplification of a somewhat more compli-

cated myocardial matrix. It now appears that the outer clockwise helix of ventricular fibers is probably continuous with and gradually merges with the inner counterclockwise helix without the presence of discrete muscle bundles. In addition to these two helical systems, the individual muscle fibers also have a twisting relationship to one another.

When a cross section of the left ventricular wall that is tangential to the epicardium (Fig 2–9) is examined, the middle 60% is found to have a nearly circumferential fiber orientation. On either side of this central zone, the fibers form increasingly oblique spirals toward the epicardium or endocardium, and the spiral turns in the opposite direction. As a result, the fiber angle is approximately +90 degrees at the endocardial surface and −90 degrees at the epicardial surface. This means that the fibers in the central zone are oriented at right angles to the fibers on either surface of the ventricle. This fiber orientation provides for maximum reduction in ventricular

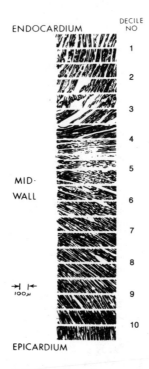

FIG 2–9.
Typical sequence of photomicrographs showing fiber angles in successive sections taken from a heart in systole. The sections are parallel to the epicardial plane. Fiber angle is +90 degrees at the endocardium, running through 0 degree at the midwall to −90 degrees at the epicardium. The sequence of numbers refers to deciles of wall thickness. (From Streeter DD, et al: *Circ Res* 1969; 24:342. Used by permission.)

volume during systole while keeping the tension between adjacent muscle fibers to a minimum. The pattern in the right ventricle appears to be similar to that described above for the left side of the heart.

In general, the ventricular architecture appears to represent a syncytium of muscle fibers that originate from the annulus fibrosus, the root of the aorta, and the pulmonary artery and terminate in the papillary muscles and trabeculae carneae. These ventricular muscle fibers ultimately insert through the chordae tendineae on the AV fibrous annuli and the other components of the cardiac skeleton. Between their origin and insertion, the myocardial fibers follow a 360-degree clockwise path down to the apex and then back on the inside of the heart to the cardiac base. This arrangement is diagrammatically shown in Figure 2–10. In addition, there are thick, relatively separate, sphincter muscle groups that surround the base of the pulmonary and aortic outflow tracts. As the same muscle syncytium encompasses both ventricles, it appears artificial to attempt to identify right or left ventricular fiber groups.

The spiral arrangement of the ventricular myocardium just described seems particularly adapted to the task of propelling blood into the aorta and pulmonary artery. During the early stages of contraction, the inflow tract from base to apex shortens and the outflow tract from apex to aorta lengthens (Fig 2–11). As a result, the left ventricle becomes more spheroid. The importance of this geometric change to cardiac energetics is discussed in

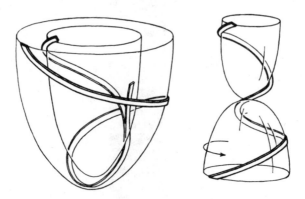

FIG 2–10.
Left, schema showing overall pathway of fiber continuity in left ventricular syncytium. This starts at the base of the heart and follows a roughly 360-degree clockwise path in the epicardial layer to the apex, and another clockwise path of roughly 360 degrees in the inner layers of the ventricle, back from the apex to the base. *Right,* a topologic eversion of the outer layers demonstrates the fiber continuity longitudinally between the two helical pathways. Lateral continuity also exists (see Fig 2–9) but is not shown in this figure. (From Grant RP: *Circulation* 1965; 32:303. Used by permission.)

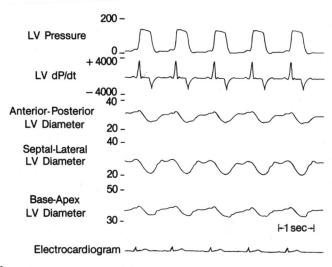

FIG 2–11.
Simultaneous plot of left ventricular pressure (mm Hg); rate of change of left ventricular pressure (dP/dt); anterior-posterior, septal-lateral, and base-apex left ventricular diameter (mm); and the electrocardiogram recorded in a conscious dog.

Chapter 8. Because of the insertion of the ventricular musculature on the cardiac skeleton, the base of the heart is pulled down, and the great vessels are stretched. The septum is depolarized early in the activation of the ventricles. As a result, it contracts first and forms a rigid prop around which the remainder of the heart "wrings out the blood" into the outflow tract. This is accompanied by a marked reduction in the internal circumference of the ventricle with very little change in the long axis of the heart. During this period the heart rotates to the right, and as a result, more of the left ventricle is brought to the front of the chest.

Physical Characteristics of the Ventricles

The size of the ventricle at the end of diastole has an important effect on the force and vigor of the contraction to follow. This relationship will be discussed in Chapter 7. It is sufficient here to point out that the end-diastolic ventricular pressure is a clinically useful indicator of the volume of blood in the ventricle. For this reason, the volume-elastic properties of the ventricle become important in evaluation of cardiac function.

Ventricular muscle, like other biologic tissues, has an exponential length (stress)-tension (strain) relationship. This usually is expressed for the intact heart by using ventricular pressure instead of myocardial tension and relating it to ventricular volume instead of myocardial length (Fig 2–12,A).

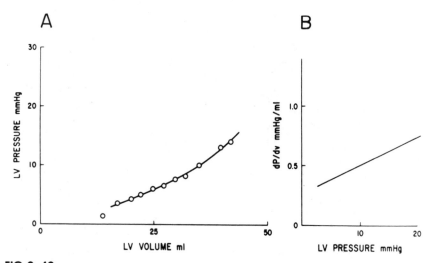

FIG 2–12.
A, relation between left ventricular diastolic pressure and left ventricular volume, expressed as an exponential function. **B,** the slope *(dP/dV)* of the stress-strain relationship plotted against left ventricular *(LV)* pressure. See text for discussion. (From Covell JW, Ross J Jr: *Am J Cardiol* 1973; 32:452. Used by permission.)

Because of its nonlinear stress-strain behavior, the heart becomes stiffer; that is, the ratio ΔP/ΔV becomes larger when the muscle length is increased. To separate the elastic behavior of the myocardium from specific changes in stiffness that accompany alteration in fiber length (or volume in the intact heart), it is usual to use the relationship between stiffness (ΔP/ ΔV) and pressure as this ratio is linearly related to internal pressure. This is shown in Figure 2–12,B. Changes in the slope of this linear relationship indicate fundamental changes in cardiac stiffness.

Specialized Conductive Tissues

The specialized conductive tissues of the heart differ structurally from the ordinary myocardium in that their cells are more variable in shape, contain fewer myofibrils, and have a characteristic pale-staining cytoplasm. Their electrophysiologic characteristics are discussed in Chapter 4. The function of these specialized tissues is to initiate and coordinate the cardiac beat. They consist of (1) the sinus or SA node (formally called the sinoatrial node), (2) the atrial internodal tracts, (3) the AV node, (4) the common AV bundle (bundle of His) and its branches, and (5) the right and left bundle branches (Purkinje system). These are diagrammatically shown in Figure 2–13.

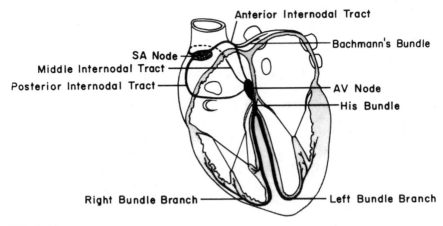

FIG 2–13.
Diagrammatic representation of major specialized conductive tissues of the heart.

Sinus Node (Node of Keith and Flack)

This is a small mass of specialized cells and collagenous tissue located at the junction of the superior vena cava and the right auricle. It has a prominent central artery, and many nerve endings occur in its vicinity. Embryologically, it is derived from the junction of the right horn of the sinus venosus and the primitive atrium. Two types of cells have been described: (1) pale, ovoid cells, with a large round nucleus, called P cells and (2) slender, elongated cells that are intermediate between the ovoid and ordinary cardiac muscle cells. The P cells are thought to be pacemaker cells, whereas the intermediate or "transitional" cells serve to conduct the impulse within and away from the node.

Internodal Tracts

Three preferential conductive pathways have been identified that extend from the area of the sinus node across the atrium and converge toward the AV node. They are the *anterior, middle,* and *posterior internodal bands.* These pathways contain a mixture of (1) closely packed, parallel myocardial fibers, (2) large pale-staining cells with a perinuclear clear zone, large nucleus, and sparse myofibrils that resemble the Purkinje cells found in the ventricular conductive tracts, (3) P cells similar to those found in the SA and AV nodes, and (4) a variety of so-called transitional cells. Those internodal bundles are sometimes difficult to demonstrate anatomically, and in the past, both their role and even their existence have been matters of dispute. Nevertheless, electrophysiologic measurements have shown that conduction proceeds more rapidly over these myocardial bundles than in less well-aligned atrial myocardium. While this preferential conduction is not necessarily evidence for a specialized conductive pathway, it is clear that specialized atrial cells are more plentiful in the area of the internodal tracts. Therefore, current thinking is to consider these tracts as a conduit with multiple cell properties and a rapid conduction rate.*

The *anterior internodal tract* curves around the superior vena cava. It then divides and sends fibers (1) to the left atrium where it merges with the ordinary myocardium (Bachmann's bundle) and (2) down through the atrial septum toward the AV node. The *middle internodal tract* (Wenckebach's tract) curves behind the superior vena cava before descending toward the AV node. The *posterior internodal tract* (Thorel's tract) continues along the terminal crest to enter the atrial septum just above the posterior margin of the AV node. The fibers from the three internodal tracts merge as they approach the AV node.

Atrioventricular Node and Common Bundle

The AV node is a small area that consists of thin specialized myocardial cells arranged in intertwining whorls. It is situated just beneath the endocardium on the right side of the atrial septum at its junction with the central fibrous body and the septal leaf of the tricuspid valve. It is just anterior to the opening of the coronary sinus. The AV node is thought to develop from one or more centers in the left horn of the primitive sinus venosus and to migrate to its present position during embryologic development. It is supplied with abundant nerve endings and vagal ganglionic cells.

At the lower end of the AV node, the parallel Purkinje cell fibers of the *common bundle* (bundle of His) penetrate the right fibrous trigone and enter the posterior inferior part of the membranous ventricular septum. As mentioned earlier, this is the only normal muscular connection between the atrial and ventricular myocardium. In some hearts an accessory muscle bundle (bundle of Kent) connects the lateral wall of the atrium and the ventricle. This anomaly has been associated with early activation of the ventricle (the Wolff-Parkinson-White syndrome). Other accessory pathways have been described between the common bundle and the upper ventricular septum.

In the ventricular septum, the conductive fibers within the common bundle begin to form the fascicle of the *left bundle branch* (Fig 2–14). These fibers separate over an area of 6.5 to 20 mm and pass to the left surface of the ventricular septum. The remainder of the fibers of the common bundle continue on the right side of the septum as a slender group, the *right bundle branch*.

---

*For a review of this subject, see Little RC (ed): *Physiology of Atrial Pacemakers and Conductive Tissues.* Mt Kisco, New York, Futura Publishing Co, 1980.

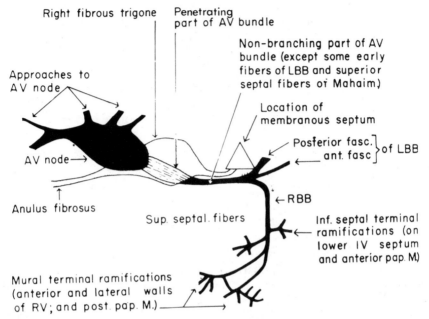

FIG 2–14.
Diagram of the atrioventricular *(AV)* conduction system as viewed from right side of the heart. Conduction tissue is shown in black. *Ant* = anterior; *fasc* = fascicle; *inf* = inferior; *IV* = interventricular; *LBB* = left bundle branch; *pap M* = papillary muscle; *post* = posterior; *RBB* = right bundle branch; *RV* = right ventricle; *sup* = superior. (From Hecht HH, Kossman CE: *Am J Cardiol* 1973; 31:233. Used by permission.)

Bundle Branches

The fibers of the left bundle branch fan out from the common bundle in a wide sheet. This soon divides into an *anterior* and a *posterior fascicle* with some intercommunication between these two divisions to form a septal fascicle. These fibers, which collectively constitute the left bundle branch, spread out under the endocardium of the left ventricle and penetrate the myocardium. The anterior fascicle goes primarily to the anterolateral wall and the anterior papillary muscle. The posterior fascicle goes to the lateral and posterior wall and the posterior papillary muscle, whereas the septal fascicle supplies primarily the lower ventricular septum and the apical wall of the left ventricle. The spread of the specialized tissues as they form the left bundle branch may permit localized pathologic lesions to interrupt only a relatively few fibers. As a result, block of a specific fascicle may take place; thus, anterior, posterior, or trifascicular blocks may occur (see Chapter 6).

The right bundle branch travels under the endocardium along the right side of the ventricular septum to the base of the anterior papillary muscle. At this point, it divides into a sheet of fibers that spread over the inside of the right ventricular wall and supply the anterior and lateral wall of that chamber, the lower ventricular septum, and the papillary muscles.

Purkinje fibers encased in connective tissue and endocardium may transverse the ventricular cavities from the septum to the free wall of the ventricle. These *pseudotendons* or *false tendons* may be quite prominent.

Innervation of the Heart

Sympathetic Fibers

The heart receives a rich supply of both sympathetic and parasympathetic nerve fibers. Preganglionic sympathetic fibers from cells in the intermediolateral columns of the upper thoracic region of the spinal cord synapse in paravertebral ganglia; postganglionic fibers then travel to the heart as superior, middle, and inferior cardiac nerves and thoracic-visceral nerves. These sympathetic fibers commingle to form an extensive epicardial plexus and are distributed to the entire heart. Some postganglionic sympathetic fibers also join the vagus nerves and are distributed to the area of the SA node, the AV node, and the atrial myocardium. As discussed in subsequent chapters, cardiac sympathetic receptors are largely of the β_1 type, and few, if any, α-adrenergic receptors are present. Stimulation of the myocardial sympathetic receptors results in an increase in both myocardial contractile force and cardiac rate and the increased mobilization of myocardial glycogen.

Parasympathetic Fibers

In contrast to the sympathetic innervation, parasympathetic fibers to the heart are primarily distributed only to the atrial myocardium and the specialized tissues of the SA and AV nodes. Preganglionic parasympathetic fibers originate in the dorsal motor nucleus of the medulla and travel in the vagus nerves. These fibers synapse with short postganglionic nerves in the wall of the atria and are distributed to the atrial myocardium and the specialized tissues of the SA and AV nodes. Stimulation of these postganglionic cholinergic fibers results in slowing of the heart rate and a decrease in the vigor of atrial contraction (see Chapter 3 for further discussion). Evidence is still incomplete regarding parasympathetic innervation of ventricular structures. Although the vagus nerve has been reported to have a negative inotropic influence on the ventricular myocardium.

Sensory Fibers

Afferent impulses from sensory endings in the wall of the heart, adventitia of the coronary arteries, and the pericardium travel in sensory nerves that accompany the sympathetic fibers. These fibers have their cell body in the thoracic dorsal ganglia and they synapse with ascending fibers in the posterior columns of the spinal cord. Sensory afferent fibers also travel with the vagus nerve.

Coronary Vascular System

Arteries

The right and left coronary arteries take their origin from the aorta at the base of the sinuses of Valsalva behind the cusps of the aortic valve. Figure 2–15 illustrates how the *right coronary artery* runs in the coronary sulcus between the right atrium and the right ventricle along the diaphrag-

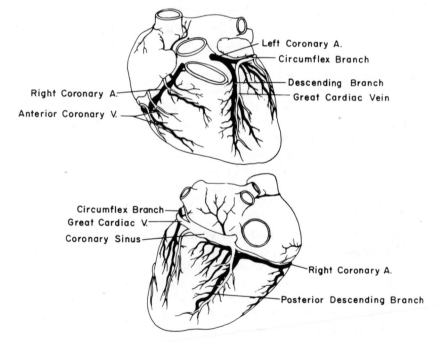

FIG 2–15.
Diagram showing location of major coronary arteries and veins on anterior *(top)* and posterior *(bottom)* surfaces of the heart.

matic surface of the heart before descending toward the apex. It gives off branches to the right atrium, to the free wall of the right ventricle, and to a variable extent to the posterior one third of the ventricular septum and posterior wall of the left ventricle. In about 70% of hearts, these latter structures receive most of their blood supply from the right coronary artery. In about one half of all hearts, an accessory coronary artery also arises from the right coronary artery. This short vessel, the *conus artery*, supplies the outflow tract of the right ventricle at about the level of the pulmonary valve. In the absence of this vessel, the pulmonary conus is supplied by the right coronary artery.

The *left coronary artery* divides soon after it leaves the aorta and forms the *left circumflex artery* and the *left anterior descending artery*. The former arises at right angles to the main vessel and travels in the AV sulcus between the left atrium and left ventricle. Its branches supply the left atrium and the lateral wall of the left ventricle. In addition, it shares with the right coronary artery the provision of blood to the posterior wall of the left ventricle. In about 10% of human hearts, the left coronary artery becomes the dominant vessel and supplies all or nearly all of this part of the heart. In 20% of hearts, the blood supply to this area is evenly distributed between the right and left coronary systems, and neither vessel predominates. The anterior descending artery continues as an extension of the main vessel before turning down in the interventricular groove toward the apex. It supplies the free wall of the left ventricle, the ventricular septum, and, to a limited extent, the anterior wall of the right ventricle.

The sinus node is supplied by a special branch of the right coronary artery in approximately 50% to 60% of hearts and in the remainder by a branch from the left circumflex artery. This artery is also the main source of blood for the atrial myocardium and atrial septum. The AV node receives its arterial supply from a branch of the right coronary artery in 90% of individuals and from the left coronary artery in the remainder.

Myocardial Capillary Bed and Venous Drainage

The coronary arteries penetrate the myocardium and proliferate in a rich network of capillaries. Arterioles and metarterioles are present. The capillary vessels lie between and run parallel to the myocardial fibers. In general, there is one capillary for each muscle fiber, with a maximum diffusion distance between them that has been calculated to be 8 to 10 μ. With cardiac hypertrophy, the diameter of each muscle fiber increases, however, there may not be a corresponding increase in vascularity. As a result, enlarged hearts have an increased vulnerability to circulatory insufficiency.

The venous drainage from the myocardial capillary bed is via three major systems: (1) the *thebesian veins*, which empty into the right and left atrium and to a limited extent into the right ventricle. These vessels may carry as much as 40% of the venous return from the atrial myocardium but probably do not carry a significant quantity of the venous outflow from the ventricles; (2) the *anterior cardiac veins*, which empty into the right atrium; (3) the *coronary sinus* and its connecting *coronary veins*, which form a series of superficial veins, particularly over the left ventricle, that drain the deeper myocardium. These vessels converge to form the coronary sinus, a large venous channel that runs in the posterior part of the coronary groove and drains into the right atrium. Approximately 85% of the coronary sinus outflow represents venous blood from the left ventricular myocardium. For this reason, blood collected from the coronary sinus is frequently used for metabolic studies of the left ventricle.

In addition to the venous channels, there are a series of sinusoidlike vessels that connect to the capillary network of the myocardium and drain directly into the ventricles. Other channels, the arterioluminal vessels, also make connections directly to the heart chambers. These relationships are summarized in Figure 2–16.

The coronary arteries act essentially as end arteries, with each perfusing its own limited capillary bed. As a result, sudden occlusion of a coronary artery results in a localized area of myocardial ischemia and/or infarction. Anastomoses between the coronary vessels are, however, easily demonstrated. For example, tracer substances injected into one coronary artery rapidly appear in the outflow from the other coronary vessels. These anastomotic connections usually are quite small and normally will not permit particles greater than 35 to 40 μ in diameter to pass. As a consequence, while anatomically present, they are not functionally significant in permitting collateral flow between vascular segments. However, if the flow in one artery is gradually decreased, as may occur with the development of local-

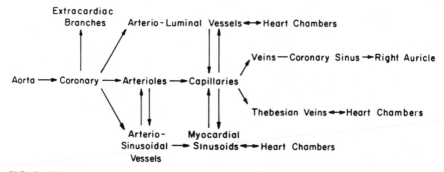

FIG 2–16.
Schematic diagram of coronary circulation. (Modified from Wearn J, et al: *Am Heart J* 1933; 9:143.)

ized occlusive coronary artery disease, these anastomotic connections will slowly enlarge. As a result, a formerly essentially nonfunctional collateral between a normal vessel and a diseased vessel may dilate sufficiently to maintain normal blood flow to the capillary bed supplied by the diseased artery. This dilation of the anastomotic vessel may result from the pressure differences across the anastomotic connection or from vasodilatory substances released from the ischemic tissue, or a combination of these effects. Because of the development of collateral vessels, it is not unusual to find localized severe arteriosclerotic heart disease at autopsy without the presence of myocardial infarction. The key, apparently, is that the arterial lesions developed slowly so that adequate anastomotic vessels had time to form.

Lymph Drainage of the Heart

The heart has a substantial lymphatic network. Fine, thin-walled lymphatic vessels are distributed throughout the myocardium and form a plexus-like layer immediately below the endocardial surface. Lymph channels follow the path of the conductive tissues, and the bundle branches have a particularly rich network. The atrial surfaces of the mitral and tricuspid valves also have an extensive lymphatic supply. Those vessels connect to the lymphatic channels that accompany the coronary arteries. The major lymph drainage is via a single large channel that joins a pretracheal node near the arch of the aorta.

Structure and Function of the Pericardium

The pericardium is a thin, fibrous sac that surrounds the heart. Superiorly it is attached to the great vessels as they enter the heart. It is fixed anteriorly to the sternum, posteriorly to the vertebral column, and the base is adherent to the central tendon of the diaphragm. The space between the serous lining of the pericardium and the epicardium of the heart normally contains a small amount of an ultrafiltrate of plasma. This fluid lubricates the heart and permits it to move freely in the pericardial cavity.

The volume of the pericardial space is adequate to permit the usual physiologic variations in the size of the heart that occur with normal living. The inelastic nature of the pericardial wall, however, puts an upper limit on the ability of the heart to enlarge. A significantly acute increase in cardiac size, for example, causes the normally negative pericardial pressure to be elevated well above atmospheric. This ability of the pericardium to contain the heart and prevent transient excessive dilation may limit right ventricular filling and prevent pulmonary engorgement under conditions of acute left ventricular enlargement due to stress. This will have the effect of protecting the pulmonary circulation from congestion. In addition, the increase in pericardial pressure that accompanies excessive cardiac enlargement acts to balance the increased diastolic pressure inside the ventricle and thus keeps the transmural pressure at a normal level. In the presence of chronic cardiac distention, the pericardial sac will slowly stretch and therefore does not interfere with the gradual enlargement of the heart.

Other important functions that have been ascribed to the pericardium include (1) the prevention of ventriculoatrial regurgitation under conditions of increased ventricular end-diastolic pressure and (2) facilitation of atrial filling due to the negative pericardial pressure, particularly during the period of ventricular systole. It is clear, however, that the pericardium is not required for normal cardiac activities, as individuals with congenital absence of this structure and patients who have had the pericardium surgically removed appear to function quite adequately.

With certain disease processes (chronic adhesive pericarditis, pericardial tamponade, or hemorrhage), cardiac filling may be restricted by the increase in pericardial pressure and/or the inelastic pericardium. As a consequence, central venous pressure is increased. In addition, the normal inspiratory increase in venous return to the right heart acts to further restrict left ventricular filling. This occurs because (1) enlargement of the right ventricle now encroaches on the pericardial space and causes a further increase in pericardial pressure, and (2) the increase in right ventricular volume displaces the ventricular septum toward the left side of the heart. As a consequence, left ventricular filling and systolic ejection are reduced. This sequence of events leads to an exaggeration of the normal inspiratory fall in arterial blood pressure. This was given the name *pulsus paradoxus* by early physicians because of the marked inspiratory weakening or even disappearance of the arterial pulse while, at the same time, the heart sounds and cardiac rhythm continued undisturbed.

COMPOSITION OF SYSTEMIC CIRCULATION

The circulation is a closed system of distensible tubes of varying diameters and physical characteristics (Table 2–1). It usually is subdivided into *arterial*, *capillary*, and *venous* components. Because the *lymphatics* serve to return fluid and other substances to the circulation that might otherwise accumulate in the interstitial space, this system is included as part of the circulatory system.

TABLE 2–1.

Approximate Physical Characteristics of Different Components of the Vascular System*

Structure	Diameter (mm)	Wall Thickness (mm)	Length (cm)	Ratio of Wall Thickness to Radius (w/r)	Wall Tension (dynes/cm)	Internal Pressure (mm Hg)
Aorta	25.0	2.000	40.0	0.16	170,000	100
Medium arteries	4.0	0.800	15.0	0.40	60,000	90
Arterioles	0.3	0.020	0.2	0.75	1,200	60
Capillaries	0.005	0.001	0.075	0.25	16	30
Venules	0.02	0.002	0.20	0.20	26	20
Medium veins	5.0	0.500	15.0	0.20	400	15
Large veins	15.0	0.800	20.0	0.10	9,750	10
Vena cava	30.0	1.500	40.0	0.10	21,000	10

*Based on data from Burton AC: Physical principles of circulatory phenomena: The physical equilibria of the heart and blood vessels. *Handbook of Physiology*, Section 2: Circulation, Vol I. Bethesda, Maryland, American Physiological Society, 1962, pp 85–106, and Burton AC: *Physiol Rev* 1954; 34:619.

Arteries

The arterial system can be subdivided into large *elastic vessels*, smaller *nutrient arteries*, and *arterioles*. The larger arteries (aorta and its major branches) have more collagen fibers and fewer smooth muscle cells in their walls than do the nutrient arteries; however, both have a prominent elastic tissue component. These elastic elements permit the proximal aorta and large arteries to be readily stretched during systole to accommodate the cardiac stroke volume. As discussed in Chapter 4, this permits much of the energy imparted to the blood by ventricular contraction to be stored as potential energy in the elastic arterial wall. This mechanism serves much the same purpose as the compression chamber on a water pump. Intermittent storage and discharge of fluid by this chamber change the pulsatile input into a more even outflow. In addition, storage of the stroke volume by expansion of the proximal aorta minimizes the cardiac afterload by reducing the increase in arterial pressure as the left ventricle ejects the stroke volume into the aorta. This chamber is called by its German name, *windkessel*, in honor of Otto Frank, who developed a mathematical analysis of the circulation using this concept. Because of the buffering function of the aorta and its main branches, they are frequently called *windkessel vessels*. The nutrient arteries arise from the large elastic windkessel vessels as a more or less parallel system of tubes that supply blood to individual organs or vascular beds (Fig 2–17).

The terminal subdivisions of the nutrient arteries are the smaller-diameter *arterioles*. These short vessels as well as some of the smaller arteries

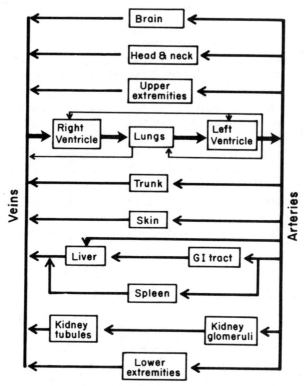

FIG 2–17.
Schematic block diagram of circulatory system showing essentially parallel arrangement of the nutrient arteries that supply blood to the various organ systems.

contain a circular layer of smooth muscle that is under a dual system of neural and chemical control. They have a rich innervation of postsynaptic sympathetic fibers that provide primarily vasoconstriction via activation of vascular muscle α-receptors. In addition, some arterioles also respond to sympathetic stimulation by varying degrees of vasodilation due to activation of vascular muscle β_2-receptors. This aspect is covered in Chapter 11. Some arterioles, particularly in skeletal muscles, also may receive cholinergic vasodilator fibers. Alterations in the tone of arteriolar smooth muscles provide a mechanism for controlling the diameter of the vessel and thereby the resistance to blood flow. The "stopcock" action of these *resistance vessels* offers a mechanism for regulating both the pressure of blood in the arterial system and the volume of local blood flow by controlling outflow. This will be discussed further in Chapters 10 and 11.

Capillary Network

The capillaries and their associated structures *(terminal arterioles* and *postcapillary venules)* constitute the microcirculation. This name originated because these structures are all less than 100 µ in diameter and can be observed only with the aid of a microscope. Thin-walled capillary vessels start, often at right angles, from the slightly larger metarterioles (Fig 2–18). If present, metarterioles act as relatively high-resistance, direct pathways through the capillary bed between an arteriole and a venule. Metarterioles are different from the short, relatively large-diameter AV *shunt vessels* that also bypass the capillary bed. These latter vessels occur in some areas of the skin where they are involved in temperature regulation.

Capillary vessels form an anastomosing network of variable configuration and density before coalescing to drain into a postcapillary venule. The microstructure of the capillary wall varies, and there is no typical organi-

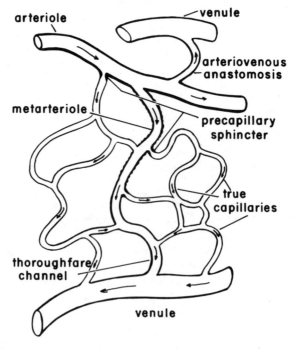

FIG 2–18.
Schematic diagram of a capillary network showing capillaries, AV shunts, and metarterioles that serve as thoroughfare channels between an arteriole and a venule. Vessel walls are thicker where smooth muscle is found. Flow through individual capillary vessels is discontinuous due to action of precapillary sphincters.

zation. In general terms, these vessels are composed of a single layer of endothelial cells with a thin basement membrane to provide support (Fig 2–19). Although some endothelial cells form tight junctions at their margin with other cells, there usually is a cleft or intercellular space about 50 to 60 A wide between each cell. These clefts apparently act as pathways for material to move into or out of the capillary lumen. The number and specific size of these pathways differ from one tissue to another. In some vessels, particularly in the kidney glomerulus and the liver, large pores or fenestrations may appear in the wall; in others, areas of the capillary wall may only become very thin and fragmented, with essentially no cytoplasm between the inner and outer cell membranes. The basement membrane is continuous in most capillaries and may play a role in limiting the movement of material into and out of the vessel; however, in some vessels, the basement membrane also contains open spaces.

The generally porous structure of the exchange vessels appears to make them ideally suited for transmural exchange of fluid and small-diameter particles between blood and interstitial fluid. In addition, small granules and vesicles are frequently observed within the endothelial cells of the capillary wall. These structures have been linked with the transport of larger molecules by micropinocytosis whereby material is engulfed by an active mechanism similar to phagocytosis. This is a slow transport process and probably does not contribute much to transcapillary exchange.

The terminal arterioles constitute the final point of neuromuscular control of capillary perfusion. These structures are also responsive to temper-

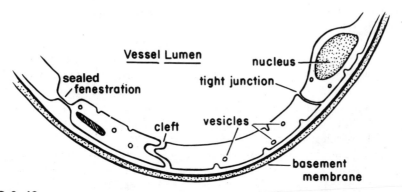

FIG 2–19.
Diagram showing two epithelial cells that make up part of the capillary wall. The cleft between the cells (about 60 A) provides for movement of fluid and solute into and out of the vessel lumen. These pores occupy less than 1% of the wall surface. Small vesicles and indentations of the surface are shown that may be involved in pinocytosis. A basement membrane made up of mucopolysaccharide surrounds the wall.

ature, pH, and levels of dissolved oxygen and carbon dioxide in the blood and neighboring fluid. In fact, they probably regulate capillary flow largely on the basis of these local conditions (see Chapter 11). Constriction and relaxation of these vessels also may be initiated by pacemaker activity within the arteriolar muscle. This rhythmic activity (vasomotion) results in an intermittent flow through individual capillaries. Because of this, only a small part of the total capillary bed is perfused at any one time. When the arteriole is relaxed, the cross-section area of the orifices leading to capillaries is less than 0.2 sq mm, and they will only permit one red blood cell at a time to pass into a capillary vessel. An individual capillary is short and averages 0.4 to 0.7 mm in length; however, their large number causes them to become a sizable structure in the aggregate. It is estimated that in the adult their total length may exceed several miles, and their total surface area may equal nearly 7,000 sq ft. Because of the large total cross-sectional area, the velocity of flow in each individual capillary is slow, averaging about 0.07 cm/second. However, because of the short length of the vessel, the average capillary transit time is only 1.5 to 2 seconds.

Veins

Blood drains from the capillaries into the venules, which constitute the first part of the venous system. These vessels are formed by the coalescence of the through channel metarterioles, capillary vessels, and, if present, the AV anastomotic shunt vessels. The venules usually are slightly larger in diameter than their companion arterioles but have a much thinner wall. In addition, clefts or openings have been observed in their endothelial lining similar to those of the capillaries. This has suggested that interchange across the venule wall between its contents and the interstitial space occurs as it does in the capillary network. For this reason, capillaries and venules usually are considered to constitute the *exchange vessels*. The venules converge to form veins of progressively larger diameter. Muscular tissue in the wall of the venules and small veins is under nervous control. However, as discussed below, changes in the tone of this circularly arranged muscle act primarily to alter the internal volume of the vessel.

There are at least two or more veins that tend to anastomose freely for each artery of the same size. This arrangement makes the total cross-sectional area of the venous system much greater than the corresponding area of the arteries (see Fig 9–7). The hemodynamic consequence of this organization will be discussed in Chapter 9. It is sufficient here to point out that the large capacity of the venous system permits it to serve as an important low-pressure storage reservoir. It is estimated, for example, that, excluding the heart and lungs, as much as 77% of the circulating blood volume at any one time is contained in the venous system, whereas approximately 16% is in the arterial vessels and the remainder in the capillaries (Table 2–2). As a result of this storage function, the veins are often called the *capacitance vessels.*

Arteries and veins both have an inner endothelial lining, a middle muscular coat, and an outer adventitial layer; however, veins have much thinner walls containing relatively fewer elastic fibers. As a result, veins are structurally much stiffer than arteries. In spite of this, the collapsible nature of veins permits them to increase their internal volume severalfold with only a small increase in pressure (Fig 2–20). This is accomplished by a change in their cross-sectional profile from a flattened ellipse to a more circular shape. As a result, over the normal range of venous pressure, veins are considerably more compliant than arteries. When filled, veins become an elastic system, and further increases in their volume can only be accomplished by stretching the wall. It is at this point that the lower distensibility of veins compared to arteries becomes apparent.

The endothelial lining of the veins is periodically formed into crescent-shaped folds with their free edge pointing toward the heart. These bicuspid valves serve an important function in preventing the retrograde flow of blood toward the tissues. Valves are more numerous in the veins of the lower extremity than elsewhere. They are not present in veins that are smaller than 1 mm in diameter or in veins in areas that are not subjected to muscular pressure such as the abdominal, thoracic, or cerebral cavities.

Lymphatics

The lymphatic vessels constitute a second circulatory system designed to collect fluid and other materials (for example, protein molecules) that might accumulate in the interstitial space and to return this material to the vascular system by way of the thoracic duct. The lymphatics also serve as

TABLE 2–2.

Distribution of Blood Volume in Man (Representative Values)

Area	Volume (ml)	% Total Blood Volume
Systemic circulation		70
Aorta and arteries (14.3%)*	565	
Arterioles (1.4%)*	57	
Capillaries (7.1%)*	282	
Venules, veins, venae cavae (77.1%)*	3,048	
Total	3,952	
Pulmonary circulation	1,016	18
Heart chambers	677	12
Total blood volume	5,645	100
*Percent of total blood in systemic circulation.		

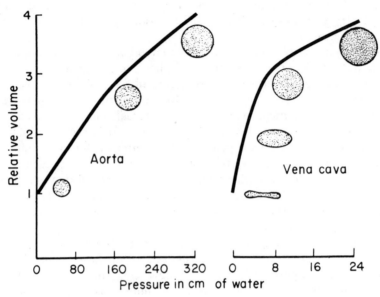

FIG 2–20.
Schematic comparison of pressure-volume curve and cross-sectional profile of the aorta and vena cava. (From Burton, AC: *Physiology and Biophysics of the Circulation,* ed 2. Chicago, Year Book Medical Publishers, 1972. Used by permission.)

an important defense mechanism. The lymph nodes that are interposed in the system contain phagocytic cells, which remove bacterial and other foreign material from the lymph. They also produce blood cells and antibodies.

The lymphatic system begins with a network of blind-ended endothelial tubes that have the same organization and relationship to the tissue cells as do the vascular capillaries. The surface areas of these two capillary systems are approximately equal. The absence of a basement membrane causes lymphatic vessels to be more permeable to large-sized particles than are the vascular capillaries. The lymphatic capillaries coalesce into larger-sized vessels that contain myogenically active smooth muscle and elastic tissue in their walls. They also have endothelial valves that permit unidirectional flow toward thoracic duct and the central veins.

RELATIONSHIP BETWEEN WALL THICKNESS AND VESSEL LUMEN

The ratio of the thickness of the vessel wall to the radius of the lumen, w/r, has physiologic significance (see Table 2–1). The arterioles have a large w/r ratio because of their prominent muscle layer and small radius. As a result, contraction of the external layer of the circular muscles in the wall of the arteriole displaces the remainder of the muscle mass toward the center of the vessel (Fig 2–21). This movement reduces the lumen out of proportion to the change in length of the circular muscle fibers. The effect is to potentiate the change in resistance to blood flow produced by the vasomotor activity of the arteriole. Their large w/r ratio permits them to close completely as a result of minimal contraction of the circular muscular elements. Vein walls are quite thin and have a w/r ratio that is relatively small. In these vessels, contraction of the muscular coat does not have nearly the effect on blood flow that it does in arterioles.

The muscular tissue in the wall of the aorta and other windkessel vessels is arranged with both a circular and longitudinal orientation so that shortening produces only a minimal effect on the diameter of the vessel. The principal action of contraction of these elements is to increase the stiffness of the artery. Recent studies suggest that the tone of this vascular muscle is under reflex control, and changes in the level of its contraction, with alterations in cardiac output, may serve to match the impedance of the vascular system with that of the cardiac pump.

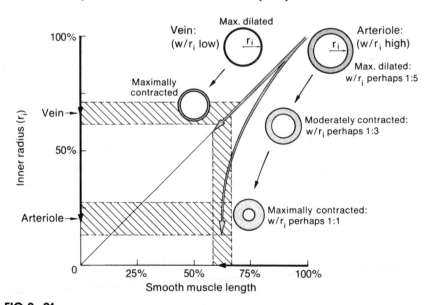

FIG 2–21.
Diagram showing in general terms how the difference in the (w/r ratio) affects the reduction in the lumen of a blood vessel due to contraction of the smooth muscle in the wall. (From Folkow B, Neil E: *Circulation.* New York, Oxford University Press, 1971, p 48. Used by permission.)

SUMMARY

The heart contains two pump systems. The right heart receives blood from the great veins and sends it on to the pulmonary vessels. The left heart receives arterial blood from the lungs and pumps it to the systemic circulation. The fibrous cardiac skeleton separates the atrial and ventricular myocardium and serves as the attachment of the AV valves. The origin and conduction of the impulse for cardiac contraction is accomplished by the specialized conductive tissues (sinus node, internodal tracts, the AV node, bundle of His, and the Purkinje fibers of the ventricular bundle branches). The heart has a rich supply of both parasympathetic and sympathetic nerve fibers. The myocardium receives its blood supply from the coronary vascular system. The heart has a substantial lymphatic network and is surrounded by the pericardial sac.

The systemic circulation can be divided into the aorta and large arteries (windkessel vessels), small arteries (nutrient vessels), arterioles (resistance vessels), capillaries and venules (exchange vessels), and veins (capacitance vessels). The vascular smooth muscle of the resistance vessels is under the dual control of local conditions and the autonomic nervous system. Lymphatic vessels return fluid and other substances from the interstitial space to the circulation.

BIBLIOGRAPHY

Ankeney JL: Further experimental evidence that pulmonary capillary pressures do not reflect cyclic changes in left atrial pressure. *Circ Res* 1958; 1:58.

Bearer EL, Orci L: Endothelial fenestral diaphragms: A quick-freeze, deep-etch study. *J Cell Biol* 1985; 100:418.

Burch GE, Roy C, Cronvich JA: Certain mechanical peculiarities of the human cardiac pump in normal and diseased states. *Circulation* 1952; 5:504.

Campeti FI, et al: Dynamics of the orifices of the vena cava studied by cineangio-cardiography. *Circulation* 1959; 19:55.

Grant RP: Notes on the muscular architecture of the left ventricle. *Circulation* 1965; 32:301.

Hawthorne EW (ed): Symposium: Dynamic geometry of the left ventricle. *Fed Proc* 1969; 28:1323.

Janes TN: The connecting pathways between the sinus node and the AV node and between the right and left atrium of the human heart. *Am Heart J* 1963; 66:498.

Licata RH: Anatomy of the heart, in Luisada AA (ed): *Cardiology: An Encyclopedia of the Cardiovascular System*, vol 1. New York, McGraw-Hill Book Co, 1959, pp 30–60.

Little RC: The physiology of atrial pacemakers and conductive tissues: Historical perspective, in Little RC (ed): *The Physiology of Atrial Pacemakers and Conductive Tissues*. Mt Kisco, NY, Futura Publishing Co, 1980.

Little RC: Volume elastic properties of the right and left atrium. *Am J Physiol* 1949; 158:237.

Little RC: Volume pressure relationships of the pulmonary left heart vascular segment. *Circ Res* 1960; 3:594.

Little RC, Weed WE: Diastolic viscoelastic properties of active and quiescent cardiac muscle. *Am J Physiol* 1971; 201:1120.

McGregor M: Pulsus paradoxus. *N Engl J Med* 1979; 301:480.

Miller AJ: Lymphatics of the heart. *Arch Intern Med* 1963; 112:501.

Permutt S, Riley RL: Hemodynamics of collapsible vessels with tone: The vascular waterfall. *J Appl Physiol* 1962; 18:924.

Pitt B: Interarterial coronary anastomoses: Occurrence in normal hearts and in certain pathological conditions. *Circulation* 1959; 20:816.

Powell EDV, Mullney JM: The Chiari network and the valve of the inferior vena cava. *Br Heart J* 1960; 22:579.

Rudolph AM, et al: Observation and sphincter mechanism at the pulmonary venous left atrial junction. *Circulation* 1961; 24:1027.

Shabetai R, Fowler NO, Guntheroth WG: The hemodynamics of cardiac tamponade and constructive pericarditis. *Am J Cardiol* 1970; 26:480.

Sherf L, James TN: Fine structure of cells and their histological organization within internodal pathways of the heart: Clinical and electrocardiographic implications. *Am J Cardiol* 1979; 44:345.

Spotnitz HM, Sonnenblick EH: Structural conditions in the hypertophied and failing heart. *Am J Cardiol* 1973; 32:398.

Titus JL: Normal anatomy of the human cardiac conduction system. *Mayo Clin Proc* 1973; 48:24.

Chapter 3 _____

Biophysics of the Cardiac Cell

_____

The fundamental electrical and mechanical properties of the myocardium and its subcellular components that are summarized in this chapter will serve as an introduction to the function of the intact heart described in subsequent sections. These cellular aspects of cardiac function underlie much of modern cardiac therapy; because of the importance of this material, it is presented as a separate unit.

ELECTRIC ACTIVITY OF CARDIAC CELLS

The resting membrane potential (E_m) of myocardial cells is in the order of -85 to -90 mV.* It can be measured, as shown in Figure 3–1, with the aid of nonpolarizing, high-impedance microelectrodes and suitable electronic amplification. The output of such a recording system usually is displayed on an oscilloscope screen or strip chart recorder in the form of a time-voltage plot.

The difference in composition of intracellular and extracellular fluid (Table 3–1) suggested to earlier physiologists that diffusional forces could separate charge and produce the resting membrane potential. Subsequent workers have confirmed and extended this basic concept to include the effects of membrane permeability and the actions of metabolic ion pumps.

_____
*The outside of the cell is assumed to be at ground (zero) potential. The magnitude of E_m is, therefore, the difference between the inside potential and zero and is a positive number. The sign indicates the polarity of the inside of the cell.

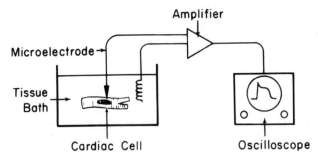

FIG 3–1.
Schematic diagram showing recording of an intracellular membrane potential from a cardiac cell. The microelectrode usually is a finely drawn glass tube filled with a solution of 3 M potassium chloride and with a tip 1 μ or less in diameter.

ELECTRIC FIELDS AND POTENTIAL DIFFERENCE

It is helpful before considering the electrophysiology of cardiac cells to first briefly review the development of an electric field when there is separation of charge in a volume conductor. Ions are charged particles that are electrically positive or negative depending on their ability to accept or donate electrons. In solutions containing electrolytes, the electrostatic attraction of particles with unlike charges and the repulsion between particles with like charges result in a strong tendency to produce ion pairs and thereby maintain electric neutrality. It is worthwhile to emphasize that, contrary to popular belief, electric neutrality in all areas of a macroscopic solution is not an absolute requirement of nature. Overall, any bulk solution must contain an equal number of positive and negative charges. However, if some force (for example, the energy contained in the higher concentration of a diffusible charged particle inside a cell) is sufficient to cause

TABLE 3–1.
Approximate Electrolyte Composition of Cardiac Intracellular and Extracellular Fluid In Vitro

Ion	Intracellular Concentration (mmol/L)	Extracellular Concentration (mmol/L)	Equilibrium Potential* (mV)
Na^+	7	144	+81
K^+	151	4	−97
Cl^-	4†	114	−90

*Calculated using the Nernst equation at body temperature.
†Calculated from membrane potential.

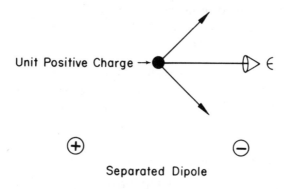

Separated Dipole

FIG 3–2.
Two-dimensional diagram showing the electrostatic attraction and repulsion of a unit positive charge placed in the electric field produced by separation of an ion pair. Intensity and direction of the field acting on the unit positive charge are shown by the vector ϵ.

an ion to move through the cell membrane and thus be separated from its ion pair, electric neutrality will no longer exist in the vicinity of the membrane. Work will be carried out in separating the ion pair according to the following relationship:

$$\text{work} = \text{force} \times \text{distance (in the direction of the force)}$$

where the distance is the amount of separation. It is important to these considerations to point out that the work term in this relationship has magnitude but not direction and is a *scalar* quantity.

Separation of an ion pair, such as described above, will set up an *electric field*. This is because the electrostatic attraction or repulsion of the separated ions will affect any other charge brought into the area. The intensity of the field at any point is defined as the electric force exerted on a unit positive charge placed at that point (Fig 3–2). In contrast to the work carried out to produce the field, the intensity of the field (ϵ) is a vector quantity, as it has both magnitude* and direction.

Work must be carried out to bring a unit positive charge from some great distance and place it in the electric field produced by the separation of an ion pair. As a result of this work, the unit positive charge obtains a certain potential energy. It follows, therefore, that the difference in the potential energy between any two points P_1 and P_2 in the field is the

---

*Defined by Coulomb's law, $F = K (q_1 \times q_2)/r^2$, where q_1 and q_2 are the values of the charged particles, r is the distance between the charges, and K is the dielectric constant.

amount of work required to move the unit positive charge from P_1 to P_2. This difference is said to equal 1 mV if it requires 10^4 ergs of work. It is more convenient in physiologic studies to use the scalar quantity E_m, discussed previously, to describe the electric field produced by the separation of charge across a cell membrane than to deal with the vector aspects of the field. In addition, the membrane potential is accessible to experimental measurement. As a result, it usually is used to quantitate the electric activity of the cell membrane.

Resting Membrane Potential

The mechanism responsible for the resting E_m of an excitable cell is complex. In discussing this phenomenon, it will be helpful to first consider two solutions of potassium chloride (KCl) (Fig 3–3) separated by a theoretical membrane that is permeable only to K^+. In this highly artificial situation, K^+ will diffuse from solution A, where it is in higher concentration,

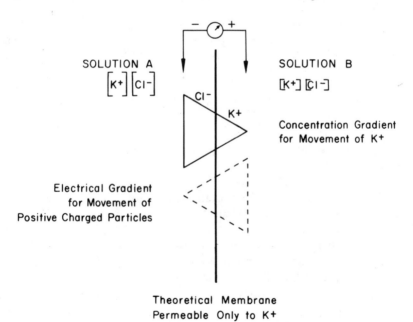

FIG 3–3.
Diagram illustrating diffusion of K^+ from solution A down its concentration gradient to solution B through a membrane permeable only to K^+. For each K^+ that diffuses through the membrane, a Cl^- is left behind. This separation of charge produces a difference in electric potential across the membrane oriented to oppose the further net diffusion of K^+. See text for discussion.

through the membrane to B, where it is present in lower concentration. Movement of the first K^+ from solution A to solution B would leave the negatively charged member of its ion pair (in this case Cl^-) behind due to its inability to penetrate the membrane. These two charged particles will still be attracted to each other; however, they will now be separated by the thickness of the membrane. The electric field produced by such a separation of charge is oriented to oppose the net movement of additional positively charged ions across the membrane. In fact, diffusion of only a relatively few K^+ particles from solution A to solution B will produce sufficient excess positive charge on the B side of the membrane to prevent further accumulation of K^+ in that area. The electric potential difference (the diffusion potential) across the membrane at this point of equilibrium (i.e., where the diffusional flux of K^+ is equal but opposite to the tendency for movement of K^+ in the electric field) can be predicted from the concentration of K^+ on each side of the membrane by use of the Nernst equation. This equation, which assumes free permeability of ions, lack of active transport, and independence of all particles in solution, is usually written as follows:

$$E_m = \frac{-RT}{ZF} \log_e \frac{[K^+]_i}{[K^+]_o} \tag{3-1}$$

where E_m is the membrane potential, R is the gas constant, T is the absolute temperature, F is Faraday's constant, and Z is the valence. Brackets indicate concentration, and the subscripts i and o indicate inside and outside of the cell, respectively. The Nernst potential in this example, as we are dealing with K^+, is also called the potassium equilibrium potential (E_K).

The Nernst equation reduces to the following more useful form for a monovalent positively charged ion such as K^+ when related to a cell membrane at body temperature:

$$E_K \text{ (in millivolts)} = 61.5 \log_{10} \frac{[K^+]_o}{[K^+]_i} \tag{3-2}$$

Note that this simplified expression uses the common log (base 10), and the negative sign has been removed by inverting the concentration ratio for K^+.

It should be emphasized that the membrane potential equals the Nernst potential only under equilibrium conditions when the diffusional and electric forces tending to move a single ion species are equal and oriented in opposing directions. In that situation, the electrochemical potential of the system is zero, and the Nernst potential for the ion in question (the equilibrium potential) represents the electric force required to counter the diffusional movement and thus maintain the ion's concentration difference across the membrane.

The approximate equilibrium potential of the major diffusible ions in cardiac tissue is listed in Table 3–1. Chloride apparently distributes itself across the cell membrane largely in accordance with the Nernst relationship as E_{Cl} is very close to E_m.* It is significant that the E_K for most cardiac cells is 5 to 10 mV higher than the resting E_m, and E_{Na} differs from the resting E_m by approximately 170 mV. This failure of the calculated equilibrium potentials for Na^+ and K^+ to agree with the measured E_m indicates that the concentrations of K^+ and Na^+ on each side of the cell membrane are not in equilibrium with the electric forces. Two conclusions are suggested: (1) the amount of K^+ inside the cell is larger than can be explained by a simple equilibrium between diffusional and electric forces, and some additional force must operate to keep K^+ inside the cell, and (2) the large concentration of Na^+ outside the cell is maintained in spite of concentration and electric gradients that are both directed into the cell. (An electric potential of 81 mV, inside of the cell positive, would be required to maintain the normal extracellular sodium concentration.) While the permeability of the resting cell membrane to sodium is low, sodium can still enter the cell. The fact that a net influx of sodium does not normally occur suggests that some additional force must also operate to keep the internal concentration of sodium low.

An active sodium-potassium transport mechanism in the cell membrane appears to supply the additional flux necessary to maintain the resting concentration of these ions on each side of the membrane. This pump utilizes energy supplied by hydrolysis of adenosine triphosphate (ATP) by the membrane enzyme Na^+-K^+ dependent adenosinetriphosphatase (ATPase) and, at least in most cells, causes the expulsion of 3 Na^+ in exchange for each two K^+ that are pumped into the cell. The Na^+-K^+ membrane pump is important for the maintenance of the resting E_m for two reasons. First, it sustains the concentration gradients necessary for the production of diffusion potentials. Second, the unequal exchange by the pump mechanism of charged particles across the cell membrane is in itself *electrogenic* and results in an electric potential difference across the cell membrane. This is discussed further below. Membrane pumps have also been reported for other ions such as unbound Ca^{2+}.

---

*Recent studies suggest that Cl^- may be transported into the cell; however, the mechanism for this movement and its functional significance is presently not understood.

Diffusion Potentials.—The cell membrane is relatively permeable to K^+, is slightly less permeable to Cl^-, and permits Na^+ to pass slowly. The diffusion potential produced by each of these ions will, therefore, have some effect on the resting E_m. Assuming an electrically neutral Na^+-K^+ pump and also that the electric field produced by the resting membrane potential is constant (as proposed by D. E. Goldman), the English electrophysiologists A. L. Hodgkin and B. Katz suggested the resting E_m could be predicted by expressing each ionic flux in terms of its electrochemical gradient and membrane permeability. This steady-state equation (sometimes called the GHK equation), as modified for cells at body temperature, becomes

$$E_m = 61.5 \log_{10} \left[\frac{P_K[K^+]_o + P_{Na}[Na^+]_o + P_{Cl}[Cl^-]_i}{P_K[K^+]_i + P_{Na}[Na^+]_i + P_{Cl}[Cl^-]_o} \right] \qquad (3-3)$$

where P represents the permeability coefficient of the membrane for the various ions.*

The GHK equation describes the resting E_m for the squid axon with considerable accuracy when the relative permeability ratio of $P_K:P_{Cl}:P_{Na}$ is assigned the value of 1.00:0.45:0.04. It is interesting that this equation reduces to the Nernst equation for K^+ if the permeability coefficients for Cl^- and Na^+ are assumed to be zero. This leads to the suggestion that the *resting* E_m is largely a "potassium potential," and because of its low permeability, sodium has only a minor effect. (The modifications in this steady state that occur in the specialized tissues of the heart during diastole will be covered later with the discussion of pacemaker activity.)

Electrogenic Pump Potentials.—As indicated above, the unequal movement of charged particles into and out of the cardiac cell due to the membrane pump leads to the accumulation of a positive charge outside the cell membrane. This has a hyperpolarizing action on the cell membrane. The contribution of this pump potential to the resting E_m in most cells is, however, small compared to that generated by the larger diffusional potentials. In cardiac cells it represents less than 5 mV. For this reason, the pump potential is often ignored in the discussion of the resting membrane potential.

---

*Conductance (g) is sometimes incorrectly substituted for P. These are similar but not identical quantities: g is the ease of movement due to an electric force, whereas P is the ease of movement due to a diffusional force.

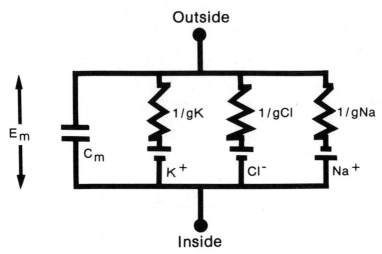

FIG 3–4.
Electrical model of an excitable membrane. The electric potential (E_m) developed across a membrane capacitor (C_m), as shown in the conductance equation, is equal to the sum of the equilibrium potentials of the ions K^+, Cl^-, and Na^+ (represented by batteries) diffusing through the membrane resistances (1/g) offered to the current developed by each ion. (Modified from Hodgkin AL, Huxley AF: *J Physiol* 1952; 117:500.)

Mechanism for Resting Membrane Potential.—The factors that combine to produce the resting membrane potential E_m can now be summarized through use of the Hodgkin-Huxley equivalent circuit (Fig 3–4). This figure assumes an electrically neutral Na^+-K^+ pump. We will consider only Na^+, K^+, and Cl^-. Each ion moves independently through the membrane under the influence of its electrochemical gradient and encounters resistance as determined by the character of its individual channel. Thus, each channel can be represented by an electromotive force (EMF) (battery) equal to the appropriate equilibrium potential (E_{Na}, E_K, or E_{Cl}) in series with a resistance. The latter represents the approximate resistance offered by the membrane to the movement of the ion in question. This is usually expressed as the conductance (g), which is the reciprocal of resistance. Thus, the circuit representing the sodium channel will, for example, have an EMF of approximately $+81$ mV and a high resistance (low conductance) reflecting the relative impermeability of the membrane for Na^+.

It can be shown that when the net current flow within the model is zero, the resting membrane potential (E_m), as shown by the sum of individual channel EMF in parallel, is given by the following conductance equation:

$$E_m = \frac{E_K g_K + E_{Cl} g_{Cl} + E_{Na} g_{Na} - I_a}{g_K + g_{Cl} + g_{Na}} \qquad (3\text{--}4)$$

This equation represents a form of weighed average and includes the contribution of the electrogenic Na^+-K^+ pump (I_a). The final result reflects the charge developed on the membrane capacitor (C_m in Fig 3–4) by the various ionic currents. At rest, the low membrane conductance for Na^+ largely removes the effect of the E_{Na} in the determination of this potential. The high g_K, on the other hand, causes the final membrane potential to be close to E_K.

To recapitulate, the resting E_m is the result of an equilibrium between two opposing forces: (1) the tendency of permeable ions, primarily K^+, to diffuse through the cell membrane down their concentration gradient and (2) the oppositely directed electric gradient produced by separation by the cell membrane of the diffusing ions from their ion pair. This equilibrium is then complicated by the Na^+ pump, which keeps Na^+ out of the cell, and by the K^+ pump, which adds K^+ to the interior of the cell. However, the net movement of ions through the membrane during the steady state is zero.

Depolarization

Ion Channels and Gates.—Before discussing the events that follow application of a threshold stimulus to a resting myocardial cell, it is necessary to summarize an additional feature of the cell membrane. It is now clearly established that ion currents selectively penetrate what appear to be specific membrane channels and that movement in these channels is regulated by voltage-dependent changes in permeability. Opening and closing of these pathways follow a complicated time course. These observations have led to the concept of *activation* and *inactivation gates*. While the physical description of these channels and gates remains theoretical, the model shown in Figure 3–5 will serve to explain their behavior.

The cell membrane appears to have individual protein-lined channels that offer priority for the movement of a specific ion or group of ions. The operation of these pathways can be illustrated by a brief description of the Na^+ channel.* Movement of Na^+ through this channel seems to be controlled by (1) a selective filter that permits only Na^+ to penetrate through the pathway and (2) two voltage-sensitive gates, called "m" and "h" gates,

---

*Recent study of individual ion channels using the patch clamp technique suggests a more complicated model with several closed and inactive states.

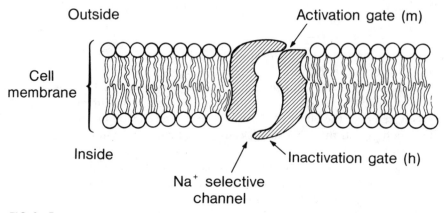

FIG 3–5.
Theoretical model of Na$^+$ selective protein channel in cell membrane. The configuration of protein gates is voltage sensitive. At resting E_m, activation gate ("m" gate) is closed; inactivation gate ("h" gate) is open.

that can open or close independently. The "m" gate is sometimes called the activation gate and the "h" gate, the inactivation gate. At a normal resting E_m, the activation (m) gate is closed and the inactivation (h) gate is open.

A reduction of 10 to 20 mV in the resting E_m appears to change the charge distribution on the peptide chains that constitute the channel gates. As a result, these proteins undergo a configuration change, and the "m" gate opens and the "h" gate closes. The "m" gate is a rapidly moving structure and completes its movement in about 0.1 msec, while the "h" gate responds more slowly. Depolarization of the cell membrane, as discussed in the next section, will, therefore, cause the Na$^+$ channel to rapidly open and then close as the slower moving "h" gate swings into position.

Ionic and Electrical Events During Depolarization.—If a resting cardiac cell is exposed to an external electric current as provided, for example, by a pair of stimulating electrodes, the outward flow of current through the cell membrane to the cathode of the stimulating electrode will reduce the value of E_m in that area. This is illustrated in Figure 3–6, which shows a schematic representation of a membrane potential recorded from a typical Purkinje cell. The reduction of the resting E_m by the external stimulating current to some critical value, e.g., -70 mV, is shown at point *A*. As described in the previous section, this sudden local reduction in E_m causes the "m" gates to open and the membrane in that area to become more permeable to Na$^+$. This change in P_{Na} upsets the complicated steady state of the resting cell membrane; Na$^+$ enters the cell, and as a result of the in-

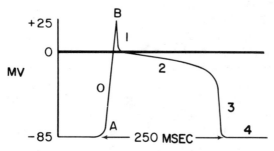

FIG 3–6.
Schematic representation of an action potential recorded from typical Purkinje cell. See text for description of the various phases.

ward movement of this positive charge, E_m is reduced even more. The local reduction in E_m with its accompanying increase in P_{Na} has a positive feedback effect on the membrane, with the result that additional "m" gates open. This leads to a rapid increase in P_{Na}, and it becomes several hundred times larger than normal. This value now so overshadows the normal P_K and P_{Cl} in the GHK equation (equation 3–3) that, in essence, this equation approaches the Nernst equilibrium equation for Na^+. This means that the E_m will be driven toward the E_{Na} of $+81$ mV by the large inward Na^+ current. This is shown as phase 0 in Figure 3–6 by the upstroke of the action potential.

The explosive increase in P_{Na}, triggered by the reduction in E_m, lasts only a brief period before the inactivation (h) gates begin to close and the increased Na^+ permeability begins to return rapidly to its normal low resting level. This process of inactivation occurs at about the time the upstroke of the action potential reaches zero on its way to a peak value in the range of $+30$ mV. At the same time, the change in the E_m from its resting level upsets the Cl^- equilibrium across the cell membrane, and Cl^- begins to move into the cell (the Cl^- channel does not appear to have gates). These two events, the reduction in P_{Na} and the inflow of Cl^-, act to prevent the E_m from reaching the equilibrium potential for Na^+ (E_{Na}), and as a result, E_m peaks at a value of about $+30$ mV. This is shown in Figure 3–6 at point *B*. The continued inflow of Cl^-, return of P_{Na} toward its low resting value, and some efflux of K^+ cause the E_m to return toward zero (phase 1).

The ionic movements that have just been described are similar to those that take place during the depolarization of most excitable cells such as nerve or skeletal muscle. The myocardium is unique, however, in that repolarization, once started, does not rapidly return the cell membrane to its normal polarized condition. Instead, a series of events takes place that keep the cardiac E_m at or near depolarization for a "plateau" of 200 to 300 msec before it begins to return to the normal resting level. This is shown in Figure 3–6 as phase 2.

Depolarization causes the myocardial cell membrane to become relatively impermeable to the outward movement of K^+, in contrast to the increased permeability for K^+ that occurs in other excitable tissues. Cardiac ventricular cells apparently have two voltage-sensitive K^+ channels that are rectifying, i.e., while permitting flow in both directions, they conduct best in only one direction. These are an X_1 channel, which conducts best in an outward direction, and a K_1 channel, which conducts best in an inward direction. Depolarization of the cell leads to immediate closure of the K_1 channel and a slower opening of the X_1 channel. The net effect is only a small outward K^+ current (I_k) during phase 2 of the ventricular action potential.

Fast and Slow Channels.—The influx of sodium into the cardiac cell occurs via two channels: (1) a *fast channel* (already discussed) that accounts for the early influx of Na^+ and the rapid phase 0 depolarization of the cell membrane and (2) a second *slower channel* that permits Ca^{2+} (and some Na^+) to move down its concentration and electrical gradients into the cell. This slow channel appears to have both activation (d) and inactivation (f) gates. In contrast to the fast Na^+ channel, these gates become activated at a lower E_m (-45 to -25 mV) and move much slower than the "m" and "h" gates. As a result, the inward Ca^{2+} current through this channel does not begin until phase 1 of the action potential and lasts for the duration of the phase 2 plateau. This inward current in combination with the influx of Cl^- and the decreased efflux of K^+ acts during this period to maintain the E_m close to zero. After 200 to 300 msec, the Ca^{2+} channel is inactivated by closure of its "f" gate. At the same time, the decreased outward flux of K^+ returns to normal as the K_1 and X_1 gates return to their resting position. (The outward flow of K^+ may also result from activation of other K^+ channels, perhaps activated by the increased intercellular Ca^{2+}.) These activities result in rapidly restoring the E_m of working myocardium to its resting position. This is shown as phase 3 of the action potential in Figure 3–6. The temporal relationships of these gate movements and ion fluxes to the electrical activity of the myocardial cell membrane are summarized in Figure 3–7. (The diastolic ionic flux in pacemaker tissue is different and is discussed below.)

Pharmacologic Action and Ion Channels.—Delineation of the ion channel concept has led to a significant step forward in cardiac therapeutics. Pharmaceutical blocking agents have been developed that selectively affect the ion channels. Several of these compounds have become important re-

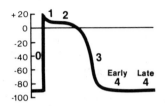

	Phase Gate	0	1	2	3	Early 4	Late 4
Na$^+$	m*	Opening	Open	Closing	Closed	Closed	Closed
	h**	Closing	Closing	Closed	Opening	Opening	Open
Ca^{++}	d*	Opening	Open	Open	Closing	Closed	Closed
	f**	Open	Closing	Closing	Opening	Opening	Open
K$^+$	x$_1$*	Opening	Opening	Open	Closing	Closing	Closed
	k$_1$*	Closing	Closing	Closed	Opening	Open	Open
Cl$^-$		Open	Open	Open	Open	Open	Open

* Activation gate

** Inactivation gate

FIG 3–7.
Relationship of a typical ventricular intracellular action potential *(above)* to the activity of various membrane ion channels and gates. See text for discussion. (Based on data by Beeler GW, Reuter H: *J Physiol* 1975; 1:251; and Ban T: *Comput Biomed Res* 1983; 16:403.)

search and treatment tools. For example, the puffer fish toxin, tetrodotoxin (TTX), acts on the outside of the cell membrane and specifically blocks the fast sodium channel, while the tetraethylammonium ion (TEA$^-$) blocks the K$^+$ channel by occupying the lumen from the inside of the membrane. A new class of drugs, the slow channel blockers (Ca^{2+} antagonists) have recently been introduced. These drugs (verapamil, nifedipine, diltiazem) specifically block the Na$^+$-Ca^{2+} channel without altering its kinetics or voltage dependence. These Ca^{2+} blocking agents are widely used clinically as antiarrhythmic agents and vasodilator drugs. They also have intercellular effects and, among other things, may block platelet serotonin release and inhibit platelet aggregation and clot formation. Adrenergic stimulation and various catecholamines act to increase the entry of Ca^{2+} through the slow channel. The mechanisms of action of these compounds are complex; however, they apparently act through stimulation of protein kinase and the production of cyclic adenosine monophosphate (cAMP) (see further discussion in Chapters 7 and 8).

It is of significance that the fast sodium channel may be altered by disease processes so that the slow inward current becomes the dominant factor leading to myocardial depolarization. In that situation, the peak of the action potential may be only 0 to $+15$ mV. This so-called slow response favors the occurrence of reentry currents and the development of cardiac arrhythmias (see Chapter 6).

Activation of the slow Na^+-Ca^{2+} channel permits the influx of Ca^{2+} into the myocardium from the extracellular fluid. This has important implications for the duration and strength of the contraction triggered by the same depolarization. These will be discussed in the next section of this chapter.

Summary.—The plateau of the cardiac action potential results from (1) a small but significant flux of Na^+ through the second slow sodium channel into the cell; (2) an inward flux of Ca^{2+}, probably through the same sodium channel, that is also important in the contraction response of the myocardium; (3) a marked decrease in the outward flux of K^+; and (4) increased inward movement of Cl^-. Thus, the repolarizing K^+ and Cl^- currents are essentially equal and opposite to the inward depolarizing Na^+ and Ca^{2+} currents. Final repolarization occurs at the end of the plateau phase with (1) inactivation of the slow Na^+-Ca^{2+} channel and (2) return of the decreased outward flux of K^+ to normal.

The description of the cardiac action potential presented in the section on depolarization made use of four channels for the movement of ions through the cell membrane. These channels are (1) Na^+ (fast), (2) Na^+-Ca^{2+} (slow), (3) Cl^-, and (4) K^+. In addition, the K^+ channel contains three subchannels, K_1 and X_1 are involved with diastolic K^+ permeability, and K_2 is apparently involved with the pacemaker activity of specialized tissues and will be described below. Studies using the voltage clamp technique suggest that other K^+ channels (X_2) may exist.

Specialized Conductive Tissues and Pacemaker Activity

The specialized conductive tissues of the heart have the ability to become pacemaker cells, i.e., they are able to spontaneously depolarize in a repetitive manner. This rhythmic activity occurs because these tissues do not have a stable resting E_m. Instead, the E_m gradually decreases with time from its maximum repolarization potential until it reaches its critical threshold and spontaneous depolarization results. Repolarization then follows in the normal manner, and the sequence starts over.

Under normal circumstances, the pacemaker function of the heart is supplied by the SA node. This is because its diastolic phase 4 depolarization—or, as it is sometimes called, the pacemaker potential or prepotential—has a faster rate of decline than the phase 4 potential of the other specialized tissues. Therefore, the SA node reaches its threshold for phase 0 depolarization first and becomes the dominant pacemaker. The resulting wave of depolarization that starts from the SA node depolarizes the remainder of the heart as it sweeps over the myocardium before the pacemaker potential from any subsidiary pacemaker can reach threshold. (This aspect of overdrive suppression is discussed more fully later in this section.) This mechanism has been extended recently by the suggestion that the rapid rate of the SA node not only discharges the slower latent pacemakers but also inhibits the rate of formation of their prepotentials by increasing the activity of their sodium pump. This is believed to shift their maximum diastolic depolarization to a more negative value. Diastolic prepotentials from various specialized tissues are schematically shown in Figure 3–8. It can be seen from this diagram that if, for some reason, the prepotential of the SA node should not develop normally, the next specialized tissue to reach its threshold level would take over the pacemaker duties. The suggestion above that overdrive of these potential pacemaker cells inhibits formation of a prepotential offers a logical explanation for the 30- to 40-second delay that frequently occurs before a lower unit takes over the pacemaker duties when the SA node is suddenly inhibited. The heart, therefore, has a large number of potential pacemakers arranged in a cascade arrangement. This provides a redundant series of "fail-safe" pacemakers.

It is worthwhile to emphasize at this point that the intrinsic rate of prepotential development decreases the farther the pacemaker tissue is from the SA node. Thus, it is not surprising that patients with a defective SA node who rely on pacemaker cells in the ventricle to drive the heart frequently have a slow heart rate (bradycardia). It is not unusual for this bradycardia to cause hemodynamic difficulties. When this happens, an ar-

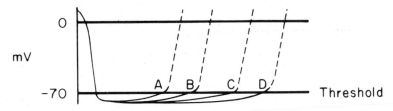

FIG 3–8.
Drawing of prepotentials as recorded from pacemaker cells in *A,* AV node; *B,* bundle of His; *C,* Purkinje fibers; and *D,* ventricular muscle. The threshold for myocardial depolarization is indicated as −70 mV. Each prepotential is shown to start from a common point at the end of ventricular repolarization.

tificial electronic pacemaker with a faster discharge rate may have to be implanted to speed up the heart.

The electrophysiology of cardiac pacemaker activity has been most intensely studied in Purkinje fibers. Recent voltage clamp studies indicate that the outward I_k current during repolarization activates a slowly developed inward Na^+ current. This I_f current utilizes a membrane channel that has different voltage-dependent and pharmacologic properties than the fast sodium channel. Diastolic depolarization and development of the prepotential (pacemaker potential) in these tissues is now thought to result from the continued slow activation of the inward I_f component during phase 4 of the action potential and not, as previously suggested, from primary deactivation of the I_k current.

Pacemaker activity by the SA node has not been as well delineated and its details remain unclear. The I_f current described above for Purkinje cells also occurs in SA node pacemaker cells (Fig 3–9). However, as it is not activated until the cell repolarizes to -50 mV, the I_f current probably does not play a major role in pacemaker function unless the SA cell is hyperpolarized. Current thinking suggests the repolarization I_k current in SA node pacemaker cells also undergoes a slow decay during phase 4 of its action potential. As a result, the cell E_m decreases with time until it reaches threshold for depolarization.

Sinus Node Pacemakers.—The SA node contains many cells that have the potential to be pacemakers. These tissues can be divided into true or *dominant pacemakers* and latent or *subsidiary pacemakers*. Dominant pacemakers differ from other specialized tissues in being more permeable to sodium and having a significant inward Na^+ current. As a result, the resting membrane potential of these cells is about -50 mV. At this potential, the fast sodium channel is inactive. As a result, prepotential development due to the reduction of gK^+ and some additional influx of Na^+ (the I_f current) (see Fig 3–9) continues until threshold is reached for the slow calcium-sodium channel. Depolarization of the dominant pacemaker cells is then accomplished by the slow inward Ca^{2+}-Na^+ current. As a consequence, these fibers show a smooth transition between diastolic depolarization and the upstroke of the action potential, the rising phase (phase 0) develops slowly, and the plateau (phase 2) is poorly sustained. Subsidiary SA node pacemaker cells, however, show characteristics of both dominant and ordinary specialized tissues. They have, for example, a rapid upstroke due to some activation of the fast sodium channel with clear demarcation between the prepotential and the spike potential. This upstroke is then followed by a slower depolarization phase.

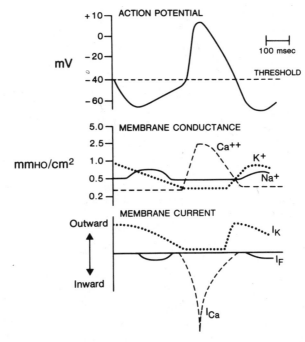

FIG 3–9.
Schematic representation of the SA node transmembrane potential *(top)*, representative conductances for the major ions *(middle)*, and membrane currents *(bottom)* for one cardiac cycle. Approximate conductances and currents are used.

Effect of Autonomic Nervous System on Pacemaker Cells.—Stimulation of the parasympathetic vagal fiber to the heart causes the heart rate to decrease, whereas sympathetic stimulation causes it to increase (Fig 3–10). These alterations in heart rate result from changes in the rate of SA node prepotential development. Increasing the rate of development, for example, will cause the prepotential to reach its threshold for depolarization more quickly and thus reduce the time interval between heartbeats.

The effects of autonomic nervous system stimulation on the heart rate is mediated through chemical transmitters liberated at the neuromuscular endings. The parasympathetic transmitter, *acetylcholine*, causes the cell membrane of the SA node to become more permeable to K^+. This has two effects: (1) the repolarization E_m is driven closer to the E_K, and (2) the rate of formation of the prepotential is reduced. The result is that it takes longer for the prepotential to reach threshold, and the heart rate is slowed. It is interesting that intense vagal stimulation, such as can reflexly result from

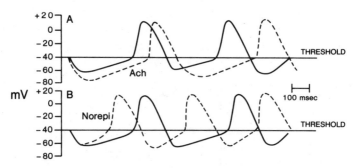

FIG 3–10.
Effect of acetylcholine *(top)* and norepinephrine *(bottom)* on the frequency of pacemaker firing. Acetylcholine *(Ach)*, the parasympathetic neurotransmitter, slows the rate by hyperpolarization the cell membrane and reducing the slope of the prepotential. Norepinephrine *(Norepi)*, the sympathetic neurotransmitter, increases the firing rate by increasing the slope of the prepotential.

vigorous massage of the carotid sinus area, may even result in cardiac standstill for an appreciable period by abolishing the prepotential altogether. *Norepinephrine*, the catecholamine transmitter of the sympathetic nervous system, increases the rate of inactivation of the K^+ outflux. In the SA node, norepinephrine increases the rate of development of the I_f current. The result in both SA node and Purkinje fiber pacemakers is a more rapid development of the prepotential and increase in the pacemaker discharge rate. Norepinephrine also causes an increased Na^+ and Ca^{2+} influx during depolarization and the plateau phase of the action potential. Sympathetic stimulation does not apparently affect the maximum E_m or the threshold for depolarization. It has been suggested that catecholamines, through a metabolic action involving cyclic $3',5'$-AMP could stimulate the inward K^+ pump (see above) and thus increase the rate of prepotential development. As a result, sympathetic stimulation leads to an increase in both heart rate and the force of cardiac contraction.

Propagation of Action Potential.—The explosive series of events that take place when a cardiac cell is depolarized are localized at first to a small area of the membrane. However, just as in nerves and other excitable tissues, these events spread to adjacent polarized areas of the cell membrane so that the excitation process, once started, is propagated down the length of the cell. This occurs because the localized depolarization segment acts as a sink for the inward flow of current from the outside of the surrounding polarized areas. The return of this current out through the resting cell membrane reduces the E_m at the margin of the depolarized zone. When this reaches threshold, the membrane in this area depolarizes, and the process is repeated. Each segment of the membrane then repolarizes so that, in effect, movement of the excitation process is followed approximately 200 to 300 msec later by a wave of repolarization. The rate of propagation of this excitation-repolarization process is a function of (1) the diameter of the myocardial cell, (2) the magnitude of the resting E_m, (3) the electric capacity and resistance of the cell membrane and cytoplasm, (4) the density of the inward depolarizing current, and (5) the rate of development of the action potential upstroke. These factors are considered in the cable properties of the cell. Further discussion of these parameters is beyond the scope of this presentation.

Cardiac muscle cells branch and interdigitate with each other to form a syncytium-like arrangement; however, electron micrographs show that the myocardium is made up of individual cells, each with its own cell membrane. The junction of one cell with another occurs at structures called *intercalated* disks. In this area, which always occurs at a Z line, the cell membranes of the adjoining cells fuse in a series of folds to form *tight junctions*. This is schematically shown in Figure 3–11. These junctions provide a low-resistance pathway (about 5 Ω/sq cm) for the spread of current be-

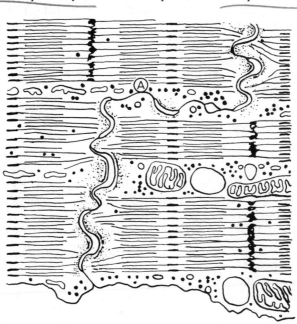

FIG 3–11.
Diagram of two adjacent myocardial cells in the area of an intercalated disk. At *A*, cell membranes of the two cells appear to fuse and form a tight junction.

tween the two cells. (The resistance of the resting cell membrane is approximately 300 Ω/sq cm.) The tight junction permits the local currents produced by depolarization of one cell to easily pass to the next cell membrane. The result is that when part of a cardiac muscle syncytium (for example, the atrial myocardium) becomes depolarized, the process will spread until it includes the entire muscle. The atrial or ventricular musculature, therefore, acts physiologically as a single muscle unit even though it is made up of many individual cells. The annulus fibrosus, described in Chapter 2, prevents electric continuity between these two muscle units, and the excitation process can only travel between them by way of the AV node and the common bundle. (See Chapter 4 for further discussion of the excitation of the heart.)

MECHANICAL ACTIVITY OF CARDIAC CELLS

Depolarization of cardiac cell membrane sets in motion a series of molecular events that results in activation of the contractile machinery. This causes sliding of the longitudinal actin and myosin filaments within the cell, and the muscle shortens or, to the degree that shortening is prevented, it develops tension. This mechanical response to stimulation is similar in many aspects to the contractile response of skeletal muscle. However, contraction of cardiac muscle has a number of unique features that are important for the function of the heart. These will be emphasized in the discussion that follows.

Structure of Cardiac Sarcomere

Each cardiac muscle fiber contains a group of branching longitudinal strands approximately 1 μ in diameter called *myofibrils*. These cross-striated units contain the contractile elements of the myocardium. Each myofibril is divided, as is skeletal muscle, into a repeating series of units every 1.5 to 2.5 μ by what appears, under the light microscope, to be a dark transverse band called a Z line. The section of myofibril between two Z lines, the *sarcomere*, is the functional unit of the myocardium. It usually is used to describe the structural aspects of contraction. Electron microscopic studies show that each sarcomere contains a middle dark zone (A band) and at each end a light zone (I band). These latter units are continuous with the I band of the sarcomere on each side. These light and dark bands result from the arrangement of the actin and myosin filaments within the myofibril. This architecture is the same for both skeletal and cardiac muscle and is shown in Figure 3–12.

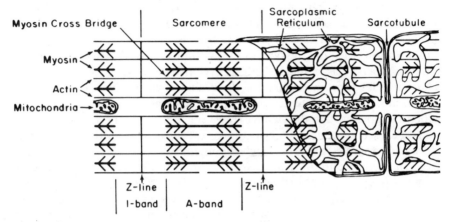

FIG 3–12.
Drawing of myocardial fiber. *Left,* ultrastructural division into interdigitating actin and myosin filaments. The organization of one sarcomere is shown containing overlapping thick (myosin) and thin (actin) filaments with cross bridges on the ends of myosin filaments. *Right,* abundant sarcoplasmic reticulum and prominent sarcotubules in the region of the Z line are shown.

The light I bands that are bisected by the Z line contain the thin, longitudinally arranged actin filaments. These extend into the dark A bands where they interdigitate with the thick, myosin filaments. These thick and thin filaments are arranged in a three-dimensional hexagonal array so that the edge of the A band of each myosin filament is surrounded by a series of six equally spaced actin filaments.

The thin filaments have recently been shown to contain at least two other proteins, *tropomyosin* and *troponin*, besides actin. The filament itself now appears to be made from two G actin monomers twisted into a single filament of F actin polymer. The spiral groove formed by the two actin strands contains the elongated strands of tropomyosin. At approximately 400-A intervals, the globular protein, troponin, is attached to the tropomyosin. The role of these proteins in contraction will be covered below.

The protein, myosin, which makes up the thick filament, is composed of two parallel α-helices of light meromyosin wound around each other with two globular heads (heavy meromyosin) attached at an angle at one end. These myosin molecules are stacked like matchsticks in an alternating arrangement. Their globular heads project outward from each end of the filament and the intertwined tails of the myosin make up the central bare region of the filament. These myosin heads have the ability to hydrolyze adenosine triphosphate. They act as cross bridges during contraction and interact with binding sites on the actin molecule.

Cardiac cells contain a longitudinal series of tubes diffusely arranged in the area of the myofilaments. This structure, the *sarcoplasmic reticulum*, is not nearly as well developed in heart cells as is its counterpart in skeletal muscle. However, the myocardium, with the possible exception of the Purkinje fibers, has a much better developed transverse tubular system. These tubules form in the area of the Z line as an invagination of the cell membrane and penetrate deeply into the cardiac fiber. They are much wider in diameter than the slender transverse tubules found in skeletal muscle and appear to offer a direct pathway for material from the extracellular space, for example, Ca^{2+}, to reach the myofibrils.

The cardiac cell also contains, in addition to the structures mentioned above, a plentiful supply of *mitochondria*. These units have an obvious role in the aerobic energy production of the cell. It is estimated that mitochondria occupy as much as 40% of the cardiac cell volume in contrast to skeletal muscle, in which 80% to 90% of the cell mass is made up of contractile myofibrils. In addition, the mitochondria have recently been implicated as an intracellular storehouse for Ca^{2+}. Glycogen and lipid stores also are found in relative abundance in cardiac cells.

Mechanism of Cardiac Contraction

The mechanism and kinetics of muscle contraction are currently a subject of active research. There is, however, general agreement on the fundamental contraction process for both skeletal and cardiac muscles whereby cross-bridge formation between the myosin heads and binding sites on the actin filaments is activated by Ca^{2+}. The method of Ca^{2+} mobilization and removal in each type of muscle is considerably different as is the duration and magnitude of the contraction state. Before discussing these fundamental differences between cardiac and skeletal muscle, the basic contraction mechanism will be briefly summarized.

Following depolarization of a muscle cell membrane, the electric activity propagates into the interior of the cell via the transverse tubules. This depolarization of the membranes of the tubular system causes the release of Ca^{2+} from intracellular stores, primarily in the sarcoplasmic reticulum. The free Ca^{2+} then combines with a troponin subunit on the thin filament. This, in turn, causes the entire troponin molecule to undergo a conformational change that is transferred to the tropomyosin molecule. The tropomyosin then moves and uncovers active binding sites for the myosin head on the actin filament. With binding between actin and myosin, the myosin head rotates and draws the thin filaments into the A band and reduces the length of the sarcomere (Fig 3–13). The binding between actin and myosin is broken in the presence of ATP, and the head returns to its original

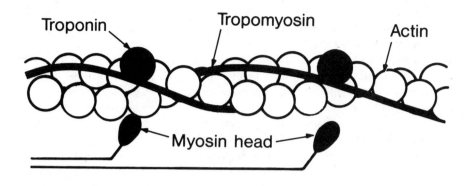

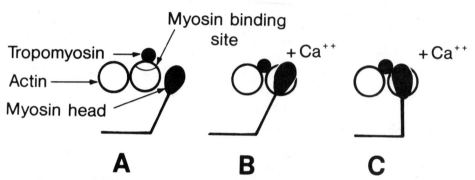

FIG 3–13.
Schematic diagram showing actin monomers *(above)* arranged into a double helix with tropomyosin filaments running near the groove between the two chains and globular troponin molecules located about 40 nm apart. Two globular heavy meromyosin heads are shown. *Below, (A)* cross section of actin helix showing relaxed muscle with myosin-binding site on actin blocked by the tropomyosin filament. *B,* binding of calcium ions by troponin causes movement of the tropomyosin filament into the groove and permits binding of the myosin head to actin. *C,* movement of the actin-myosin cross bridge causes sliding of the actin filament and muscle contraction.

position. It then reattaches to another actin-binding site, and the cycle repeats. Coincident with repolarization of the cell membrane there is active pumping of Ca^{2+} into the longitudinal portion of the sarcoplasmic reticulum. Removal of the intracellular Ca^{2+} in contact with the myofibrils to a level below 10^{-7} M results in loss of Ca^{2+} from the troponin-binding sites. This causes the tropomyosin to recover the actin-myosin binding sites, and muscle relaxation takes place.

This basic contraction process just described is somewhat modified in cardiac muscle. The relative paucity of the sarcoplasmic reticulum in the myocardium suggests that this structure may not be as efficient in supplying Ca^{2+} for contraction as is its counterpart in skeletal muscle. As shown diagrammatically in Figure 3–14, it now appears that the inward Ca^{2+} current via the slow Na^+-Ca^{2+} channel during the plateau phase of the action potential adds a significant amount of Ca^{2+} to that which is delivered from the sarcoplasmic reticulum during the depolarization process. It has recently been suggested that entry of extracellular Ca^{2+} triggers the subsequent release of Ca^{2+} from the sarcoplasmic reticulum. Thus, if insufficient Ca^{2+} enters from the outside, little or no Ca^{2+} is released from the sarcoplasmic reticulum. The results are (1) that the period of contraction, the active state, of cardiac muscle lasts much longer than in skeletal muscle and (2) that the intensity of the contractile response can be modified by factors that regulate the inward Ca^{2+} current. For example, the increase in cardiac contractility due to epinephrine may result in part from the effect of that substance on the permeability of the membrane for calcium during the plateau phase of the action potential.

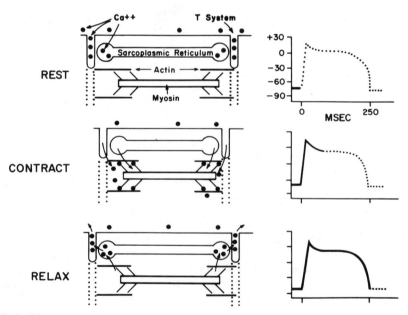

FIG 3–14.
Diagram of electric events and movement of Ca^{2+} during contraction of cardiac muscle. Following depolarization and during plateau phase of the action potential, there is a movement of Ca^{2+} from the sarcoplasmic reticulum and interstitial fluid within the transverse tubules *(T)* into the area of the contractile proteins. Role of the mitochondria (not shown) in this process is unclear. During repolarization (relaxation), there is an active pumping of Ca^{2+} back into the sarcoplasmic reticulum and perhaps the mitochondria. (Modified from Chidsey CA III: *Hosp Pract [off]* 1972; 7:65.)

The role of cardiac mitochondria as a source of activator calcium is currently under study. These structures contain ample stores of Ca^{2+}; however, it appears that its release is too slow to be effectively used to trigger contraction. It may serve as a buffer for other intracellular storage sites for calcium.

At the end of the plateau phase of cardiac action potential, repolarization of the cell membrane is associated with relaxation of the muscle. During this period there is recapture of the intracellular calcium by the sarcoplasmic reticulum. This inward pumping requires utilization of energy from the splitting of ATP. Much of the trapped Ca^{2+} within the sarcoplasmic reticulum has been postulated to then move out through the cell membrane during diastole either via an electroneutral Na^{+}-Ca^{2+} exchange or perhaps by an energy-utilizing Ca^{2+}-Na^{+} pump. Sufficient Ca^{2+} does remain in the sarcoplasmic reticulum to initiate the next contraction; however, it is not sufficient by itself to produce a maximal contraction for that sarcomere length.

Contractile Response of Cardiac Muscle

Activation of the contractile elements in cardiac muscle by the release of stored intracellular Ca^{2+} combined with the influx of extracellular Ca^{2+} produces a twitch contraction that is grossly similar to the contraction of skeletal muscle. However, as shown in Figure 3–15, peak tension usually is reached during the last third of the plateau phase of the accompanying electric response. As a result of the long period of depolarization, the muscle is refractory to a second stimulus until late in the relaxation phase. Because of this *refractory period*, cardiac muscle cannot produce a tetanic type of contraction such as occurs in skeletal muscle, and it has only a limited ability to show summation. The syncytial arrangement of cardiac muscle and the lack of motor innervation and myoneural endings means that cardiac muscle does not have motor units such as are found in skeletal muscle.

The mechanical energy produced by the contraction of cardiac or skeletal muscle is a function of its sarcomere length just before contraction. It is customary to refer to this length in terms of the force or *preload* required to stretch the muscle to its precontraction length. The energy output of a muscle increases with an increase in its initial length or preload up to a critical point. Extension of the muscle beyond this length then results in a decrease in the vigor of the contraction. This fundamental property of muscle was first described for skeletal muscle in 1893 by Blix and was then extended to the heart by Frank, Starling and co-workers, and others (see Chapter 7). The molecular basis of this length-tension relationship has become clearer as understanding of the contractile process has developed. It

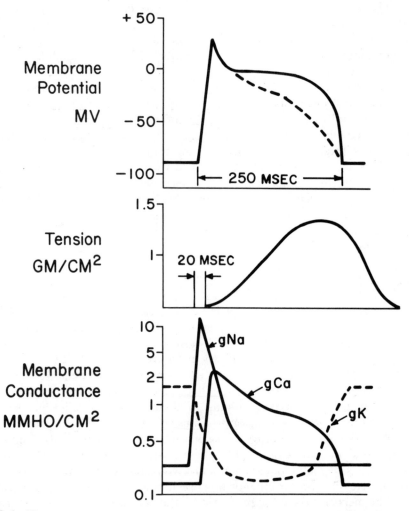

FIG 3–15.
Temporal relationships between electric events and development of myocardial tension following stimulation of a cardiac muscle cell. Approximate changes in membrane conductance *(g)* for the major ions are shown.

is now understood that the resting degree of interdigitation of the contractile fibrils depends on the tension applied to the ends of the muscle fiber (Fig 3–16). Thus, under a large preload, that is, the load supported by the muscle before the onset of contraction, the actin filaments may be pulled out from the myosin filaments so that many of the myosin cross bridges cannot make contact with binding sites on the thin filaments. Activation of

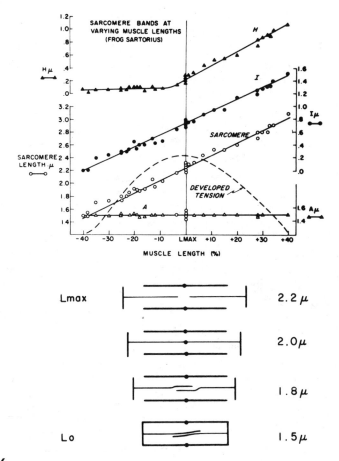

FIG 3–16.
Top, relationship between muscle length and sarcomere length; developed tension; and A-band, I-band, and H-zone width. *Bottom,* schematic diagram of relationship between thick and thin filaments at different sarcomere lengths. (Modified from Spiro D, Sonnenblick EH: *Prog Cardiovasc Dis* 1965; 7:295. Used by permission.)

the muscle at this long initial length will then result in fewer force-generating combinations, and the tension developed will not be very strong. At a low degree of muscle stretch and muscle length, overinterdigitation of the contractile filaments will also cause a cross-bridge-binding site mismatch. Recent studies suggest that binding of Ca^{2+} by troponin may also be modulated by sarcomere length. Thus at the optimal length of 2.2 μ, maximal cross-bridge binding takes place, and the maximal contractile tension results.

When cardiac muscle is stretched, it shows the property of elasticity; that is, it acts like a spring and resists attempts to change its length. In this regard it is stiffer than skeletal muscle. For example, at the optimal length for the development of tension, cardiac muscle develops a significant passive tension; the resting tension in skeletal muscle under the same conditions is usually much smaller. If a muscle (cardiac or skeletal) is prevented from shortening during contraction by fixing its ends (i.e., isometric contraction), some internal structure in series with the contractile elements must elongate in order that the contractile elements may shorten. These considerations led A. V. Hill to propose a muscle model that in its simple form contained two elastic elements, one in parallel and a second in series with the contractile unit (Fig 3–17). This model, which may take several configurations, is helpful in considering the contractile response of the heart. For example, when a papillary muscle is arranged so that it is *afterloaded* (i.e., it must pick up a load or weight from a support), activation will cause the contractile unit to begin to shorten. This reduction in the length of the contractile unit will stretch the series elastic element until it develops sufficient internal tension to lift the afterload. At this point, the muscle changes its mode of contraction from isometric to isotonic. The remainder of the active state of the muscle, which fortunately is quite long in cardiac muscle, will then be expended in shortening the muscle and lifting the afterload away from its support (Fig 3–18).

In the above situation, increasing the afterload will cause a greater amount of the total contractile energy to be utilized during the isometric phase of the contraction to develop tension, and less will be available for

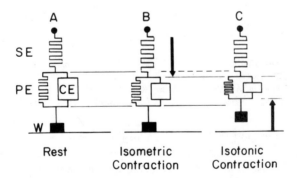

FIG 3–17.
Three-component model of papillary muscle: *A*, at rest; *B*, during isometric contraction in a preloaded mode with shortening of contractile unit and lengthening of series elastic unit; *C*, isotonic contraction with further shortening of contractile unit as it picks up the afterload *(W)*. SE = series elastic element; PE = parallel elastic element; CE = contractile element. See text for further discussion.

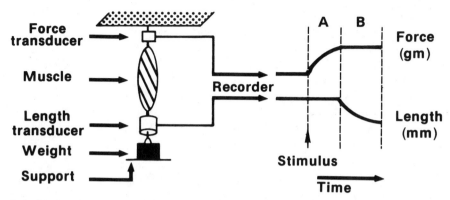

FIG 3–18.
Left, afterloaded papillary muscle, i.e., muscle load (weight) is supported during rest. *Right,* simultaneous records of muscle force and length. Muscle stimulated to contract at *arrow.* *A,* period of isometric contraction, *B,* period of isotonic muscle shortening. (From Little RC, Little WC: *Arch Intern Med* 1982; 142:819. Used by permission.)

lifting the weight. As a result, the larger the afterload, the shorter the distance the weight is moved and the slower the rate of movement. (The effect of afterload on cardiac output is discussed further in Chapter 7.) It is of interest to examine the maximum rate of muscle shortening and relate it to the size of the afterload. This is accomplished, as shown in Figure 3–19, by plotting a *force-velocity* curve.

The force-velocity curve can be used to illustrate a number of facets of the biophysics of cardiac contraction. It shows, for example, that the smaller the tension (i.e., the load), the faster the rate of shortening. On a molecular level, this finding can be interpreted to show that rapid sliding of the contractile filaments gives less time for individual cross-bridge formation and development of tension.

The maximum velocity (V_{max}) of shortening will occur when the muscle does not develop any force (i.e., the load is zero). This would represent a pure isotonic contraction and, as such, cannot be experimentally measured. However, this point (V_{max}) can be estimated by extrapolation of the force-velocity curve back to a zero load. This concept, particularly when it is extended to the intact heart, is somewhat controversial, and the validity of using it to compute V_{max} continues to be questioned. Nevertheless, the concept of V_{max} has proved a useful construct in understanding cardiac mechanics.

The V_{max} is a measure of the rate of actin-myosin interactions and represents the maximum rate at which energy is converted to mechanical shortening. As discussed below, the value of V_{max} has been related along with

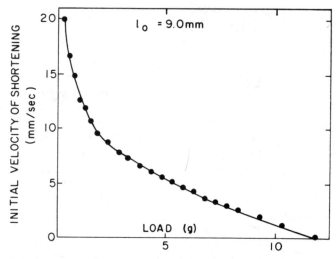

FIG 3–19.
Force-velocity curve for cat papillary muscle obtained by plotting initial velocity of muscle shortening for different afterloads. (From Sonnenblick EH: *Fed Proc* 1965; 24:1396. Used by permission.)

the maximal amount of tension produced by a true isometric contraction (the P_o tension in the force-velocity plot) to the contractile state, or "contractility" of the myocardium. The maximal of P_o tension is a measure of the number of active cross-bridge interactions.

This relationship between the contractile state of the myocardium (V_{max}) and the number of active cross-bridge interactions (P_o) can be illustrated by examining the results of two different interventions: (1) changing the initial muscle length and (2) changing muscle contractility by administering the inotropic drug, norepinephrine.

When the initial muscle length is increased, the contractile response also is augmented according to the length-tension relationship. However, the force-velocity relationship (Fig 3–20) plotted for different initial muscle lengths shows only an increase in P_o without change in V_{max}. In these experiments, increasing the initial muscle length caused the contractile filaments to move to a more optimal position for cross-bridge formation. As a result, contraction resulted in a larger number of effective interactions, and more force developed. However, the maximum rate of force development was not changed. Therefore, the velocity of shortening as plotted in the force-velocity plot will show some increase with increases in muscle length at all loads except at a zero load.

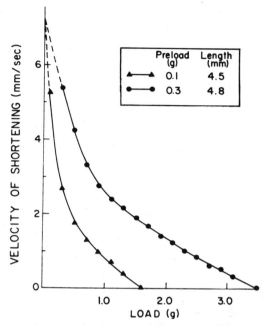

FIG 3–20.
Effect of increasing initial muscle length on force-velocity relationship of cat papillary muscle. The initial velocity of shortening is plotted against the afterload for each curve. Preload and initial muscle length for each curve is shown in the inset. Increasing initial muscle length increases maximum force of contraction *(P$_0$)* with no change in maximum velocity of shortening *(V$_{max}$)*. (From Sonnenblick EH: *Fed Proc* 1965; 24:1396. Used by permission.)

While studies of the type just described appeared unambiguous, the assumption that V_{max} is independent of muscle length has recently been questioned. This uncertainty occurred when it was shown that the amount of intercellular calcium released during excitation may be length-dependent. This suggested that the level of activation is a function of muscle length and that the preload may not be an independent regulator of myocardial performance. This matter is still under investigation.

When cardiac muscle is exposed to an *inotropic* influence such as the administration of norepinephrine, the contractile force produced for a given muscle length is increased. This results in a shift in the length-work relationship to the left (Sarnoff effect). This is illustrated in Figure 3–21. However, at the same time the force-velocity curve shifts to the right under the influence of norepinephrine with an increase in both V_{max} and P_o (Fig

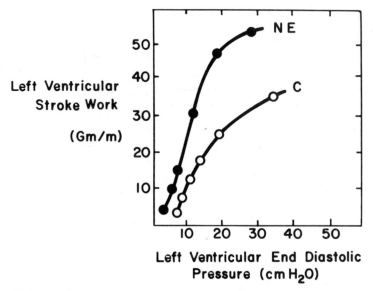

FIG 3–21.
Length-stroke work curves obtained before and after administration of norepinephrine *(NE)* showing shift of the curve due to inotropic influence of the drug. C = control. (From Sarnoff SJ, Mitchell JH, in Hamilton WF, Dow P [eds]: *Handbook of Physiology,* vol 1. Washington, DC, American Physiological Society, 1962. Used by permission.)

3–22). In this case, the inotropic drug apparently caused an increase in both the rate of energy conversion and the number of force-generating sites. The latter effect probably resulted, as explained above, because of the increased inward flux of Ca^{2+} during contraction, with activation of more binding sites. It has become popular to attribute this type of increased contractile activity to increased muscle *"contractility"* without a further definition of the term.

The experimental work on which the cardiac force-velocity relationship is based was carried out in isolated papillary muscles. However, the results of these basic studies can be transferred to the three-dimensional human heart. The initial muscle length of the ventricular myocardium is determined by the end-diastolic volume and the compliance of the left ventricular wall. The afterload is the aortic pressure head. Obviously the complex geometry of the ventricle and the changes that take place during contraction make the determination of force-velocity relationships such as V_{max} difficult in the clinical situation. Nevertheless, the principles regulating the contractile response of the isolated heart muscle that were discussed in the preceding sections agree very well with the results obtained in patient studies.

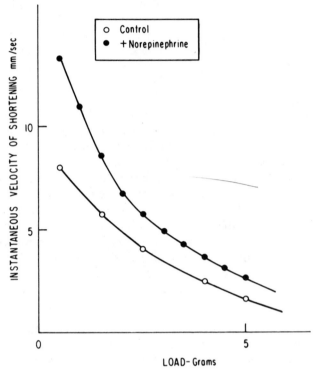

FIG 3–22.
Effect of norepinephrine on force-velocity relationship of cat papillary muscle. Initial length was constant at 9 mm with a preload of 0.5 gm for both determinations. (From Sonnenblick EH: *Fed Proc* 1965; 24:1396. Used by permission.)

SUMMARY

Electrical Properties of Cardiac Cells.—Resting myocardial cells are electrically polarized due to the separation of charged particles across the cell membrane. This results from the complex interaction of diffusional forces, electric fields, selective permeability of the cell membrane to ions, active transport of charged particles, and voltage-sensitive membrane channels. These factors can be summarized by the Hodgkin-Huxley-Katz equation and the conductance equation. Ion currents selectively penetrate the cell membrane via specific channels with voltage-dependent gates. Depolarization and subsequent repolarization follow the flux of charged particles through the voltage-sensitive gates in the membrane. The specialized conductive tissues and pacemaker cells have the ability to develop an unstable resting membrane potential (the pacemaker potential). Depolarization of pacemaker cells in the SA node and cells in the upper AV node result from the influx of Ca^{2+} through the "slow calcium channel." The rate of this prepotential development can be modified by autonomic nervous system control.

Mechanical Activity of Cardiac Cells.—Depolarization of cardiac cells result in activation of the contractile machinery. The resulting cross-bridge formation between myosin- and actin-binding sites in the presence of Ca^{2+} is similar to the contraction process of skeletal muscle. However, the cardiac active state is prolonged due to the influx of Ca^{2+} via the slow channel and by an isoelectric interchange of intracellular Na^+ for extracellular Ca^{2+}. This permits modulation of the contractile response by the regulation of intracellular Ca^{2+}. Repolarization is associated with recapture of intracellular calcium by the sarcoplasmic reticulum and relaxation. The mechanical response to contraction in cardiac muscle follows length-tension and preload and afterload mechanisms similar to skeletal muscle.

BIBLIOGRAPHY

Baumgarten CM, Fozzard HA: The resting and pacemaker potential, in Fozzard HA, Jenning RB, Harber E, et al (eds): *The Heart and Cardiovascular System. Scientific Foundation*. New York, Raven Press, 1986, pp 601–626.

Beder SP: Cellular electrophysiology of the sinus node, in Yabek SM, Gillette PC, Kugler JD (eds): *The Sinus Node in Pediatrics*. New York, Churchill Livingstone, Inc, 1984.

Bozler E: The initiation of impulses on cardiac muscle. *Am J Physiol* 1943; 138:273.

Braunwald E: Mechanism of action of calcium-channel blocking drugs. *N Engl J Med* 1982; 307:1618–1627.

Braunwald E, Ross J Jr, Sonnenblick EH: Mechanism of contraction of the normal and failing heart. *N Engl J Med* 1967; 277:794.

Chidsey CA III: Calcium metabolism in the normal and failing heart. *Hosp Pract [Off]* 1972; 7:65.

Coraboeuf E, Deroubaix E, Hoerter J: Control of ionic permeabilities in normal and ischemic hearts. *Circ Res* 1976; 38:92.

Davis RE: Biochemical processes in cardiac function. *Hosp Pract [Off]* 1970; 5:49.

Entman ML, Levey GS, Epstein SE: Mechanisms of action of epinephrine and glucagon on the canine heart: Evidence for increase in sarcotubular calcium stores mediated by cyclic 3′,5′-AMP. *Circ Res* 1969; 25:429.

Fawcett DW, McNutt NS: The ultrastructure of the cat myocardium: Ventricular papillary muscle. *J Cell Biol* 1969; 42:1.

Fozzard HA, Arnsdorf MF: Cardiac electrophysiology, in Fozzard HA, Jenning RB, Harber E, et al (eds): *The Heart and Cardiovascular System. Scientific Foundation*. New York, Raven Press, 1986, pp 1–30.

Fozzard HA, Gibbons WR: Action potential and contraction of heart muscle. *Am J Cardiol* 1973; 31:182.

Hodgkin AL, Huxley AF: A quantitative description of membrane current and its application to conduction and excitation in nerve. *J Physiol* 1952; 117:500.

Hodgkin AL, Katz B: The effect of sodium ions on the electrical activity of the giant axon of the squid. *J Physiol* 1949; 108:37.

Hoffman F: Origin of the heart beat, in Luisada AA (ed): *Cardiology: An Encyclopedia of the Cardiovascular System*. New York, McGraw-Hill Book Co, 1959, pp 2–41.

Hutter OF, Noble D: Rectifying properties of heart muscle. *Nature* 1960; 188:495.

Hutter OF, Trautwein W: Vagal and sympathetic effects on the pacemaker fibers in the sinus venosus of the heart. *J Gen Physiol* 1956; 39:715.

Jewell BR: A reexamination of the influence of muscle length on myocardial performance. *Circ Res* 1977; 40:221.

Junge D: *Nerve and Muscle Excitation*, ed 2. Sunderland, Mass, Sinauer Associates, Inc, 1981.

Katz AM: Contractile proteins in normal and failing myocardium. *Hosp Pract* [*Off*] 1972; 7:57.

Lakatta EG: Starling's law of the heart is explained by an intimate interaction of muscle length and myofilament calcium activation. *J Am Coll Cardiol* 1987; 10:1157–1164.

Mullins LJ: *Ion Transport in Heart*. New York, Raven Press, 1981.

New W, Trautwein W: The ionic nature of slow inward current and its relation to contraction. *Pflugers Arch* 1972; 334:24.

Noble D, Powell T: *Electrophysiology of Single Cardiac Cells*. London, Academic Press, 1987.

Noble D: Application of Hodgkin-Huxley equation to excitable tissues. *Physiol Rev* 1966; 46:1.

Noble D: *The Initiation of the Heartbeat*, ed 2. New York, Oxford University Press, 1979.

Noble D, Tsion RW: The kinetics and rectifier properties of the slow potassium current in cardiac Purkinje fibers. *J Physiol* 1968; 195:185.

Randall JE: *Elements of Biophysics*, ed 2. Chicago, Year Book Medical Publishers, 1962.

Reuter H, Beeler GW: Calcium current and activation of contraction in ventricular myocardial fibers. *Science* 1969; 163:399.

Rosen K (ed): Cardiac electrophysiology symposium. *Arch Intern Med* 1975; 135:387.

Ruegg JC: Dependence of cardiac contraction on myofibrillar calcium sensitivity. *News in Physiol Sci* 1987; 2:179.

Schultz SG: *Basic Principles of Membrane Transport*. Cambridge, Cambridge University Press, 1980.

Schwartz A: Symposium on cardiovascular disease and calcium antagonists. *Am J Cardiol* 1982; 49:497.

Sperelakis N: Origin of the cardiac resting potential, in Berne RC, et al (eds): *Handbook of Physiology, Section 2: The Cardiovascular System*, vol 1. Bethesda, Maryland, American Physiological Society, 1979.

Trautwein W: Membrane currents in cardiac muscle fibers. *Physiol Rev* 1973; 53:793.

Vanhoute PM: Symposium. Calcium entry blockers and the cardiovascular system. *Fed Proc* 1981; 40:2851.

Vassalle M: Automaticity and automatic rhythms. *Am J Cardiol* 1971; 28:245.

Vassalle M: Effect of pharmacological interventions on atrial pacemakers, in Little RC (ed): *The Physiology of Atrial Pacemakers and Conductive Tissues*. Mt Kisco, NY, Futura Publishing Co, 1980, pp 315–338.

West TC: Electrophysiology of the sinoatrial node, in De Mello WC (ed): *Electrical Phenomena in the Heart*. New York, Academic Press, 1972, pp 191–218.

Wit AL, Friedman PL: Basis for the ventricular arrhythmias accompanying myocardial infarction. *Arch Intern Med* 1975; 135:459.

Chapter 4 _____

Dynamics of the Heartbeat

_____

The ionic mechanisms involved in the excitation and contraction of the isolated myocardium have been discussed in Chapter 3. This section will cover the activation and contraction of the intact heart and will analyze the sequence of events that take place during one cardiac cycle, i.e., one contraction *(systole)* followed by the period before the next contraction *(diastole).* This discussion is divided into three sections: (1) activation of the heart, (2) mechanical and pressure events of the cardiac cycle, and (3) normal heart sounds.

ACTIVATION OF THE HEART

The biophysical factors that underlie the pacemaker function of the sinoatrial (SA) node have been summarized in Chapter 3. Before turning to the details of cardiac activation, it may be helpful to trace the sequential spread of the depolarization process from its origin at the SA node to its termination at the atrial and ventricular myocardium. Following activation of the pacemaker cells in the SA node (see Chapter 2), depolarization of the cardiac cells follows the atrial conductive pathways and sweeps out across the atrial myocardium much as "ripples spread when a stone is thrown into a still pond." The excitation wave travels slowly through the atrioventricular (AV) node and then is rapidly distributed to the ventricular endocardium via the bundle of His and the specialized conductive fasciculi of the right and left bundle branches. Final activation of the ventricles is achieved by spread of the depolarized process through the ventricular muscle to the epicardium.

Atrial Activation

It is now generally recognized that, in addition to the rather slow radial spread of the depolarization process over the atrial myocardium referred to above, the excitation process also travels over the atrial conductive fibers described in Chapter 2. The conduction velocity in these tissues (0.9 to 1.8 m/sec) is much faster than that of the ordinary atrial myocardium (Table 4–1). This is due in part to (1) the presence of parallel myocardial fibers that permit a faster propagation of the excitation wave front than is possible in the less well-aligned ordinary myocardium and (2) the large number of specialized atrial cells in the internodal tracts. For these reasons the conductive tissues can be considered to be the "freeways" of the heart. In this analogy, the specialized tissues rapidly transmit the wave of the excitation to distant parts of the heart, whereas the ordinary muscle fibers serve as the "secondary roads" for final distribution of the stimulus to the contractile elements of the myocardium. The rapid transmission via the atrial conductive tissues and Bachmann's bundle permits the excitation process to reach the left atrium quickly. After its rapid propagation over the specialized tissues, the activation wave leaves the conductive tissues and travels over the ordinary atrial myocardium. This dual system permits the depolarization process to spread almost simultaneously over both the right and left atria, and as a result, the entire atrial musculature is depolarized within approximately 0.08 second after activation of the SA node.

TABLE 4–1.

Average Conduction Velocity of Cardiac Impulse*

Tissue	Velocity (m/sec)
SA node	0.05
Atrial myocardium	0.3–0.5
Specialized atrial fibers	0.9–1.8
Junctional tissue	0.02–0.05
AV node	0.12
Purkinje fibers	2.0–4.0
Ventricular myocardium	0.3–0.5

*Data from Scher AM, et al: *Circ Res* 1959; 7:54; Scher AM, et al: *Circ Res* 1955; 3:56; Wagner ML, et al: *Circ Res* 1966; 18:502; Draper MH, Weidmann S: *J Physiol* 1951; 115:74.

Conduction in the specialized tissues is vulnerable to blockage by scar tissue or other pathologic lesions. In *interatrial block*, for example, the activation process must reach the left atrium through the slower conducting ordinary myocardium because of interference with propagation of the excitation process in Bachmann's bundle. The result in this condition is that left atrial depolarization is delayed. This can be detected clinically by a change in the form and duration of the P wave in the electrocardiogram (ECG) (see Chapter 5).

Atrioventricular Node

Because of the rapid conduction velocity in the atrial specialized tissues, the AV node depolarization begins well in advance of final activation of the atrial myocardium. In fact, AV node depolarization usually begins when activation of the atria is approximately two thirds complete. However, the slow conduction through the junctional cells of the upper AV node provides adequate time for atrial activation and the subsequent atrial contraction to be completed before the excitation wave penetrates the AV node on its way to the ventricle.

The fibers in the marginal zone at the upper end of the AV node have special electrophysiologic features. As shown in Figure 4–1, the resting membrane potential of the upper AV node has a lower magnitude than that of the atrial or His bundle fibers. In addition, the action potential recorded in these fibers has a characteristically slow upstroke, a rounded peak, and a decreased or absent overshoot.

A number of explanations have been proposed to explain the slow conduction velocity of the cells in the upper AV node. These have included the small diameter of the fibers and the possibility of long conductive pathways due to folding of the fibers within the node itself. Recent electrophys-

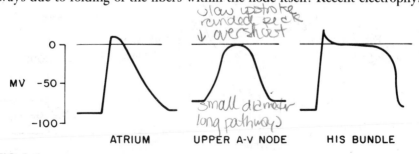

FIG 4–1.
Diagrammatic representation of transmembrane action potentials recorded from fibers of the atrium, upper AV node, and atrial portion of His (common) bundle. (Modified from Hoffman BF, et al: *Circ Res* 1959; 7:11.)

ical data suggest, however, that the conduction pathways are of normal length. In addition, the slow onset and decreased size of the action potential in these marginal cells, along with the change in their cable properties due to their small diameter, offer strong evidence for a decremental type of conduction through this area. The decreased electric activity produced in these tissues during depolarization because of their lower resting membrane potential also reduces the margin of safety that normally ensures the propagation of the action potential. It is not unexpected, therefore, that this area of the AV node may be vulnerable to block (see Chapter 6).

Anatomical studies suggest that the internodal conductive tissues make connections with the AV node at more than one location. This finding is in agreement with electrophysiologic observations that the upper AV node functions as a multilevel transmission system with different conductive velocities and refractory characteristics. Two parallel pathways, an α path that conducts rapidly and a β path with a slower conduction velocity and a shorter refractory period, have been postulated. This is illustrated in Figure 4–2. In this model, the excitation process is considered, under normal conditions, to enter both the α and β pathways from the atrium. The impulse conducted over the slower β path will be blocked near the junction of the two pathways by the antidromic (i.e., moving back toward the atrium) impulse that enters the β pathway from the fast α pathway. As a result, conduction to the lower AV node and common bundle is via only the α fibers and the final common pathway of the lower node and bundle of His.

A dual transmission mechanism in the AV node offers an explanation for echo beats and other types of coupled contractions that occur clinically. For example, if the excitation process from the atrium is blocked for some

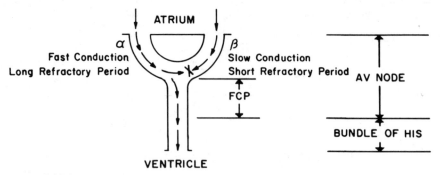

FIG 4–2.
Schematic representation of a model dual transmission system through the upper AV node. *FCP* = final common path. (Modified from Mendez C, Moe GK: *Circ Res* 1966; 19:378.)

reason from entering the β pathway, it would be conducted to the ventricle over the α pathway and common final pathway; however, this same wave of activation could return to the atrium by retrograde conduction through the unused β pathway. Due to the slower conduction in the β pathway, the atrial myocardium would have had time to complete the refractory period that follows its first depolarization by the time the retrograde excitation wave returned to the atrium. As shown in Figure 4–3, this sequence of events would result in the production of an echo or second depolarization of the atrium. This reentry mechanism also can lead to other abnormalities of cardiac rate and rhythm. These will be discussed in Chapter 6.

The AV node has been functionally subdivided into a junctional and a subjunctional area. The junctional region can be further divided into an

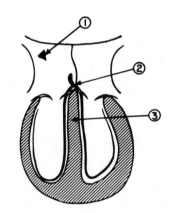

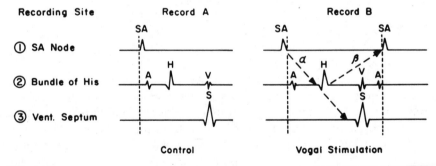

FIG 4–3.

Electric recordings from the dog heart. In *Record B* the AV nodal delay (*A–H* interval) is prolonged, and the atrium is reactivated by retrograde conduction, as shown by reversal in the order of depolarization in the second atrial depolarization. *SA* = SA node; *A* = atrial septum; *H* = bundle of His; *S* = ventricular septum. (Modified from Wallace AG, Dagett WM: *Am Heart J* 1974; 68:661.)

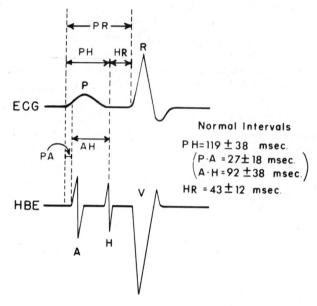

FIG 4–4.
Drawing of a simultaneous ECG and His bundle electrogram *(HBE)* showing subdivisions of the P–R interval. (From Hecht HH, Kossmann CE: *Am J Cardiol* 1973; 31:232. Used by permission.)

upper, atrial portion, which is under autonomic nervous system control, and a lower, ventricular portion, which is essentially autonomous. Conduction disturbances, particularly within the junctional region, can be localized with considerable precision by means of intracardiac ECG recordings. The clinical ECG will be covered in the next chapter. It is worthwhile here, however, to anticipate this discussion and briefly describe the *His bundle recordings.*

An electrode can be positioned inside the heart in the area of the tricuspid valve by means of right heart cardiac catheterization* so that with proper frequency filtering, depolarization of the common bundle (His bundle) will result in a biphasic or triphasic deflection. Recently these His-bundle recordings have been noninvasively obtained using high-resolution external chest recordings and electronic averaging of a large number of cardiac cycles. The *His bundle* (H) *deflection* occurs (Fig 4–4) between the deflection representing atrial *(A)* and ventricular *(V)* depolarizations. The H deflection permits subdivision of the P–R interval of the ECG, i.e., the time

*This procedure involves introducing a flexible tube into a peripheral vein and then advancing it under fluoroscopic control into the chambers of the right heart.

between onset of atrial and ventricular depolarization into two subintervals designated P–H and H–R. These deflections are shown in Figure 4–4 with their normal values. The P–H interval is the time required for the excitation wave to travel across the atrium and through the AV node, whereas the H–R interval is a measure of the conduction time from the point of the recording in the His bundle through the distal common bundle and bundle branches to the ventricular myocardium. Clinical electrophysiologists frequently use the term A–H and H–V for these intervals. Measurement of these periods from the His bundle recording may be of diagnostic value to the cardiologist when confronted with a complicated case of disturbed AV conduction.

An important physiologic feature of the AV node is that under normal conditions it shows unidirectional conduction. Orthograde conduction, i.e., conduction from the atrium to the ventricles, occurs easily whereas retrograde conduction takes place only under exceptional circumstances such as with reentry activation (see Chapter 6). This property of unidirectional conduction appears to reside in a small group of cells in the distal common bundle. These cells conduct orthograde impulses normally but respond to retrograde activation with only a localized nonpropagated response.

Ventricles

Since the atriums and ventricles are separated by the annuli fibrosi, the AV node and common bundle offer the only normal pathway for the excitation process to reach the ventricle (see Chapter 2). The depolarization wave is rapidly distributed by the bundle branches to the extensive network of subendocardial Purkinje fibers that line each ventricle. These fibers turn inward and merge with the ordinary cardiac muscle of the myocardium. As a result, activation of the ventricle wall is from inside to outside. Each Purkinje fiber appears to activate a distinct area of the myocardium. This anatomical finding offers an explanation for some of the clinical features associated with disturbed conduction in the ventricle. For example, if a disease process blocks transmission over some of the rapidly conducting fibers (such as a bundle branch or one of its major fasciculi), the myocardium supplied by these fibers will be activated from adjoining areas of the ventricular wall by the slow transmission of the depolarization process over the ordinary muscle fibers. As a result, the time required to complete the depolarization of the ventricles will be prolonged. This change in activation time, plus alterations in the normal order of activation, will lead to characteristic changes in the ECG. This will be discussed further in Chapter 5.

Activation of the ventricular myocardium follows a definite sequence.

The first part to be activated is on the left side of the ventricular septum near the origin of the anterior papillary muscle. The depolarization process travels from this location into the septum from left to right. A similar area on the right side of the septum is activated from the right bundle branch about 5 msec later. Most of the septum, however, is excited from the left side, and only a thin subendocardial layer is activated from the right bundle branch. Within 5 to 10 msec after onset of septal depolarization, the wave of excitation is distributed to the inside of each ventricle. From here it moves through the free wall of the ventricles with final depolarization of the posterobasal area of the left ventricle, the pulmonary conus, and the basilar part of the ventricular septum.

MECHANICAL EVENTS OF THE CARDIAC CYCLE

Activation of the myocardium is followed by cardiac contraction. In the intact heart, this leads to a series of events that are associated with its function as a pump. It is convenient to relate these activities to the changes in pressure that take place inside the chambers of the heart and the great vessels during the cardiac cycle. Representative pressure pulses from the left atrium, left ventricle, and aorta are diagrammatically shown in Figure 4–5, along with a graphic representation of the electric activity of the heart (ECG). The temporal phases of the cardiac cycle are indicated by vertical lines. The left heart pressure relationships and their association with the mechanical events of the cardiac cycle are discussed first. These relationships will then be summarized for the right heart.

Left Heart Events

Atrial Systole.—A contraction wave follows closely behind the sequential activation of the left atrial myocardium. This local reduction in the size of the atrial cavity pushes the atrial contents ahead of it as it sweeps across the atrium toward the mitral valve orifice. As a result, atrial blood is forced through the open mitral valve into the ventricle (see Chapter 2). This activity is accompanied by an increase in atrial pressure. This increase is the *A wave* of the atrial pressure pulse (see Fig 4–5; also Fig 4–6). The volume of blood contributed to ventricular filling by atrial contraction varies inversely with the duration of the previous diastole and directly with the vigor of atrial systole. At slow heart rates, the long diastolic interval permits major ventricular filling to take place before the onset of atrial contraction. As a result, when diastole is prolonged, the contribution of atrial systole may

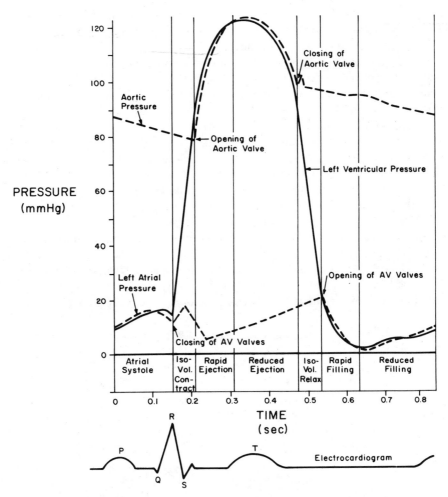

FIG 4–5.
Diagram showing a representative pressure pulse from aorta, left ventricle, and left atrium. An ECG also is shown. See text for discussion.

be minor. The contribution of atrial systole to ventricular filling is reported to increase with age. At normal heart rates in young adults it adds about 20% of the left ventricular end-diastolic volume. This increases to as much as 43% by ages 51 to 68 years.

Closure of the Mitral Valve.—A number of events contribute to closure and tensing of the mitral (and tricuspid) valve. Probably the most important is the change in the AV pressure gradient that follows atrial contraction and that accompanies ventricular contraction. The increase in ventricular volume produced by atrial systole causes a small increase in ventricular pressure. This so-called *atrial kick* is slightly delayed in its onset due to transmission through the open mitral valve. As a result, the atrial A wave has started to decline when ventricular pressure reaches its peak. This may cause the normal atrioventricular pressure gradient to be briefly reduced or even reversed (see Fig 4–6). Reduction or reversal of this AV pressure gradient will slow and may temporarily reverse the forward flow of blood into the ventricle. It has been suggested that these "atriogenic" changes in the inflow pattern of the ventricle permit the open mitral valve cusps to float upward to or toward a closed position. Under these circumstances, final closure and tensing of the valves is then promptly achieved by the "ventriculogenic" increase in ventricular pressure due to ventricular contraction. This mechanism for the presystole positioning of the valve cusps is illustrated in Figure 4–7. In addition to the reversal in the AV pressure gradient, the presystolic positioning of the valve cusps also may be helped by eddy currents set up behind the open valve cusps during atrial systole, by contraction of the atrial-like muscle at the base of the valve, and perhaps by a reduction in lateral pressure in the valve area by the faster

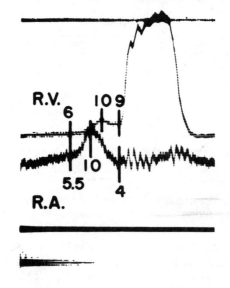

FIG 4–6.
Record of simultaneously recorded right ventricular *(RV)* and right atrial *(RA)* pressure pulses from the dog. Pressures are given in millimeters of mercury. During atrial contraction (A wave in the atrial pressure pulse), the pressure rose from 5.5 to 10 mm Hg. After atrial relaxation, atrial pressure is 4 mm Hg, whereas ventricular pressure is 9 mm Hg. (From Little RC: *Am J Physiol* 1951; 166:289. Used by permission.)

A. ATRIUM CONTRACTING   B. ATRIUM RELAXING

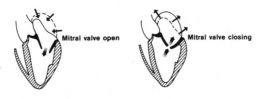

Mitral valve open   Mitral valve closing

C. VENTRICLE STARTING TO CONTRACT

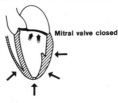

Mitral valve closed

FIG 4–7.

Diagrammatic representation of effect of atrial contraction **(A)**, atrial relaxation **(B)**, and ventricular contraction **(C)** on closure of the mitral valve. See text for further discussion. (From Little RC: Physiological basis for mitral valve function, in Boudoulas H, Wooley CF, (eds): *Mitral Valve Prolapse and Mitral Valve Prolapse Syndrome.* Mt Kisko, NY, Futura Publishing Co, 1988. Used by permission.)

velocity of flow through the valve orifice (Bernoulli effect) or the production of vortices between the valve cusps. Closure of the AV valves will be discussed further in the next section in connection with the heart sounds.

The prompt closure of the mitral valves following atrial systole causes most of the atrial stroke volume to be retained in the ventricle. At the same time, relaxation of the atrium allows the pressure in that chamber to quickly return to a lower level. This pumping function permits the atria to convert a relatively continuous inflow from the vena cava or the pulmonary veins to an intermittent outflow while interposing the minimal interference to venous return and, at the same time, providing for maximal ventricular filling (Fig 4–8). This mechanism also allows ventricular end-diastolic pressure, which is a function of ventricular volume, to be maintained at a higher level than mean atrial pressure. The importance of this mechanism in the control of cardiac output will be discussed later.

Ventricular Systole.—The onset of ventricular contraction and the associated rapid increase in ventricular pressure promptly close the mitral valves if the presystolic positioning described above has not already done

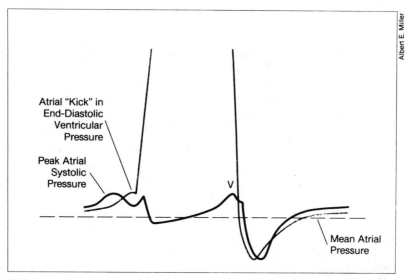

Albert E. Miller

FIG 4–8.
Typical atrial and ventricular pressure curves showing the effect of atrial systole on ventricular end-diastolic pressure (the atrial "kick"). Peak atrial systolic pressure and ventricular end-diastolic pressure are higher than mean atrial pressure. See text for details. (From Little RC, Downes TR: *Cardiologic Consultation* 1987 (summer); 8:1–6. Used by permission.)

so. Under the influence of the rapidly increasing ventricular pressure, the AV valve cusps bulge into the atrium even though the chordae tendineae prevent eversion of the edge. This encroachment on the atrial volume produces a small upstroke, the *C wave*, in the atrial pressure pulse. The continuing development of tension by the ventricular myocardium pulls the annulus fibrosus and the AV ring toward the apex (see Chapter 2). This descent of the atrial base stretches the atrial walls and increases its internal volume. As a result, there is an abrupt fall in atrial pressure. The nadir of this fall is the *X point*. Atrial pressure then rises during the remainder of ventricular systole, the *V wave*, as venous return pools behind the closed AV valve.

Left ventricular pressure rises rapidly as the contraction process begins to squeeze the blood contained inside the ventricle against the closed valves. During this period, the circumference of the left ventricle increases, the apex-to-base length decreases, and the ventricle becomes more spheroid (see Fig 2–11). As a result of these dimensional changes, myocardial fiber length may undergo some alterations during this phase of contraction. These events have led to changing the name of this segment of the cardiac cycle from the older term, isometric contraction, to *isovolumic contraction.* In spite of these dimensional changes, ventricular contraction in the main is still essentially isometric, and most of the contractile energy is used to quickly increase ventricular pressure to the level of aortic diastolic pressure. Under normal circumstances, this is accomplished within approximately 0.06 to 0.08 second after the onset of contraction. Thus the rate of ventricular pressure change (dp/dt) is about 70 mm Hg in 0.07 second or 1,000 mm of Hg per second. Ventricular pressure continues to increase, and as it rises above aortic pressure, the aortic valve cusps are forced open, and the period of *rapid cardiac ejection* begins.

With opening of the aortic valve and ejection of blood, the ventricular myocardium is able to shorten, and the heart shifts from its essentially isometric form of contraction to a more isotonic type. The ejected blood quickly reaches a maximum velocity, which in the dog may be as high as 150 cm/second, and within 0.10 to 0.11 second from the onset of ejection, 80% to 85% of the stroke volume leaves the heart. This period is called the phase of *rapid cardiac ejection.* Inertia and resistance factors make it difficult for this ejected volume to quickly push the blood already present in the aorta into the periphery. As a result, most of the stroke volume is accommodated by stretching the elastic wall and increasing the internal volume of the proximal aorta. This windkessel mechanism permits much of the kinetic energy imparted to the blood by ventricular contraction to be stored in the elastic tissue as potential energy. This stretch energy is then available to maintain aortic pressure during diastole and thus permits a continuous forward flow of blood. This aspect will be covered in more detail in later chapters. Near the end of the period of rapid cardiac ejection, ventricular pressure peaks and begins to fall. The beginning of the phase of *reduced ventricular ejection* occurs when aortic and ventricular pressure momentarily equilibrate.

Closure of Aortic Valve.—During the remainder of ventricular systole, ventricular pressure falls below aortic pressure, and a negative pressure gradient develops across the aortic valve. This is shown in Figure 4–9. Due to its forward momentum, blood continues to be ejected from the ventricle during this period in spite of the reversed pressure gradient, but the rate of ejection decreases rapidly. The fact that blood continues to move forward during this period appears paradoxical to some students. It should be recalled that energy exists in several forms, and even though aortic pressure is higher than ventricular pressure during this period, the total energy of the ventricular blood, i.e., pressure energy plus the kinetic energy, is still higher than the total energy level of the blood in the aorta. Approximately 0.17 second after onset of the phase of reduced ejection, forward movement of blood out of the ventricle stops, and flow then momentarily reverses as blood attempts to regurgitate into the ventricle. This backflow will catch the open aortic valve cusps, and they are promptly closed (see Chapter 2). This closure abruptly stops the regurgitant flow. The rapid deceleration of the fluid column, as a result of the valve closure, produces a sharp oscillation in the aortic pressure. This prominent feature of the aortic pressure pulse, the *incisura* is frequently used to mark aortic valve closure and the end of ventricular systole (see Fig 4–9).

Aortic pressure then continues to fall slowly during the remainder of the cardiac cycle as blood moves out of the arterial system through the capillaries and into the veins. During this period, the energy that had been stored during systole in the stretched elastic tissues of the aortic wall is converted back into pressure and drives the blood through the body. A small wave may occur in the aortic pressure during this period. This results

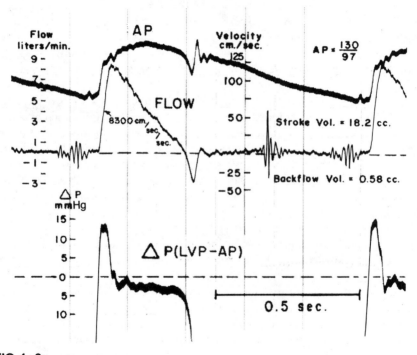

FIG 4–9.
Relationship between pressure gradient *(ΔP)* and flow through aortic valve of the dog. *Top,* aortic pressure; *middle,* flow; and *bottom,* pressure gradient between ventricle and aorta. *AP* = aortic pressure; *LVP* = left ventricular pressure. (Modified from Spencer MP, Greiss FC: *Circ Res* 1962; 10:274. Used by permission.)

from reflected pressure waves from regions downstream where narrowing or branching of the arterial system takes place. This is discussed further in Chapter 9.

Opening of Mitral Valve.—During the 0.06 to 0.08 second after closure of the aortic valve, ventricular volume remains constant as the mitral valve is still closed, and blood can neither enter nor leave the ventricle. This is the period of *isovolumic relaxation*. During this interval, ventricular pressure falls rapidly as tension goes out of the myocardium. Coincident with this drop in pressure, the curve of the mitral valve cusps toward the atrium first begins to flatten, and then when ventricular pressure falls below atrial pressure, it begins to bulge toward the ventricle. At the same time, the valve annulus abruptly terminates its descent toward the ventricle. This event is reflected in the atrial pressure pulse by a small notch that occurs just after the peak of the V wave. Approximately 0.036 second after atrial and ventricular pressure cross, the AV valve cusps are forced open.

It has been generally assumed that the mitral valve is forced open at the end of the period of *isovolumic relaxation* by the developing AV pressure gradient as ventricular pressure falls below atrial pressure. Recent echocardiographic studies suggest that traction on the valve cusps via the chordae tendineae due to late relaxation of the papillary muscle may also play a role in valve opening, and this event may not be entirely a passive one. Opening of the mitral valve permits the blood that had pooled in the atrium during ventricular systole to rush into the relaxing ventricle. The pressure relationships during this period of *rapid ventricular filling* are illustrated in Figure 4–10. The ventricle continues to relax during this period so that its capacity increases more rapidly than it is filled from the atrium. Thus, ventricular pressure falls in spite of the inrush of blood. This has suggested to some that relaxation of the ventricle at this point may literally "suck" blood from the atria. During this period atrial pressure falls rapidly. This drop is called the Y descent.

As the contraction tension leaves the ventricle and it begins to fill, the annulus fibrosus moves back toward its rest position. The upward movement probably represents the counterpart of the descent of the cardiac base during the *isovolumic phase* of ventricular contraction. This movement is completed by the end of the rapid phase of ventricular filling.

Approximately 0.06 second after opening of the mitral valve, the rapid rate of ventricular filling is suddenly reduced. This occurs at the transition point between the end of ventricular relaxation and the beginning of passive distention. At this point, ventricular pressure reaches its lowest level and begins a rapid upward swing. This rebound, which may be palpable under some circumstances on the chest wall as an outward thrust, probably re-

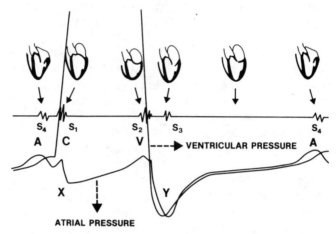

FIG 4–10.
Relationship between left atrial and left ventricular pressure during the cardiac cycle.
The *A, C, V, X,* and *Y* waves of the atrial pressure pulse are shown. *Top,* diagrammatic
representation of the mitral valve position. *Middle, phonocardiogram. S₁–S₄* = first
through fourth heart sounds. (From Little RC: Physiologic basis for mitral valve function,
in Boudoulas H, Wooley CF (ed): *Mitral Valve Prolapse and Mitral Valve Prolapse Syndrome,* Mt Kisco, NY, Futura Publishing Co, 1988. Used by permission.)

sults (1) from overfilling due to the inertial forces set up during the period
of rapid ventricular filling and (2) from the change from a relaxing chamber
to a distensible organ. At this time, atrial pressure may momentarily fall
below ventricular pressure, and the mitral valve may float to or toward
reclosure. Shortly thereafter, however, the normal AV pressure gradient
is reestablished, and the mitral valve reopens. Following this period, the
valve cusps may drift toward a midposition if venous return is not unduly
elevated. In any event, they are once again opened wide by the increased
flow into the ventricle that accompanies onset of the next atrial contraction.

Echocardiography

A noninvasive procedure for following changes in cardiac geometry and
recording the position and movement of the heart valves has evolved from
techniques developed during World War II to detect underwater objects.
Echocardiography utilizes pulses of sound energy and measures the time
required for that energy to be reflected from objects in its path back to the
energy source. In clinical usage, a train of 1-μsec pulses of 2- to 20-MHz
sound is emitted at a rate of 1,000 pulses per second by a transducer placed
on the chest (Fig 4–11). The ultrasonic energy is concentrated into a narrow

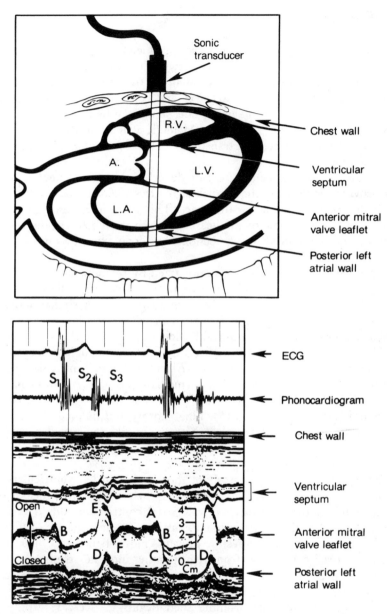

FIG 4–11.

Top, procedure for recording echocardiogram of anterior mitral valve leaflet. Sonic transducer is placed on chest wall, and the sound beam is directed into the chest as shown. A = aorta; *RV* = right ventricle; *LV* = left ventricle; *LA* = left atrium. *Bottom,* record of echo that results when sound is reflected from structures within the chest. From the top, ECG, phonocardiogram showing the heart sounds, and echocardiogram. S_1, S_2, S_3 = first, second, and third heart sounds, respectively. See text for discussion.

beam directed into the thorax. Echoes are produced when the sound energy travels through an interface, such as between tissue and blood, that presents a change in acoustic impedance. During the interval between sound bursts, the transducer acts as a receiver and converts the reflected sound energy back into an electrical signal. This signal can be calibrated and displayed on an oscilloscope and in the M mode will show the distance between the reflecting surface and transducer. This trace can be photographed or recorded on a strip chart.

In addition to the standard M-mode echocardiogram, newer procedures provide for viewing the cardiac structures many times a second by moving the sound beam across the heart. This two-dimensional technique provides a triangular view of the heart in which movement of the cardiac structures can be followed. Cross-sectional and long-axis views of the heart are also easily obtained.

Mitral valve dynamics can be summarized by reference to the M-mode echocardiographic tracing of the anterior mitral valve leaflet shown in Figure 4–11. The posterior mitral valve leaflet undergoes a similar series of movements. By the end of the period of *isovolumic relaxation*, the fall in ventricular pressure causes the mitral leaflets to bulge into the left ventricle *(D)*. This is immediately followed by rapid separation of the cusps, and they open to their maximum position *(E)* during rapid ventricular filling. The valve cusps then return to an intermediate position *(F)* until they are again opened as a result of atrial systole *(A)*. The mitral valve then begins to close during atrial relaxation *(B)*. Final closure and bulging of the valve cusps into the atrium *(C)* takes place with the onset of ventricular contraction.

Ventricular Volume.—Analysis of the changes in left ventricular volume during the cardiac cycle (Fig 4–12) may help clarify the previous discussion of the cardiac pressure pulses. Atrial contraction adds a variable amount of blood to the partially filled ventricle. Prompt closure of the mitral valve at the end of atrial systole prevents most of the extra blood contributed by atrial contraction from regurgitating into the atrium. As a result, ventricular volume stabilizes during the phase of isovolumic contraction at a higher level than before atrial contraction. With opening of the aortic valve, ventricular volume then begins to decrease rapidly as blood is ejected into the aorta. After about 0.10 second, this rate of decrease is slowed as aortic pressure rises above ventricular pressure, and the volume stabilizes at its lowest value.

It is important to point out that the left ventricle does not normally empty itself completely. The diastolic remainder left in the ventricle at the

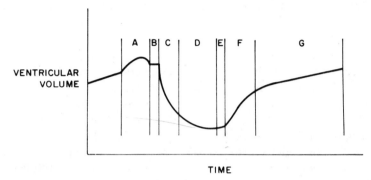

FIG 4–12.
Schematic plot of left ventricular volume during one cardiac cycle. *A* = atrial systole; *B* = isovolumic contraction; *C* = rapid cardiac ejection; *D* = reduced cardiac ejection; *E* = isovolumic relaxation; *F* = rapid ventricular filling; and *G* = reduced ventricular filling.

end of ejection does, however, constitute a reserve blood supply that can be mobilized to increase the stroke volume by increasing the vigor of ventricular contraction.

Opening of mitral valve permits the blood that collected in the atrium during ventricular contraction to fill the ventricle. During this period, ventricular volume increases very rapidly. This increase continues but at a reduced rate during the period of reduced filling as the heart is gradually distended by venous return.

Right Heart Events

In general, the pressure relationships of the right side of the heart are qualitatively similar to those described above for the left heart, and opening and closing of the tricuspid and pulmonary valves follow the same dynamic events as the mitral and aortic valves on the left side. While these events are similar, the pressure levels are lower. The average capacity of the adult right atrium is about 160 ml, or 20 ml larger than the left atrium, and the wall is slightly more distensible. As the same volume of blood travels through each chamber per minute, it is not surprising that the average right atrial pressure is about one half that of the left atrium (see Table 7–1).

The low right atrial pressure results in a normal right ventricular end diastolic pressure that is 3 to 4 mm Hg lower than the left ventricular preload. However, as the resistance to blood flow through the lungs is roughly one fifth that of the systemic circulation, a right ventricular systolic pressure of 24 mm Hg is normally sufficient to move the cardiac output through the pulmonary circulation.

Venous Pulse.—A type of pulsation that differs from the pressure pulse so far described appears in the low-pressure venous system during the cardiac cycle. This venous pulse can be demonstrated by placing a subject in a supine position with the head slightly raised and turned to one side. When the skin over the jugular bulb is observed, it can be seen to rise and fall in a ripple of three waves during each heartbeat. The walls of the veins are normally not under tension, and the vein has a flattened cross section. However, if the forward flow of blood is impeded, the volume inside the vein increases; the vessel assumes a more elliptic shape, and the change in volume is visible as a *volume pulse* (see Fig. 2–6).

The three waves of the venous pulse, *A*, *C*, and *V*, represent the change in venous volume produced by the variable resistance to venous return presented by right atrial pressure. Thus, the normal venous pulse, as illustrated in Figure 4–13, is a backward transmission of the right atrial pressure pulse transformed into a volume pulse. Careful study of this volume pulse offers the physician a look at events in the right heart in the same manner as the components of the aortic pulse reflect left ventricular events. The *A* wave is due to the increase in right atrial pressure produced by atrial contraction. The *C* wave occurs during early ventricular contraction and may represent bulging of the tricuspid valve back into the right atrium. The *V* wave represents the increase in right atrial pressure as it fills while the tricuspid valve remains closed during right ventricular systole.

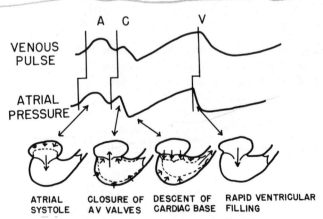

FIG 4–13.
Simultaneous plot of venous volume pulse and right atrial pressure during the cardiac cycle, indicating time lag between the two events. The major cardiac events associated with each wave are indicated at the bottom.

NORMAL HEART SOUNDS

A series of sound vibrations is associated with the cardiac cycle. These sounds usually can be heard by careful auscultation over the heart. The normal heart sounds and their relationship to the pressure changes within the heart are shown in Figure 4–14.

First Heart Sound

The *first heart sound* (S_1) occurs at the time of closure of the AV (mitral and tricuspid) valves. It has three components (Fig 4–15): (1) a few preliminary low-frequency vibrations that originate in the ventricular myocardium at the onset of contraction, (2) a louder middle component associated with closure and tensing of the AV valves, and (3) a terminal set of low-intensity vibrations produced by opening of the pulmonic and aortic valves and the onset of ventricular ejection. The first component is at or near the limit of audibility and usually is not heard. The third component also is normally not audible but may be accentuated in some abnormal conditions. In such cases, it may be perceived as an extra ejection sound.

The middle of valvular component of S_1 is frequently split into two closely spaced subdivisions, M_1 and T_1 (Fig 4–16). Current evidence

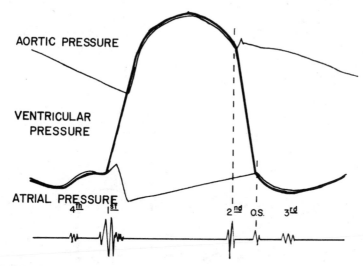

FIG 4–14.
Relation of heart sounds to aortic pressure *(top)*, ventricular pressure *(middle)*, and atrial pressure *(bottom)*. (Modified from Schwartz ML, Little RC: *N Engl J Med* 1961; 264:280. Used by permission.)

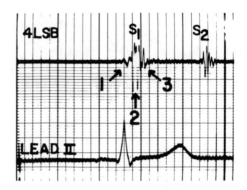

FIG 4–15.
Phonocardiogram recorded from fourth intercostal space to the left of the sternum and labeled to show the three phases of the first sound: *(1)* initial muscular component, *(2)* valvular component, and *(3)* ejection component. *4LSB* = fourth intercostal space, left sternal border; S_1, S_2 = first and second heart sounds, respectively. Lead II of the ECG is included for timing. (From Little RC: *Ohio State Med J* 1969; 65:483. Used by permission.)

strongly suggests that M_1 is associated with closure of the mitral valve and T_1 results from the forces that close the tricuspid valve. The separation between these sounds results from a combination of the asynchronous contraction of the two ventricles and the more vigorous contraction of the left ventricle. The latter events cause left ventricular pressure to rise more abruptly than right ventricular pressure. The result is that the mitral valve usually closes before the tricuspid. Thus, M_1 may normally lead T_1 by as much as 0.04 second.

The etiology of the middle component of S_1 has been controversial. It

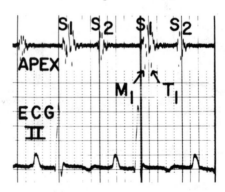

FIG 4–16.
Apex phonocardiogram showing normal splitting of the first sound *(S₁)*. Mitral *(M)* and tricuspid *(T)* components of the first sound are labeled. (From Little RC: *Ohio State Med J* 1969; 65:483. Used by permission.)

now appears clear, however, that it occurs as a by-product of AV valve closure. The presystolic positioning of the AV valves discussed in the previous section limits the amount of regurgitation that accompanies final closure. There is, nevertheless, a tendency for this backflow to occur as the valve leaflets swing together and bulge into the atrium. Coincident with production of S_1, this eversion of the valve leaflets is terminated abruptly. This sudden deceleration of the at least potentially regurgitant column of blood apparently liberates sufficient force to set the valve cusps and their supporting tissues into vibration.

The intensity of S_1 is related to the position of the AV valves at the onset of ventricular contraction and to the vigor of that contraction. Optimal time for the presystolic positioning of the valve cusps is provided by an interval between atrial and ventricular contraction that is slightly longer than normal. In this situation the valve cusps are closed, or nearly closed, at the onset of ventricular contraction. As a result, the regurgitant flow during final closure is minimal, and S_1 is soft. If the interval between atrial and ventricular contraction (this is the same as the P–R interval in the ECG) is too short, there will be insufficient time for presystolic positioning to take place. If this interval is too long, the AV valves will reopen. In both cases, the valve will be closed from an open position by ventricular contraction, much as an open door is closed by the wind. This will result in the maximum regurgitant flow during closure and a loud S_1. This relationship between the duration of P–R intervals and intensity of S_1 is shown in Figure 4–17.

Second Heart Sound

The second heart sound (S_2) occurs at the end of cardiac ejection and marks the dynamic events associated with closure of the aortic and pulmonary valves. It is divided into an aortic and pulmonic component (A_2 and P_2) (Fig 4–18). Recent studies utilizing high-fidelity intracardiac sound and pressure recordings indicate that these sounds occur immediately after valve closure and coincident with the respective incisura in the aortic and pulmonary artery pressure pulse (see earlier discussion regarding aortic valve closure). Production of S_2 results when forces liberated during the rapid deceleration of the regurgitant flow toward the heart set the aortic and pulmonary valve cusps and their surrounding structures into vibration.

Normally A_2 precedes P_2 due to the difference in the time of closure of the aortic and pulmonary valve. This separation may be as much as 50 msec during inspiration and is usually reduced to 20 or 30 msec during expiration. With auscultation it is difficult or impossible to identify two sounds that are separated by less than 25 msec; therefore, normal or *physiologic splitting* of S_2 is recognized clinically by the separation of S_2 during

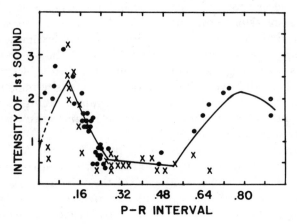

FIG 4–17.
Plot of relative intensity of the first heart sound taken from phonocardiograms of two patients with complete AV block and varying PR intervals. (From Little RC: *Ohio State Med J* 1969; 65:483. Used by permission.)

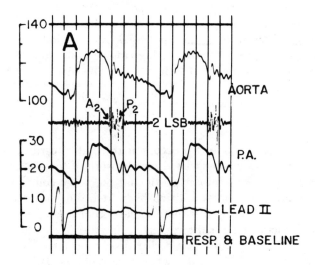

FIG 4–18.
Pressure pulses recorded from the aorta *(first tracing)*; pulmonary artery *(P.A., third tracing)*; phonocardiogram recorded from the second left sternal border *(LSB, second tracing)*; and ECG *(fourth tracing)* in an anesthetized dog. A_2 is associated with the incisura of the aortic pulse, P_2 with the incisura of the pulmonary pulse. (From Boyle J III, Little RC: *Am Heart J* 1964; 68:91. Used by permission.)

inspiration into its A_2 and P_2 components, while S_2 is perceived as a single sound (Fig 4–19) during expiration.

Ejection into the pulmonary artery continues for a short period after the end of left ventricular ejection even though mechanical systole ends essentially simultaneously in both the right and the left ventricle. In addition, the reversal of flow at the time of the incisura lasts somewhat longer in the pulmonary artery than in the aorta. The mechanism responsible for these events is poorly understood, but it appears to be related to the lower input impedance of the pulmonary artery compared to the aortic outflow tract. The interval between the end of mechanical systole and the nadir of the incisura has been called the "hangout time." It is normally about 15 msec for the aorta and 35 to 115 msec for the pulmonary artery.

These findings provide an explanation for the inspiratory splitting of S_2 that was described earlier. Pulmonary arterial impedance decreases during lung inflation because of changes in both pulmonary vascular resistance and capacitance. This causes the hangout time in the pulmonary artery to increase. As a result, during inspiration, the pulmonary incisura is delayed further, and the separation between A_2 and P_2 is increased.

Understanding of the relationship between cardiovascular events and the timing of S_2 is important for the clinical diagnosis of disease states. For example, *paradoxical* or *reverse splitting* of S_2 (that is, P_2 before A_2) occurs in pathologic conditions where left ventricular ejection is prolonged, such as left bundle-branch block or severe arterial hypertension. In such situations, the delay in A_2 can be recognized by an inspiratory decrease in the separation between A_2 and P_2 as P_2 moves closer to A_2.

Third Heart Sound

The *third heart sound* (S_3) is a short, low-intensity sound that may occur early in diastole. It was considered for many years to result from reclosure of the mitral valve (and in some cases of the tricuspid valve) at the end of

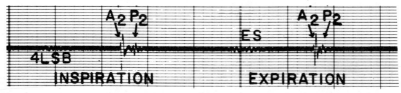

FIG 4–19.
Phonocardiogram showing physiologic (normal) split of the second heart sound. *4LSB* = fourth intercostal space, left sternal border; *ES* = ejection sound. (Modified from Schwartz ML, Little RC: *N Engl J Med* 1961; 264:280. Used by permission.)

the period of rapid ventricular filling. However, it is now generally accepted that S₃ results instead from the sudden tensing of the chordae tendineae and AV ring as the relaxing ventricle pulls these structures taut at the end of its rapid filling. This mechanism is most apt to occur when the ventricle is dilated or when ventricular filling is unusually large. For this reason, S₃ is a normal finding in healthy children and young adults. If not previously present, it will also develop in a large proportion of normal pregnant women during the last trimester as a consequence of their larger fluid volume and increased cardiac output. In older adults, S₃ is usually considered a pathologic sound and is frequently associated with heart failure or conditions such as anemia or thyrotoxicosis, which produce increased ventricular filling early in diastole. A third heart sound is frequently associated with a sharp break in the outward movement of the ventricle and a palpable impulse at the apex at the time of the extra sound.

Fourth Heart Sound

A soft low-frequency sound may occur about 0.01 to 0.02 second after the peak of the A wave in the atrial pressure pulse. The *fourth heart sound* (S₄) originates in the ventricle during the rise in ventricular pressure produced by atrial contraction. It is frequently near the limits of audibility but may become much louder if ventricular compliance is reduced or if ventricular diastolic pressure is elevated.

SUMMARY

Activation of the Heart.—Cardiac depolarization normally starts with the pacemaker cells of the SA node. It follows the atrial conductive tissues as it spreads out over the atria and is then delayed in the upper AV node before being rapidly distributed to the ventricles via the bundle of His and the Purkinje fibers in the ventricular bundle branches.

Mechanical Pressure Events.—Contraction of the myocardium follows electrical activation and produces characteristic alterations in the pressure in each cardiac chamber. Following atrial relaxation, the AV valves move toward closure; final apposition results from the rapid increase in ventricular pressure with the onset of ventricular systole. The pulmonary and aortic valves open with the onset of ventricular ejection as ventricular pressure rises above pulmonary and aortic pressure. Following a period of rapid and reduced ejection, ventricular pressure falls, and the aortic and pulmonic valves close as the ventricles begin to relax. At the end of the period of isovolumic relaxation, the AV valves are forced open as ventricular pressure becomes less than atrial pressure and ventricular filling begins.

Heart Sounds.—A series of normal sound vibrations is associated with the cardiac cycle. The first sound (S_1) is associated with closure of the AV valves. The second sound (S_2) results from closure of the pulmonary and aortic valves. The aortic component (A_2) of S_2 usually precedes the pulmonary component (P_2). A third sound (S_3) may occur early in diastole as a result of ventricular filling and a soft fourth sound (S_4) due to the increase in ventricular pressure following atrial systole may be heard in late diastole.

BIBLIOGRAPHY

Abrams J: Current concepts of the genesis of heart sounds: I. First and second sounds. *JAMA* 1978; 239:2787.

Benchimol A, Desser KB, Gartian JL: Bidirectional blood flow velocity in the cardiac chambers and great vessels studied with the Doppler ultrasonic flowmeter. *Am J Med* 1972; 52:467.

Braunwald E, Frahm CJ: Studies on Starling's law of the heart: IV. Observations on the hemodynamic function of the left atrium in man. *Circulation* 1961; 24:633.

Brecher GA: Critical review of recent work on ventricular diastolic suction. *Circ Res* 1958; 6:554.

Bryg RJ, Williams GA, Labovits AR: Effect of aging on left ventricular diastolic filling in normal subjects. *Am J Cardiol* 1987; 59:971.

Burggrof GW, Craige E: The first heart sound in complete heart block: Phono-echocardiographic correlation. *Circulation* 1974; 50:17.

Durrer D, et al: Total excitation of the isolated human heart. *Circulation* 1970; 41:899.

Feigenbaum H: *Echocardiography*, ed 2. Philadelphia, Lea & Febiger, 1976.

Fowler NO, Adolph RJ: Fourth sound gallop or split first sound. *Am J Cardiol* 1972; 30:441.

Hawthorne EW: Instantaneous dimensional changes of the left ventricle in dogs. *Circ Res* 1961; 9:110.

Hecht HH: The irregular heart 1971: New techniques and concepts. *Circulation* 1971; 4:944.

James TN: The connecting pathways between the sinus node and the AV node and between the right and the left atrium in the human heart. *Am Heart J* 1963; 66:498.

Laniado S, et al: Temporal relation of the first heart sound to closure of the mitral valve. *Circulation* 1973; 47:1006.

Lewis T, Meakins J, White PD: The excitatory process in the dog's heart: I. The auricles. *Philos Trans R Soc Lond [Biol]* 1914; 205:375.

Little RC: Effect of atrial systole on ventricular pressure and closure of the A-V valves. *Am J Physiol* 1951; 166:289.

Little RC: The mechanism of closure of the mitral valve: A continuing controversy. *Circulation* 1979; 59:615.

Little RC: The physiology of atrial pacemakers and conductive tissues: Historical perspective, in Little RC (ed): *The Physiology of Atrial Pacemakers and Conductive Tissues*. Mt Kisco, NY, Futura Publishing Co, 1980.

Little RC: Physiological basis for mitral valve function, in Boudoulas H, Wooley CR (ed): *Mitral Valve Prolapse and Mitral Valve Prolapse Syndrome*. Mt Kisco, NY, Futura Publishing Co, 1988, pp 67–88.

Little RC, Downes TR: Atrial transport and its importance to cardiovascular function. *Cardiologic Consultation* 1987 (Summer); 8:1.

Moe GK, Preston JB, Burlington H: Physiologic evidence for a dual A-V transmission system. *Circ Res* 1956; 4:357.

Nixon PGF: The genesis of the third heart sound. *Am Heart J* 1963; 65:712.

Sano T, Ohtsuka E, Shimamoto T: "Unidirectional" atrioventricular conduction studied by microelectrodes. *Circ Res* 1960; 8:600.

Shaver JA, O'Toole JD: The second heart sound: Newer concepts. *Mod Conc Cardiovasc Dis* 1977; 66:7.

Spencer MP, Greiss FC: Dynamics of ventricular ejection. *Circ Res* 1962; 10:274.

Stefadouros MA, Little RC: The etiology and clinical significance of the diastolic heart sounds. *Arch Intern Med* 1980; 140:600.

Steffens TG, Hagan AD: Role of chordae tendineae in mitral valve opening: Two-dimensional echocardiographic evidence. *Am J Cardiol* 1984; 53:153.

Wooley CF, et al: Left atrial and left ventricular sound and pressure in mitral stenosis. *Circulation* 1968; 38:295.

Chapter 5 _____

Fundamentals of Electrocardiography

Useful information about the electric events of the cardiac cycle can be obtained by recording the voltage produced by the beating heart at the surface of the body. When used clinically, the electrocardiogram (ECG) is recorded from specific sites on the body in the form of a graph showing the variation in voltage with time. Interpretation of these ECGs is, however, complicated by the three-dimensional character of the body and the distance between the heart and the recording electrodes. To handle these considerations, early workers made the simplifying assumption that the body is a homogeneous volume conductor with a standard geometry. A body of theory based on this assumption has developed that supplies a field of reference for the ECG and permits the subject to be approached in an analytic fashion. These basic principles will be covered in a descriptive manner in this chapter and related to the physiology of the heart.* This information will then be utilized in the discussion of the disturbances of cardiac rhythm that follows in the next chapter.

*This discussion will treat the heart as a single equivalent dipole. Consideration of multidipole models and a rigorous mathematical treatment of ECG theory are both beyond the scope of this book.

THE BODY AS VOLUME CONDUCTOR

The body can be considered to have electric properties similar to those of an infinitely large container of saline (Fig 5–1). The heart is represented in this model by two electrodes placed close together at the center of the tank and connected to a source of electric current such as a battery. As a result, the electrode pair becomes a dipole with a positive and a negative pole. An electric current will flow from the positive pole through the saline to the negative pole. The lines shown in the cross-sectional diagram of the tank in the lower part of Figure 5–1 represent an infinite number of such current pathways. Most of the current will take the direct path between the electrodes, and the density of current flow will be progressively less as the conductive pathway lengthens. It should also be kept in mind that, in a three-dimensional volume conductor, the current paths are, in reality, conductive surfaces, and in the cross-sectional view of the tank, the cut edges of these surfaces appear as lines.

The nomenclature used to describe an electric potential is relative. For example, if the electromotive force delivered to the dipole in the tank is of a low value, such as 4 V, the potential at the negative pole can be assigned the value of -2 V and the potential of the positive pole $+2$ V. Under

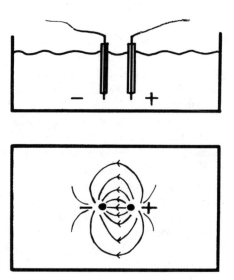

FIG 5–1.
Top, diagrammatic representation of an electric dipole placed at center of a large tank of saline. *Bottom,* cross section through tank at level of dipole showing representative lines of current flow.

these circumstances, the value of 0 V can be defined in terms of the dipole as being halfway between the potential at each pole. It follows from this that a point on any current flow line halfway between the positive and the negative pole will have a potential that will satisfy the above definition of 0 V. If all of the points in the volume conductor where the electric potential, as determined by the dipole, is zero are connected (Fig 5–2), a zero isopotential line (or surface in the three-dimensional tank) will be defined. In the two-dimensional diagram (see Fig 5–2), this zero isopotential line is *at right angles to and bisects a line connecting the poles of the dipole* (i.e., at right angles to the axis of the dipole).

The establishment of a zero isopotential line (or surface) will determine the sign of the potential produced at any point in the volume conductor by the dipole. For example, if the point at which the potential is measured is on the side of the zero isopotential line toward the positive pole of the dipole, that point will have a positive sign. A new isopotential line (surface) that has the value of the potential at that point, for example, + 1½ V, can be constructed by connecting all points in the volume conductor with that voltage (see Fig 5–2). This fact will be helpful later in visualizing the effect of the cardiac dipole on the electric potential at specific body locations.

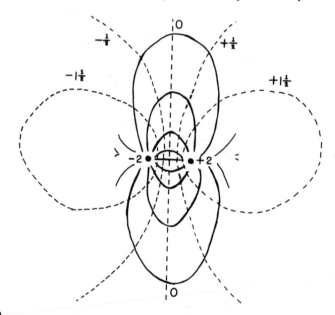

FIG 5–2.
Plot of representative lines of current flow *(solid lines)* and isopotential lines *(dashed lines)* in a two-dimensional volume conductor as produced by a potential of 4 V applied to the center dipole. See text for discussion.

The absolute magnitude and sign of the potential at any point P in the two-dimensional cross-sectional diagram (see Fig 5–2) can be calculated using the diagram shown in Figure 5–3 and the equation

$$E_P = \frac{KQ \text{ cosine } \theta}{d^2} \qquad (5\text{--}1)$$

where K is the conductivity constant, Q the dipole moment (i.e., the charge times the distance between the dipole), d the distance between point P and the dipole center, and θ the angle between the axis of the dipole and a line connecting point P and the dipole center.

If for illustrative purposes the conductivity constant (K) in equation 5–1 is assigned a value of 1, the electrical potential anywhere on a line that bisects the dipole shown in Figure 5–3 and is at a right angle to its axis will be zero, i.e., the zero isopotential line. This follows because the cosine of 90 degrees is zero. Similarly, as the cosine of 0 degrees is 1, the potential generated by the dipole at any point on its axis will be inversely proportional to the square of the distance from the dipole center.

The magnitude of the potential at any point in the volume conductor can be experimentally measured with the use of a reference electrode. For simplicity, this principle will be illustrated using a two-dimensional volume conductor (Fig 5–4). When a third electrode is placed in the volume conductor, it will fall on some isopotential line generated as a result of the dipole voltage. The greater the distance between this electrode and the dipole, the smaller the value of the electric potential. In fact, as the distance between the electrode and the dipole becomes infinitely great, the electric voltage, as determined by equation 5–1, will become zero. For this reason, if the third electrode is a *great distance* from the dipole, its electric potential will be close to zero and *can be considered to be zero.*

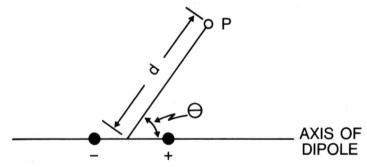

FIG 5–3.
Diagram to be used with equation 5–1. See text for discussion.

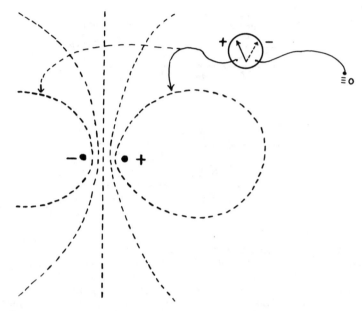

FIG 5–4.
Representative isopotential lines as produced in a two-dimensional volume conductor containing a dipole *(left)* and an indifferent reference electrode *(right)* placed a great distance from the dipole. The potential of the reference electrode is assumed to be zero. This electrode is connected through a voltmeter to an exploring electrode *(arrow)*.

This distant electrode (sometimes called an indifferent electrode because its value is not affected by the orientation of the dipole or by moderate changes in its intensity) can be used as a reference point (zero) for measurement of the voltage at any point in the volume conductor that is near the dipole. For example, in this situation if a voltmeter is connected to the reference electrode and its other lead is used as an exploring electrode (see Fig 5–4), the voltmeter will record the potential of the exploring electrode. The principle of a zero, or essentially zero, reference electrode underlies the clinical recording of the unipolar ECG from the body surface. This will be discussed later in this section.

EQUIVALENT DIPOLE

Myocardial cells are electrically polarized at rest so that the inside is negatively charged in regard to the outside (see Chapter 3). Such a cell can be considered, as shown in the upper part of Figure 5–5, to consist of a

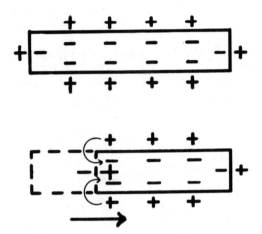

FIG 5–5.
Top, representation of a polarized muscle cell. *Bottom,* the left end of the muscle has been depolarized. A local current flows from outside of the polarized segment into the cell (*small arrow*) at the margin between polarized and depolarized areas. A symbolic dipole equivalent to this electric activity has been placed at the margin between depolarized and polarized areas. The *large arrow* shows direction of movement of the depolarization process. See text.

series of dipoles separated by an insulating membrane. In this model there is no net flow of current as long as the cell remains at rest. For this reason, lines of current flow will not occur in a volume conductor if the resting cardiac muscle cell is substituted for the dipole in the experimental setup described above. Furthermore, as there is no current flow, different iso-potential lines cannot be constructed and an exploring electrode placed in the tank near the resting muscle cell will not record a potential (Fig 5–6, top). However, if the myocardial cell is depolarized at one end, as shown in the lower part of Figure 5–5, a local current will flow into the cell all along the margin between the polarized and depolarized portion. This current flow can be considered to result, at least on the outside of the cell, from a ring of individual dipoles oriented with their positive pole toward the polarized segment of the membrane. It is convenient to consolidate this ring of electric activity into a single representative dipole equivalent to the total strength and average orientation of all the individual dipoles. In Figure 5–5 such an *equivalent dipole* has been placed at the boundary between the polarized and depolarized membrane and oriented with the positive pole toward the polarized area. It is important to emphasize that this equivalent dipole represents the net magnitude and orientation of the electric activity produced on the outside of the myocardial cell by the depolarization wave as it propagates over the fiber.

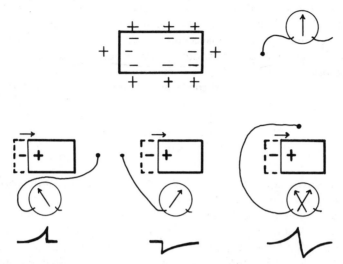

FIG 5–6.
Schematic representation of effect of a polarized muscle cell on an exploring electrode placed at various positions in the volume conductor. *Top,* muscle at rest. *Bottom,* effect of depolarization of the muscle from left to right.

If an exploring electrode is placed in the volume conductor close to the strip of cardiac muscle undergoing depolarization, the electrode will fall on an isopotential line produced as a result of the electric activity at the area of depolarization. The polarity of this potential will depend on the location of both the zero isopotential line (see above) and the electrode. As indicated in Figure 5–6, if the exploring electrode is near the polarized end of the muscle, it will have a positive charge, whereas if it is near the depolarized end, it will have a negative value. In addition, as the depolarization process propagates down the length of the muscle, the distance between the area of electric activity (the equivalent dipole) and the electrode will change. As a result, the voltage of the exploring electrode will either increase or decrease as the distance changes in conformity with equation 5–1. When the depolarization process reaches the end of the muscle, all electric activity will stop, as the muscle will be completely depolarized and the potential of the exploring electrode will return to zero. Repolarization of the muscle will then result in a similar series of potential changes in the volume conductor.

RECORDING THE CLINICAL ELECTROCARDIOGRAM

The basic principles of volume conductors discussed above can now be applied to the recording of the ECG. The *standard limb leads,* i.e., *leads I,*

II, and *III*, are recorded from electrodes placed on the right arm *(RA)*, the left arm *(LA)*, and the left leg *(LL)* (in clinical usage, an electrode connected to ground is usually placed on the right leg to reduce electrical interference). The limbs act as binding posts for leading the electric potential off the thorax so that, in effect, the electrodes might as well be placed on the right and left shoulder and the pelvis. The leads are defined as follows:

$$\text{lead I} = \text{LA} - \text{RA}$$
$$\text{lead II} = \text{LL} - \text{RA}$$
$$\text{lead III} = \text{LL} - \text{LA}$$

When lead I is recorded, the voltmeter measures the difference in the electric potential produced at the right and left arm by the heart. For example, if at some instant during the cardiac cycle, the potential of the right arm is $+1$ mV and the left arm is -1 mV, lead I will show a deflection equal to 2 mV. However, the direction of this deflection, i.e., upward (positive) or downward (negative), will depend on the direction of current flow through the voltmeter. Therefore, to give meaning to the direction of the ECG deflection, a standard procedure for attaching the voltmeter has been established. This convention is indicated in the definition of the limb leads given above. It can be explicitly stated as follows: The deflection will be upright when the following conditions are present: (1) lead I, the left arm is positive in regard to the right arm; (2) lead II, the left leg is positive in regard to the right arm; and (3) lead III, the left leg is positive in regard to the left arm. Commercial ECG equipment has the lead wires labeled to ensure that attachment to the patient will follow these conventions.

It is helpful to consider that the right and left shoulder and the pelvis form the apexes of an equilateral triangle even though this, anatomically, is clearly not true (Fig 5–7). This triangle is named the *Einthoven triangle* in honor of the Dutch physiologist who first proposed its use. (Other, non-equilateral triangles based on lead field concepts have been more recently proposed as a field of reference. They will not be discussed here.) It is further assumed that the electric activity of the heart, as represented by the equivalent dipole, is concentrated at the center of the Einthoven triangle. As a result, this dipole will change its magnitude and orientation during the cardiac cycle but will not move from its central position.

The sides of the triangle represent the axes *of the three standard limb leads*. Thus, each lead is oriented, as shown in Figure 5–7, at a 60-degree angle from the other. This arrangement provides a conceptual triaxial frame of reference for relating the various leads. This will be discussed later.

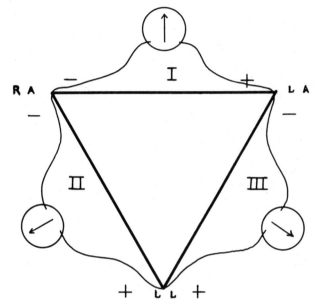

FIG 5–7.
The Einthoven equilateral triangle labeled to show the three standard limb leads and polarity that will result in an upward (positive) deflection. *RA* = right arm; *LA* = left arm; *LL* = left leg.

The Heart as Polarized Cell

The ventricular myocardium forms a W-shaped shell with the middle portion representing the ventricular septum and the open ends representing the atrioventricular (AV) ring. For the purpose of this discussion, the ventricles are considered to act as a single polarized cell. Activation of the ventricular myocardium follows the pathways that are described in Chapter 4. This process of depolarization can be divided into a number of arbitrary time intervals. This is shown in Figure 5–8. The average direction of the advancing wave of depolarization during each of the four periods used in this illustration is indicated by an arrow. The magnitude of the electric activity is shown by the length of the shaft. These arrows, therefore, are *vectors*, as they show the direction and magnitude of the electric activity of the equivalent dipole during each interval of ventricular depolarization. Vector I shows that the average direction of depolarization through the ventricular septum is from the left ventricle to the right ventricle. It should be remembered that the heart is normally rotated so that the right ventricle

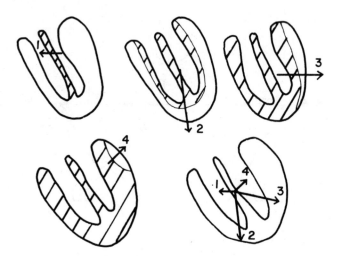

FIG 5–8.
Diagrammatic representation of the ventricle showing process of depolarization divided into four periods. Depolarized portion is shown by *diagonal lines*. Direction and magnitude of the electric activity during each period are indicated by *arrows*. See text for further discussion.

is behind the sternum; as a result, vector 1, when related to the body, points anteriorly and to the right. Only a limited amount of muscle is involved in this procedure so the magnitude of the electric force during that period, as indicated by the length of the vector, will be small. Vector 2 indicates the average direction and magnitude of the wave of depolarization as it travels through the myocardium from the inside to the outside of the heart. Vectors 3 and 4 represent these same quantities during the terminal phases of ventricular depolarization. As all the electric activity of the heart is assumed to reside at the center of the Einthoven triangle, these vectors have been moved, as shown in the lower right side of Figure 5–8, to a common origin at that point.

To summarize, the cardiac vectors define the average direction and magnitude of the electric events during successive periods of ventricular depolarization. The positive pole of the equivalent dipole is oriented toward the head of the electric vector during depolarization of a muscle cell. The electric activity of the heart, and therefore the equivalent dipole, is assumed to be fixed at the center of the heart, and the composite vector diagram indicates its orientation and magnitude during each phase of depolarization.

SCALAR AND VECTOR ELECTROCARDIOGRAMS

The heart is a three-dimensional object that lies inside the chest. The chest can be represented by a cube (or similar structure). As illustrated in Figure 5–9, the direction and magnitude of the electric activity of the heart—the *spatial vector*—can be resolved into a frontal, horizontal, and sagittal component by drawing lines from each end of the spatial vector that are perpendicular to the appropriate side of the cube and constructing a new vector—the *manifest vector*. For example, the spatial vector AB shown in Figure 5–9 that is directed upward and to the back is resolved into a frontal plane manifest vector A'B' that shows only an upward direction. The limb leads of the electrocardiogram, as discussed below, are resolved from the frontal plane manifest vector, and the *chest* or *V-leads* are determined from the horizontal component. A record of the electric potential change during the cardiac cycle as reflected in each lead can then be made using a voltmeter and a strip chart recorder. This record is the *scalar ECG*. Clinically, the processes just described are reversed, and the frontal and horizontal scalar leads are used to reconstruct the spatial orientation of the cardiac electric activity.

Vectorcardiogram

Division of the time required for ventricular depolarization into four equal segments, as described above, permits construction of vectors that

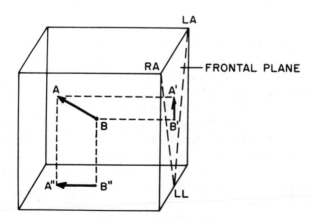

FIG 5–9.
Diagrammatic representation of the chest as a cube containing a spatial cardiac vector. The projection of the spatial vector *AB* onto the frontal and horizontal plane is shown as manifest vectors *A'B'* and *A"B"*. RA = right arm; LA = left arm; LL = left leg.

show the average magnitude and direction of the electric activity during each of these periods. Ventricular depolarization could be subdivided into a larger number of periods and an average vector constructed for each interval. In that case, each vector would indicate the average magnitude and direction of the electric activity developed during a smaller segment of the total time required for ventricular depolarization. Using this procedure, a progression of instantaneous vectors could be constructed that would indicate the electric activity during the total period of depolarization. The locus, in the frontal plane, of the head of all these possible vectors is indicated in Figure 5–10 by a line that starts at the origin of the vectors and connects the heads of vectors 1, 2, 3, and 4 before returning to the center of the triangle. The closed loop produced by this procedure is the *vectorcardiogram*. As oriented in the figure, the frontal plane vectorcardiogram would develop in a counterclockwise direction, as each part of the ventricle is activated in turn. (Depending on the degree of rotation of the heart on its longitudinal axis, the frontal projection of the spatial vector loop may appear to rotate in either direction.)

It should be clear at this point that the vectocardiogram, as just described, is an abstract representation of the instantaneous average magnitude and direction of the electric activity of the ventricle during depolarization (similar vector loops can be described for cardiac repolarization). As the vectorcardiogram is a theoretical construct, it cannot be directly recorded. However, as described in the next section, it can be synthesized from orthogonal scalar ECG leads.

Scalar ECG

Before considering the effect of the vectorcardiogram on scalar ECG leads I, II, and III, it will be helpful to discuss the effect of the forces represented by the manifest vector 1 in Figure 5–11. As indicated earlier, vector 1 is the frontal plane projection of the spatial vector that represents the electric activity of the equivalent dipole at that instant. The tail of vector 1 is at the center of Einthoven's triangle. During depolarization, the vector head indicates the orientation of the positive pole of the dipole. For the reasons described earlier, the zero isopotential line will make a right angle with the manifest vector at the center of Einthoven's triangle. Thus, as a result of the electric activity represented by vector 1, the right apex of the Einthoven triangle will fall on a positive isopotential line, and the left apex will fall on a negative isopotential line as generated in the frontal plane by the equivalent dipole. This polarity will produce a downward deflection in lead I if the ECG electrodes are attached according to the standard con-

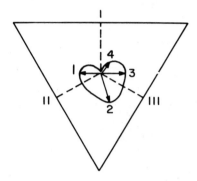

FIG 5–10.
Plot of locus of heads of the instantaneous cardiac vectors during ventricular depolarization. The vectorcardiogram for four vectors from Figure 5–8 is shown.

vention. The effect of vector 1 on the other leads, as discussed below, can be predicted using this same procedure.

Prediction of the effect of a cardiac vector on a scalar ECG lead also can be done by means of a geometric construction. This involves resolving the cardiac vector into the axis of the lead. This is accomplished for lead I by dropping perpendicular lines from the topside of the Einthoven triangle to the origin and tip of vector 1. The resolved vector in the axis of lead I (M in Fig 5–11) is then constructed between these lines on the side of the triangle with the head of the constructed (i.e., resolved) vector pointing toward the right apex. The magnitude of the lead I deflection produced by

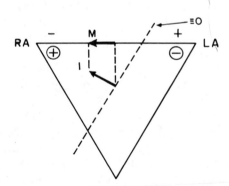

FIG 5–11.
Effect of cardiac vector *1* on polarity of the right arm *(RA)* and left arm *(LA)* apexes of the Einthoven triangle is shown in the two *circles*. Vector *M* is the resolution of vector *1* in the plane of lead I. See text.

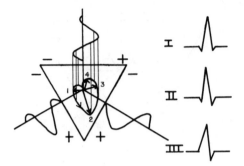

FIG 5–12.
Schematic diagram showing projections of the vectorcardiogram on the sides of the Einthoven triangle. The deflection that will occur in leads I, II, and III is shown on the *right.* See discussion in text.

the original cardiac vector I will be proportional to the length of this resolved vector. The standard conditions required for an upward deflection in lead I, i.e., right arm negative and left arm positive, are indicated by placing the appropriate plus or minus sign at the end of the lead axis. When this is done, the resolved vector in the axis of the lead will point to the sign of the deflection. In the example shown in Figure 5–11, this deflection in lead I will be down (negative).

The geometric procedure just discussed can now be generalized by using the vectorcardiogram to include all possible vectors as they are produced during the depolarization process. This is illustrated in Figure 5–12. A perpendicular line is constructed from the lead involved to the head of the instantaneous vectors as they develop in sequence. The "footprint" or pattern of this series of perpendicular lines as they move up and down the side of the triangle is then examined. This is accomplished visually, as shown in Figure 5–12, by "pulling" the overlapping footprint out along the extended diagonal of the triangle. The orientation of the resulting deflection in the ECG is determined as described above.

The technique just outlined for predicting the configuration of the scalar limb leads can be utilized in a reverse sense to construct the cardiac vector loop. This procedure is used in the clinical recording of the vectorcardiogram.* This can be accomplished by supplying the electrical signal from orthogonal leads in the plane under study (i.e., frontal, sagittal, or

*Various geometric reference systems have been proposed. A cube is used in this discussion.

horizontal) to the corresponding deflection plates of an oscilloscope. For example, for the frontal plane, the horizontal lead I and vertical lead aV_F can be used. The vector loop for the plane under study then appears on the face of the oscilloscope, as the potential change in one lead is plotted by the oscilloscope beam against the simultaneous potential change in the other lead.

Atrial Depolarization

A vectorcardiogram representing the electric forces involved during atrial depolarization also can be constructed. These forces, as discussed in Chapter 4, are primarily oriented so that they face toward the AV ring. Thus (Fig 5–13), when they are combined to form a vector loop, it will be oriented downward toward the bottom apex of the Einthoven triangle. Atrial depolarization involves a relatively small muscle mass; therefore, the vectors and vector loop will not be very large.

The result of the projections of the atrial vector loop on the axis of the standard limb leads (see Fig 5–13) will result typically in a small upward deflection in leads I, II, and III. This is the P wave of the ECG. (Rotation of the mean axis of the atrial vector loop a few degrees in a counterclockwise manner so that the loop extends into the right upper quadrant will result in this deflection in lead III becoming diphasic or inverted.)

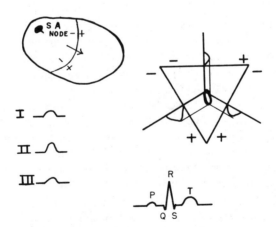

FIG 5–13.
Depolarization of the atrium *(top left)* is directed from the SA node toward the AV ring. The resulting vectorcardiogram *(top right)* is shown. This will result in a small upward deflection (the P wave) in leads I, II, and III *(bottom left)*. A typical scalar ECG record shows the normal relationship of the P, QRS, and T waves *(bottom right)*.

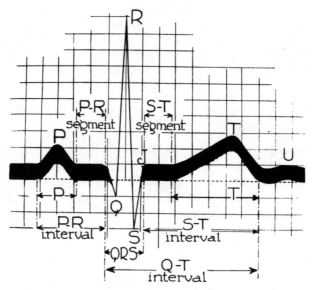

FIG 5–14.
The standard nomenclature for waves of the ECG. (From Burch G, Winsor T: *A Primer of Electrocardiography*, ed 6. Philadelphia, Lea & Febiger, 1972. Used by permission.)

Cardiac Repolarization

The electric forces involved in the repolarization process have so far not been discussed. Repolarization of the ventricle occurs largely from the outside toward the inside so that the last part depolarized is repolarized early. The repolarization process is somewhat slower than depolarization; however, the same total electric energy is expended during both events. Ventricular depolarization typically progresses from the inside of the ventricle toward the outside; however, repolarization usually but not always occurs in the opposite direction.* As a result, the electric forces representing ventricular repolarization result in a vector loop that is typically directed downward and to the right. These repolarization forces typically produce a broad upward deflection in leads I, II, and III.

The ECG deflections caused by atrial and ventricular depolarization and repolarization, when placed in their proper time sequence in a scalar record, result in a typical configuration, as shown in the right corner of Figure 5–13. The standard nomenclature makes use of the letters P, QRS, and T to describe these deflections (Fig 5–14). The physiologic meaning of

---

*As the path of depolarization and repolarization within the heart are different, the area under the QRS and T waves will also be different in any single lead.

TABLE 5–1.

Major Deflections and Intervals of the Normal Adult ECG

Deflection or Interval	Normal Duration (sec)	Physiologic Meaning
P	0.06–0.11	Depolarization of atrium
P–R interval (P–Q)	0.12–0.21	Time from onset of atrial depolarization to onset of ventricular depolarization
QRS	0.03–0.10	Depolarization of ventricle
T	Varies	Repolarization of ventricle
Q–T (measured from onset of Q to end of T)	0.26–0.49	Time from onset of ventricular depolarization to end of ventricular repolarization

these components is shown in Table 5–1. It should be apparent at this point that the configuration of each ECG lead will be different depending on the axis of the lead and how the vector forces are oriented. For example, a QRS complex in a specific lead may or may not contain a Q, an R, or an S deflection. However, no matter what deflections are present in that lead, the deflections resulting from ventricular depolarization are called the QRS complex. In a similar manner, the interval between onset of the P wave and the beginning of the QRS complex is called the P–R interval even if the QRS complex starts with a Q wave.

Atrial repolarization forces result in a deflection, the P_T wave; this deflection is small, and it is normally lost in the simultaneously occurring QRS complex. The U wave, a small deflection of uncertain origin, may follow the T wave.

The time axis of the ECG record is supplied by a series of vertical lines 0.04 seconds apart (every fifth line is darker). A series of horizontal lines 1 mm apart is also printed on the record. The voltmeter is standardized so that a 1-mV signal will produce a deflection of 10 mm; however, if the ECG deflection is unusually large, a one-half standardization may be used.

UNIPOLAR ELECTROCARDIOGRAPHIC LEADS

V Leads

The standard limb leads so far discussed measure the difference between the potential generated by the cardiac forces at two specific points on the frontal plane of the body. The concept of a zero reference electrode discussed earlier in this chapter can be applied to the body so that the electric potential at a single surface point can be measured. F. N. Wilson and his co-workers devised an electric network that supplied this reference point by connecting the RA, the LA, and the LL electrodes together through 5,000-Ω resistors (Fig 5–15). The potential at this central connection, the *central terminal of Wilson*, is considered to be zero, as defined by the cardiac dipole (or at least to be so close to zero that it can be considered to be zero). The 5,000-Ω resistors are used to minimize the effect of small differences in skin resistance under the ECG electrodes. This central terminal is connected to the negative pole of the voltmeter, and an exploring electrode is attached to the other pole. When this exploring electrode is placed on the surface of the body, the resulting ECG deflection reflects the potential generated by cardiac forces at that point. This type of recording is referred to as a unipolar or V lead.

The unipolar V leads are used clinically to record the potential on the chest wall at various points across the precordium. These positions are shown in Figure 5–16. The records obtained with these leads reflect the projections of the cardiac vectors onto the horizontal plane of the body. An upward deflection is produced when the positive pole of the equivalent dipole is facing toward the exploring electrode, and a downward deflection results when this pole faces away. The ECG deflections produced in the V_1 to V_6 unipolar chest leads by the cardiac vector loop are shown in Figure 5–17.

Augmented Unipolar Limb Leads

The potential produced at the apexes of the Einthoven triangle by the cardiac vector loop can be recorded by using the V-exploring electrode described above. The resulting deflections are small because, in essence, the

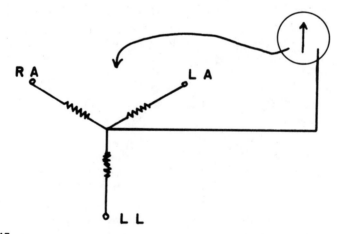

FIG 5–15.
Schematic diagram of the connections for the Wilson central terminal used in recording the V leads. *RA* = right arm; *LA* = left arm; *LL* = left leg.

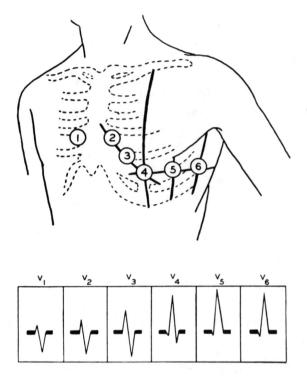

FIG 5–16.
Top, positions on the chest for recording conventional precordial V leads and, *bottom*, the typical QRS complexes in V_1 to V_6. (From Lipman BS, Massie E, Kleiger RE: *Clinical Scalar Electrocardiography*, ed 6. Chicago, Year Book Medical Publishers, 1972. Used by permission.)

potential measured at the apex is also being added to the central terminal. E. Goldberger suggested that the size of these records could be augmented by 50% without significantly changing their configuration by interrupting the connection between the central terminal and the apex of the triangle where the potential is to be determined. These aV leads (augmented unipolar extremity leads) are designated aV_R, and aV_L, and aV_F for the potential recorded, respectively, from the RA, LA, and LL.

The axis of the unipolar limb leads are the appropriate diagonals of the Einthoven triangle just as the limb lead axes are defined by the sides of the triangle. Thus, the deflection in a unipolar limb lead can be predicted by projecting the head of the cardiac vector onto the appropriate diagonal as the head of successive vectors follow the path of the vectorcardiogram.*

---

*Due to the difference in amplitude of the V and aV leads and the length of their lead axis, a slightly different calibration is required for these leads in the hexaxial system. For example, lead $I = (LA - RA) = (V_L - V_R) \times 1.7 = (aV_L - aV_R) \times 1.15$.

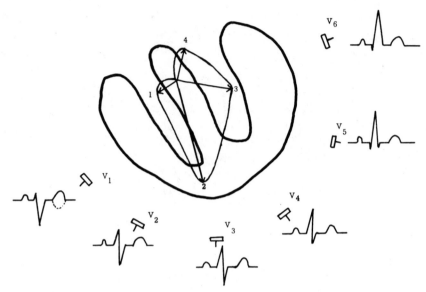

FIG 5–17.
Orientation of precordial leads to cardiac vector loop and the ECG deflections produced in V_1 to V_6.

This is illustrated in Figure 5–18. The deflection will be upright (positive) when the perpendicular from the head of the vector falls on the diagonal between the center of the triangle and the apex where the potential is measured.

AXIAL REFERENCE SYSTEM

Earlier in this chapter, it was pointed out that the sides of the Einthoven triangle represent the axes of the standard limb leads. If these axes are moved so that they cross a common midpoint without changing their orientation, they will form a triaxial reference system (Fig 5–19). The axes of the unipolar limb leads bisect the angle between adjacent limb leads. When these axes are added, the triaxial diagram becomes a hexaxial system. This diagram shows the orientation and interrelationship of all the frontal plane lead axes.

In the hexaxial reference system, the positive end of the lead I axis is assigned the value of 0 degrees on a circle divided into an upper negative 180 degrees and a lower positive 180 degrees (Fig 5–20). In this diagram, the orientation of any lead is defined by the angle that the positive end of

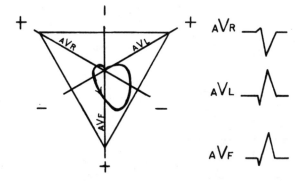

FIG 5–18.
Orientation of frontal cardiac vector loop to axis of unipolar extremity leads and the typical configurations of aV_R, aV_L, and aV_F.

its axis makes with the horizontal I axis. For example, lead II has a value of +60 degrees, aV_F has an angle of +90 degrees, and aV_L has an angle of −30 degrees.

ELECTRIC AXIS OF QRS COMPLEX

So far, we have divided the electric activity during ventricular depolarization into a number of instantaneous vectors. The same principle can be applied to construct a single vector that represents the average magnitude and direction of the *entire* depolarization process. The orientation of this

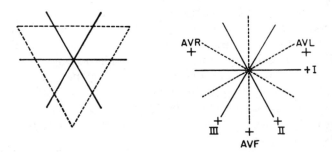

FIG 5–19.
Hexaxial reference system produced by transposing sides and three diagonals of the Einthoven triangle to a common central point. (Modified from Lipman BS, Massie E, Kleiger, RE: *Clinical Scalar Electrocardiography*, ed 6. Chicago, Year Book Medical Publishers, 1972. Used by permission.)

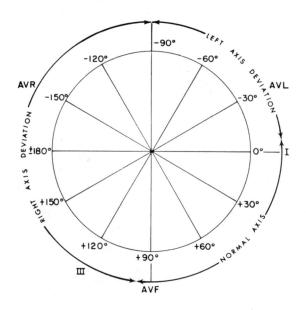

FIG 5–20.
Hexaxial reference system showing orientation of the lead axes, which are labeled on their positive end, and the usual range of the mean axis deviation. A mean axis between −10 degrees and −30 degrees is now considered borderline and −30 degrees or greater to show left axis deviation. (Modified from Lipman BS, Massie E, Kleiger RE: *Clinical Scalar Electrocardiography,* ed 6. Chicago, Year Book Medical Publishers, 1972. Used by permission.)

mean vector, expressed in terms of the angle it makes with the lead I axis, is called the *electric axis* or *mean axis of the QRS complex.*

This mean axis can be determined by measuring the algebraic sum of the area under each deflection in the QRS complex in two leads. These sums are then plotted on the appropriate lead axis in the axial reference system. The mean axis is then found by dropping perpendicular lines from the point plotted on the lead axis and connecting the center of the axial system with the intersection of the perpendiculars. A hypothetical example is shown in Figure 5–21 in which the QRS area of lead I is +3 units and of lead III is +2 units. The mean electric axis of the QRS complex in this example is +53 degrees.

In clinical practice, it usually is not necessary to determine the mean electric axis with extreme accuracy. Rather, a gross determination is made by observing the configuration of the QRS complex in the standard leads and visualizing the results in terms of the hexaxial reference system. For example, the standard limb lead axis that is at right angles to the mean

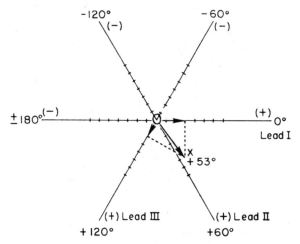

FIG 5–21.
Determination of mean QRS axis utilizing triaxial reference system. See text. (From Lipman BS, Massie E, Kleiger RE: *Clinical Scalar Electrocardiography*, ed 6. Chicago, Year Book Medical Publishers, 1972. Used by permission.)

electrical axis will have a net QRS deflection of zero. Thus, when the mean electrical axis is + 30 degrees, the algebraic sum of the QRS deflection in lead III will be zero. An example of extreme right (+ 130 degrees) and left axis (− 40 degrees) deviation is shown in Figure 5–22.

So far, only the frontal plane projection of the mean spatial direction of ventricular depolarization has been considered. It is sometimes of value clinically to determine the anterior-posterior orientation of this spatial vector. This can be accomplished by simply calculating the average direction of the QRS deflection in the V_2 precordial lead. This lead has an axis that runs from the back to the front of the chest (i.e., − 90 degrees to + 90 degrees in the horizontal plane). If the mean spatial vector, for example, is directed anteriorly (Fig 5–23), the resolved vector in the V_2 lead axis in the horizontal plane will point toward the V_2 electrode, and the average direction of the deflection in V_2 will be upward, whereas a posteriorly directed mean spatial vector will produce a vector in the axis of lead V_2 that points away from the V_2 electrode, and the average deflection in that situation will be down.

Finally, application of the concept of the zero isopotential line discussed earlier in this chapter can be applied to the determination of the spatial orientation of the mean QRS vector. Just as the potential on a perpendicular plane that bisects the axis of the equivalent dipole will have a potential of zero, everywhere on the body surface where a perpendicular

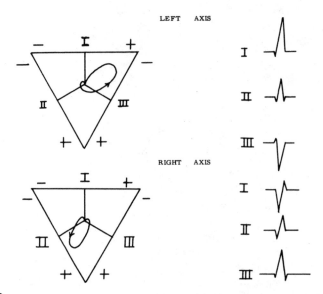

FIG 5–22.

Effect of deviation of mean electric axis on a typical vector loop and the QRS complexes, as recorded by standard limb leads.

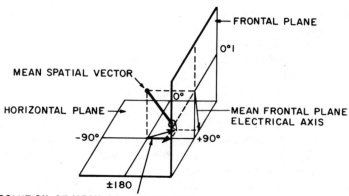

FIG 5–23.

Diagram of frontal and horizontal reference planes showing projection of an anteriorly directed spatial vector onto the horizontal plane with resolution of the projected vector into the lead axis of V_2 chest lead. Frontal plane projection of the spatial vector also is shown. See text for further discussion.

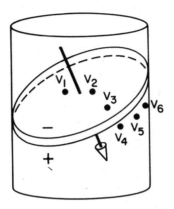

FIG 5–24.
Diagram showing transition zone produced on the surface of the thorax cylinder by a posteriorly directed mean spatial vector. The position of the V chest leads is indicated. (Redrawn from Grant RP: *Circulation* 1950; 1:878.)

plane that bisects the axis of the mean QRS vector cuts the torso, the deflection will be equiphasic (equal value of R and S deflections) and will have a net value of zero. This line of intersection on the chest wall, sometimes called the transition zone or null contour, usually comes close to the V₃ or V₄ electrode position (Fig 5–24). All areas on the chest toward the head of the mean cardiac vector from this transition zone will have a net positive (larger R than S) deflection, and all areas between the transition zone and the tail of the mean cardiac vector will have a net negative (larger S than R) deflection.

SUMMARY

The average instantaneous electric activity during myocardial depolarization and repolarization can each be represented by an equivalent dipole placed at the center of the chest. The magnitude and direction of the dipole can be shown by a vector. Projection of the head of this vector onto the frontal plane of the chest as the vector changes during the cardiac cycle constitutes the vectorcardiogram. Resolution of these manifest vectors into the axis of the various electrocardiographic leads will predict the form of the ECG record. The P and QRS deflections represent, in turn, depolarization of the atria and then depolarization of the ventricle. The T wave represents repolarization of the ventricle. Use of a triaxial or hexaxial reference system permits determination of the mean electric axis of atrial or ventricular activation or repolarization.

BIBLIOGRAPHY

Burch G, Winsor T: *A Primer of Electrocardiography*, ed 6. Philadelphia, Lea & Febiger, 1972.

Burger HC, van Milaan JB: Heart-vector and leads. *Br Heart J* 1946; 8:157.

Craib WH: A study of the electrical field surrounding active heart muscles. *Heart* 1927; 14:71.

Einthoven W, Fahn G, de Waart A: On the direction and manifest size of the variations of potential in the human heart and on the influence of the position of the heart on the form of the electrocardiogram, Hoff HE, Sekelj P (trans). *Am Heart J* 1950; 40:163.

Goldberger E: A simple, indifferent electrocardiographic electrode of zero potential and a technique of obtaining augmented unipolar leads. *Am Heart J* 1942; 23:483.

Goldman MJ: *Principles of Clinical Electrocardiography*, ed 12. Los Altos, Calif, Lange Medical Publications, 1986.

Graettinger JS, Pack JM, Graybiel A: A new method of equating and presenting bipolar and unipolar extremity leads of the electrocardiogram. *Am J Med* 1951; 11:3.

Lipman BS, Dunn D, Massie E: *Clinical Electrocardiography*, ed 7. Chicago, Year Book Medical Publishers, 1984.

Wilson FN, et al: Electrocardiograms that represent the potential variations of a single electrode. *Am Heart J* 1934; 9:477.

Witham AC: *A System of Vectorcardiographic Interpretation*. Chicago, Year Book Medical Publishers, 1975.

Zipes DP, Julife J: *Cardiac Electrophysiology and Arrhythmias*. Orlando, Fla, Grune & Stratton, Inc, 1985.

Chapter 6 _____

Alterations in Cardiac Rate, Rhythm, and Conduction Pathways

The rhythm of the heart can be modified by a number of physiologic, pharmacologic, and disease processes. In this chapter, normal variations in cardiac rate and rhythm are analyzed and related to the scalar electrocardiogram (ECG). In addition, the mechanism of some of the more common arrhythmias and conduction disturbances are discussed and their ECG abnormalities summarized. A detailed analysis of ECG diagnosis of cardiac arrhythmias is, however, beyond the scope of this chapter.

NOMENCLATURE

The nomenclature used to describe the rate and rhythm of the heart is derived from the cardiac mechanism. The terminology lists the location of the pacemaker, describes any conductive abnormalities, and classifies the rate or rhythm. For example, a regular rate of 60 to 100 beats per minute with the sinoatrial (SA) node serving as the pacemaker and without conduction defects is called a *normal sinus rhythm*. The pacemaker location is sometimes omitted if it is the SA node. Thus, the above rhythm is also called a *sinus rhythm* or a *normal rhythm*. A *tachycardia* is a rhythm with a rate above 100 beats per minute and a *bradycardia* has a rate below 60 beats per minute.

NORMAL SINUS MECHANISM

The normal sequence of atrial and ventricular activation, discussed in Chapter 4, is summarized in Figure 6–1 and related to the deflection produced in a typical scalar ECG. Each P wave is followed by a normal QRS complex and T wave. All QRS complexes are preceded by P waves, and the P–R and Q–T intervals are within normal limits (Table 6–1). The R–R interval is regular.

The SA node normally receives sufficient inhibitory parasympathetic impulses from the vagus nerve to keep the heart rate well below the intrinsic discharge rate of the pacemaker cells. In fact, most of the heart rate changes produced by ordinary activity are achieved by increasing or decreasing this vagal tone. (The reflex nature of this inhibitory input to the SA node will be discussed in Chapter 10.) If the usual level of this inhibitory vagal discharge to the SA node is increased, the heart rate will slow even further and a *sinus bradycardia* will result. A slow rate of this type is frequently a normal occurrence in trained athletes and in many individuals during sleep.

Cessation of the vagal input to the heart will permit the heart rate to increase up to the intrinsic rate of the SA node. Studies in patients in

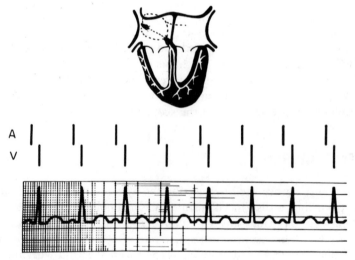

FIG 6–1.
Normal sinus rhythm. *Top,* schematic diagram of major conductive pathways in the heart. *Middle,* top line of each pair represents atrial depolarization; the bottom line, ventricular depolarization. The interval between lines represents conduction delay at the AV node. *Bottom,* representation of typicl ECG.

TABLE 6–1.

Heart Rate, Cycle Length, Upper Limits of Q–T and P–R Intervals*

Heart Rate (beats/min)	Cycle Length (sec)	Upper Limit Q–T Interval (sec)	Upper Limit P–R Interval (sec)		
			Infant	Youth	Adult
40	1.50	0.49 ⎫			
45	1.33	0.47 ⎪			
50	1.20	0.45 ⎬	0.18	0.19	0.22
55	1.09	0.44 ⎪			
60	1.00	0.42 ⎭			
65	0.92	0.40 ⎫			
70	0.85	0.38 ⎪			
75	0.81	0.38 ⎬	0.17	0.18	0.21
80	0.75	0.37 ⎭			
85	0.71	0.36 ⎫			
90	0.67	0.35 ⎪	0.16	0.16	0.20
95	0.63	0.35 ⎬			
100	0.60	0.34 ⎭	0.15	0.16	0.19
120	0.50	0.31			
150	0.40	0.28 ⎫			
170	0.35	0.26 ⎭	0.15	0.16	0.18

*Data from Zeigler RF: *Electrocardiographic Studies in Normal Infants and Children.* Springfield, Ill, Charles C Thomas Publishers, 1951, and Burch G, Winsor T: *A Primer of Electrocardiography.* Philadelphia, Lea & Febiger, 1947.

whom all nervous influences to the SA node were removed by pharmacologic blocking agents suggest that this intrinsic discharge rate is age dependent: the very young have a basic rate of approximately 117 beats per minute; this slows to about 104 beats per minute at 20 to 30 years of age and is reduced to nearly 92 beats per minute by 45 to 50 years of age. Heart rates in excess of these values are achieved by sympathetic stimulation. In older adults, the maximum *sinus tachycardia* produced by this mechanism usually does not exceed 180 beats per minute. This may be slightly higher in children and young adults.

ECTOPIC CARDIAC FOCI

An *ectopic beat* results when the pacemaker function of the heart is assumed for one beat by cells other than those in the SA node. These isolated events are also sometimes called *premature beats* or *extra systoles* because they occur early in diastole before the SA node is normally scheduled to discharge. The new pacemaker is called an *ectopic focus*. Depending on the location of the ectopic focus, ectopic beats may be premature atrial beats (PACs) or premature ventricular beats (PVCs). When this focus fires repeatedly and takes over the pacemaker duties for a period of time, the cardiac mechanism is called an *ectopic rhythm*.

Ectopic Beats

Under conditions of emotional stress, excessive ingestion of coffee or other stimulants, or abnormalities of the atrial myocardium, latent atrial pacemaker cells may depolarize early and produce an atrial ectopic beat (Fig 6–2). Because of the location of the focus, activation of the atrium does not follow the normal path. Hence, the P wave produced in the ECG by the ectopic beat usually has a different configuration than the P wave of a normal beat. The activation process from the ectopic focus spreads through the atrial myocardium and, depending somewhat on its location, usually causes the SA node to be prematurely depolarized before its normal prepotential has reached threshold. When this occurs, the SA node promptly repolarizes and then reaches its next firing threshold earlier than if it had not been prematurely discharged. As a result, if the ectopic focus does not continue to fire, the SA node will resume its pacemaker activity slightly in advance of the predicted time, and the heart rate will be shifted.

The ectopic atrial impulse is conducted to the ventricle over the usual pathways and results in a normal sequence of ventricular depolarization and repolarization. As a result, the ectopic QRS and T wave will be of normal configuration and duration.

When the ectopic focus is in or near the AV node, the activation proc-

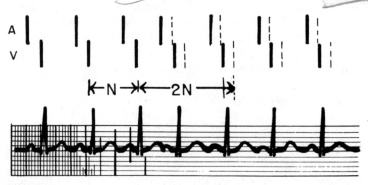

FIG 6–2.
Ectopic atrial beat. *Top,* pairs of lines representing atrial and ventricular depolarizations, as in Figure 6–1. *Dashed lines* show expected occurrence of depolarizations if ectopic beat did not occur. *Bottom,* representation of typical ECG. (*N* = interval between normal beats.)

ess can quickly reach the ventricle. In this situation, depending on the presence or absence of retrograde conduction, the ectopic focus may or may not also activate the atrium. An *ectopic nodal beat*, or as it is usually called, an *ectopic junctional beat*, without retrograde conduction, as shown on the left in Figure 6–3, results in an early QRS complex and T wave. Again, ventricular conduction is over the normal pathways so that these deflections will be normal in appearance. Depolarization of the SA node at its regular time will lead to a normal P wave. This may either be superimposed on the QRS complex, or it may appear slightly before the QRS complex or during the Q–T interval, depending on how early the ectopic beat came in the cardiac cycle. This normal atrial depolarization process will be blocked from reaching the ventricle by the refractory atrioventricular (AV) node. Control of the heartbeat will then be regained by the next normal atrial depolarization, and the cardiac rhythm will not be shifted. In this case, the time between the ectopic beat and the next normal beat is sufficient to make up for the short interval between the last normal beat and the ectopic beat. This space between the ectopic and normal beat is called a *compensatory pause.*

If the ectopic junctional (nodal) impulse is conducted in a retrograde fashion to the atrium, the typical sequence of events shown on the right of Figure 6–3 will take place. The retrograde activation of the atrium usually causes the P wave to have a different configuration and, depending on the location of the ectopic focus in the node or upper bundle, to occur slightly before, during, or after the QRS deflection. If retrograde activation reaches the SA node before it is ready to fire, it will be prematurely depolarized.

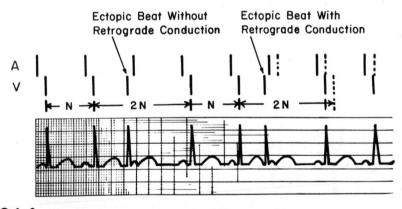

FIG 6–3.
Ectopic nodal beats with and without retrograde conduction. Diagram is the same as in Figure 6–1. (*N* = interval between normal beats.)

This will cause it to start its depolarization cycle early; a compensatory pause will not occur, and the cardiac rhythm will be shifted.

Ectopic beats can be initiated from a focus in either ventricle (Fig 6–4). In such an *ectopic ventricular beat*, the excitation process does not follow the normal ventricular conduction pathways. For example, activation from a focus in the right ventricle may be distributed locally over the slow-conducting ventricular myocardium before it travels through the septum and is distributed to the left ventricle over the regular Purkinje system. Depolarization will take longer than normal, and the vector loop for that beat will have an abnormal configuration. As a result, the QRS complex typically is slurred, notched, and wider than normal. Secondary T-wave changes also may occur. This follows because of the abnormal depolarization; repolarization will also be over a different pathway.

The position of the ectopic focus in the ventricle may be determined with considerable accuracy by considering the direction of the early, middle, and late ventricular depolarization vectors. This procedure will be described later in this section in connection with the discussion of bundle-branch blocks.

In the absence of retrograde conduction from an ectopic ventricular beat, the P wave produced by normal activation of the atria is usually lost in the early, wide, and bizarre-appearing QRS complex. Conduction of this normal atrial depolarization to the ventricle is, however, blocked, as the ventricle is already depolarized and will be refractory due to its earlier activation. The continued rhythmic activity of the SA node then results in the next atrial depolarization appearing on schedule, and the cardiac rhythm will pick up after a full compensatory pause.

Ectopic Rhythms

An ectopic focus will take over the pacemaker duties under two sets of circumstances: (1) when the ectopic rate is faster than the normal discharge

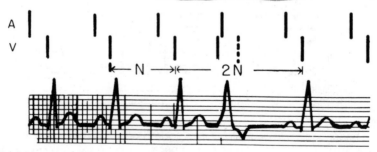

FIG 6–4.
Ectopic ventricular beat. See text for discussion. (*N* = interval between normal beats.)

rate of the SA node (in this circumstance an *ectopic tachycardia* usually will result [see below]) and (2) when the SA node for some reason either fails to develop a prepotential or its propagation is blocked. In this case the next most irritable focus will be activated to run the heart. Under these circumstances, the heart rate usually is slow. In general, the farther the substitute pacemaker is from the SA node, the slower the rate. A typical value for a junctional [AV nodal] pacemaker is 40 to 60 beats per minute; a ventricular pacemaker may be as slow as 15 to 40 beats per minute. When the SA node fails for some reason to serve as the cardiac pacemaker and a lower pacemaker takes over its task, the rhythm is called an *escape rhythm*.

Ectopic Atrial Tachycardia.—A rapid heart rate can result from the repetitive discharge of an atrial ectopic focus. These attacks usually start suddenly, last for a variable period, and then stop just as quickly. For this reason, the rapid rate is often called *paroxysmal atrial tachycardia* (PAT). It was previously thought that these attacks were caused by the ectopic pacemaker's overdriving the SA node and taking over control of the heart rate. Recent electrophysiologic studies have suggested that a second mechanism, the *reentry phenomenon*, is frequently the cause of this arrhythmia and that enhanced automaticity of an ectopic focus probably occurs in only a small number of cases.

The reentry mechanism requires that, at some point, conduction through the heart takes parallel pathways, each path having a different conduction speed and refractory characteristics. For example, such an arrangement has been postulated for the AV node (see discussion of echo beats in Chapter 4), and similar dual pathways have been demonstrated in the SA node, atrial or ventricular myocardium, and perhaps in the bundle of His.

Longitudinal dissociation of conduction, such as described above, may occur if transmission through one of two parallel myocardial fibers is slowed (Fig 6–5). Several possibilities present themselves in this situation; for example, a premature impulse may find the faster-conducting pathway (which may also have a longer refractory period) still refractory from the passage of the last normal impulse. The slower-conducting pathway, with its short refractory period, is, however, able to accept the excitation wave. While this impulse is traveling through the slower-conducting pathway, the previously blocked fast fibers will recover their ability to conduct. If the two parallel paths connect to some common area of excitable myocardium, the depolarization process from the slower path can enter the now nonrefractory faster-conducting pathway and travel in a retrograde manner back to the area where the excitation process had its origin. By this time, the slower pathway will have recovered and be ready to again conduct the excitation wave. This mechanism, once initiated, can become a self-perpetu-

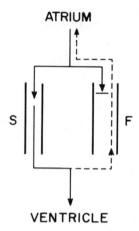

ATRIUM

VENTRICLE

FIG 6–5.
Schematic diagram of parallel pathways for conduction of the cardiac impulse that can lead to a circus movement of the excitation wave. *S* = slow pathway; *F* = fast pathway; *solid line* = orthodromic conduction; *dashed line* = retrograde conduction.

ating *circus movement* that will cause repetitive depolarizations of the atrial myocardium.

As a result of either a repetitively firing ectopic atrial pacemaker or of a reentry circus movement, each cardiac beat during an attack of PAT starts with depolarization of the atria. Thus, each ECG cycle will start with a P wave. Due to their abnormal origin, they usually are abnormal in form, and because of the rapid cardiac rate, they are sometimes difficult to identify (Fig 6–6). Typically, ventricular conduction is not affected so that the QRS and T deflections will be essentially normal. However, under some circumstances, the rapid cardiac rate may cause conduction problems due to differences in the refractory period of various parts of the ventricle.

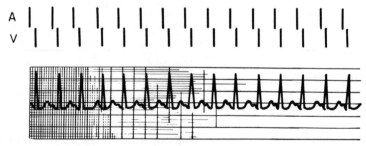

FIG 6–6.
Atrial tachycardia.

If *ventricular aberration* of this type occurs, the ECG diagnosis of an atrial pacemaker is more difficult as the QRS complexes may resemble those seen with an ectopic ventricular pacemaker.

When the ectopic pacemaker is in the AV node, each beat will have the ECG characteristics described above for a nodal ectopic beat. If the rate is rapid and the P waves are obscured, it may not be possible to differentiate a *junctional nodal tachycardia* from an *atrial tachycardia*. In this situation, the cardiac mechanism is classified as a *supraventricular tachycardia* to indicate that the pacemaker is "above" the ventricle.

Ventricular Tachycardia.—The rapid discharge of an ectopic ventricular focus causes a *ventricular tachycardia* (Fig 6–7). The ventricular rate in this arrhythmia usually varies between 150 and 250 beats per minute, but in some cases it may be slower. Because of the aberrant conduction in the ventricles, the QRS complexes are slurred, notched, and wide. If the regular sinus rhythm is intact and retrograde conduction to the atria does not occur, the P waves in the ECG will not be disturbed, and they will appear at their regular place. As the discharge rate of the SA node usually is much slower than the ectopic ventricular pacemaker, the P waves will be independent of the ventricular events. In fact, they will often be hidden in the more frequently appearing QRS and T deflections and a careful search may be required to find them.

As with supraventricular tachycardia, a reentry mechanism may operate to produce a ventricular tachycardia. This mechanism appears to be of particular importance in the production of ventricular arrhythmias after occlusion of a coronary artery as well as in disease processes that interfere with energy transfer in the cell membrane. It is postulated that in these patients the explosive increase in sodium conductance that leads to the rapid depolarization of the myocardial cell membrane may be reduced or abol-

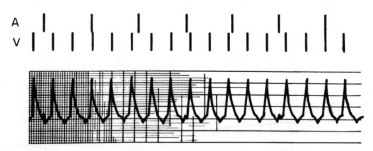

FIG 6–7.
Ectopic ventricular tachycardia without retrograde conduction to the atrium. The SA node depolarizes at its normal rate. See text for further discussion.

ished in some areas. In these membranes the inward movement of sodium
and calcium through the "slower" channel normally associated with the plateau phase of the action potential (see Chapter 3) causes a slower form of
depolarization. As a result, the rate of change of the depolarization process
is reduced, and the action potential may reach a peak value of only 0 to 15
mV (Fig 6–8). The slow rate of upstroke and low amplitude of the action
potential results in a slow conduction velocity, a prolongation of the refractory period, and production of areas of functional unidirectional block at
the interface between normal and refractory myocardium. This provides
the necessary requirements of reentry.

A model of a reentry mechanism proposed for the ventricle is shown
in Figure 6–9. In this diagram, the excitation wave traveling in a Purkinje
fiber divides, and one part enters a depressed section, which shows the
combining of slow conduction and unidirectional block described above.

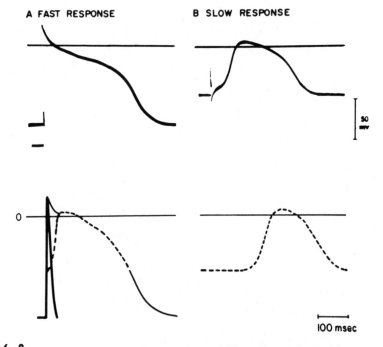

FIG 6–8.
Comparison of transmembrane action potential recorded from dog Purkinje fibers when
perfused with normal Tyrode's solution **(A)** and when Tyrode's solution contains added
K$^+$ and epinephrine **(B).** Action potential in panel **A** is a fast response, whereas panel
B shows a slow response. Diagram at bottom of each panel shows the relative time
course of Na$^+$ *(dark line)* and Ca^{2+} *(dashed line)* currents. (Modified from Witt AL, Friedman PL: *Arch Intern Med* 1975; 135:459.)

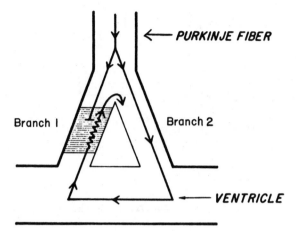

FIG 6–9.
Schematic model of reentry mechanism in a peripheral Purkinje fiber and its adjacent ventricular muscle. *Branch 1* exhibits slow conduction and unidirectional block. *Branch 2* shows normal conduction. See text for discussion. (Modified from Giardina EV, Bigger JT Jr: *Circulation* 1973; 48:959. Used by permission.)

The other part of the excitation wave travels at its normal velocity in the unaffected fiber and enters the myocardium at a lower level. This excitation wave is then able to enter the lower end of the depressed section of Purkinje fiber and spread slowly back toward the bifurcation. With a proper balance between the velocity of the retrograde conduction and the rate of recovery of the normal fiber, a *reentry circus movement* may become established.

FLUTTER AND FIBRILLATION

When an ectopic atrial focus or reentry mechanism causes the atria to be discharged at a uniform rate in excess of about 250 beats per minute, the condition is called *atrial flutter*. At these rapid rates, the AV node and ventricular tissues may not be able to respond to each depolarization. As a result, a physiologic AV block may be present, and the ventricular rate will be one half, one third, or some smaller multiple of the atrial rate. The ECG record (Fig 6–10) characteristically contains a regular series of closely spaced P waves, sometimes called *flutter waves*. As the pacemaker is in the atrium, conduction to the ventricles is via the regular pathways and the QRS and T deflections are normal. The ventricular rate is regular unless the degree of functional block is changing. In that case, the ventricular rate

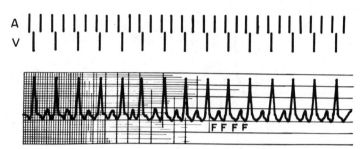

FIG 6–10.
Atrial flutter.

may be grossly irregular, and it may resemble the rhythm of *atrial fibrillation*.

The cause of atrial fibrillation is unsettled. Two mechanisms are proposed. The first suggests that a series of ectopic atrial foci discharge in a rapid and uncoordinated fashion. The second postulates a reentry mechanism similar to that described above, where a continuous depolarization wave travels in a circular fashion in the atrium and sends off secondary waves into the atrial myocardium. The result with either of these mechanisms is that different areas of the atrial myocardium are simultaneously depolarized and repolarized in a chaotic fashion. Because of this irregular electric activity, the excitation process no longer travels as a coordinated front through the myocardium. The result is that the atria lose their ability to form a contraction wave, and the dynamic effect of atrial systole is lost. In this situation, the dilated atria have been described as having the appearance of a "bag of worms" due to the small fibrillating waves that travel in all directions over the surface. As a consequence of the uncoordinated electric activity, *P waves do not appear in the ECG*. Instead, there usually is an irregular undulation of the base line; these are called *fibrillation* or *f waves*.

In atrial fibrillation the AV node is bombarded with stimuli that arrive in a rapid and random fashion from the atria. These impulses are transmitted to the ventricle whenever the AV node is able to conduct the depolarization process. The result is that the ventricular response is *irregularly irregular* (Fig 6–11). This total irregularity of the heartbeat is a prominent clinical feature of atrial fibrillation and helps to distinguish it from regular irregularity of a second-degree heart block or a run of regularly occurring premature beats. The pacemaker in atrial fibrillation is supraventricular so that the form of the QRS and T deflections will be normal. Characteristically, the rate is rapid; however, after treatment with digitalis or a similar cardiac glycoside that increases the refractory phase of the AV node, the

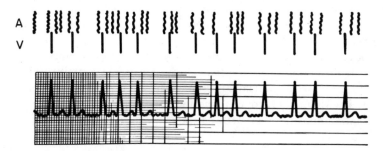

FIG 6–11.
Atrial fibrillation. P waves are absent. The chaotic electric activity of atrium is indicated by an irregular baseline between ECG complexes. Due to the random nature of the arrival of these excitation waves at the AV node, the ventricular response is totally irregular.

ventricular rate may be reduced due to the conduction of fewer impulses through the AV node.

Ventricular fibrillation, in which chaotic electric activity similar to that just described for atrial fibrillation occurs in the ventricle. Once established, the irregular electric activity of ventricular fibrillation prevents the development of a coordinated heartbeat. Instead, the ventricles undergo an irregular twitching movement that is not effective in pumping blood, and the cardiac output falls to zero. This uncoordinated electric activity of the ventricle leads to a bizarre irregular pattern of rapid ECG deflections without any discernible rhythm. It is a serious arrhythmia that will result in death within a few minutes unless cardiopulmonary resuscitation is initiated and a normal cardiac mechanism is restored. Ventricular fibrillation may be triggered by such events as myocardial ischemia, electric shock, or an ectopic ventricular pacemaker. A diseased heart is particularly susceptible to develop this arrhythmia if stimulated during a short interval at the end of its repolarization period. An ectopic ventricular beat occurring during this vulnerable period may be sufficient to cause a reentry circus movement or a repetitive firing ectopic focus to develop in the ventricle. For this reason, the development of ectopic ventricular rhythms following a myocardial infarction may indicate an increased risk of developing ventricular fibrillation.

Electric defibrillation is accomplished by exposing the heart to a brief burst of an external electric current of the proper density and duration. This causes the entire myocardium to be depolarized. Hopefully, the myocardium will then repolarize as a unit without restarting the fibrillation process. Development of a pacemaker will then permit the heartbeat to be reestablished. A variation of this procedure is utilized to abolish other arrhythmias such as atrial fibrillation. This is called *cardioversion*. Because of the vulnerable period described above, defibrillation and electric pacing equipment are usually synchronized with the ECG so that this stimulus does not coincide with the T wave. A proper diagnosis is imperative before electric defibrillation is attempted, as the treatment usually will produce fibrillation if it is not already present. The procedure should also not be attempted without the proper resuscitation equipment at hand, along with trained individuals familiar with its use.

ATRIOVENTRICULAR BLOCK

The electric characteristics of the marginal tissues in the AV node and upper bundle of His described earlier in Chapter 3 make this area susceptible to conduction disturbances and blockage.

In *first-degree AV block*, conduction through the AV node is prolonged. This is shown in Figure 6–12,A by a longer than normal P–R interval. His

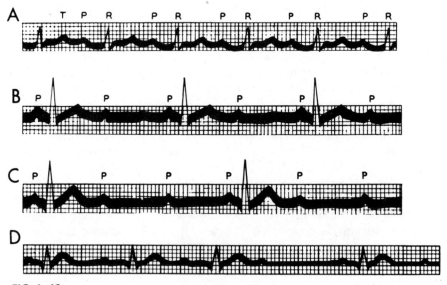

FIG 6–12.
ECG records showing **A,** prolonged AV conduction (first-degree heart block) with a P–R interval of 0.27 second; **B,** second-degree heart block (2:1); **C,** 3:1 AV block; **D,** Wenckebach type of AV block. (From Lipman BS, Massie E, Kleiger RE: *Clinical Scalar Electrocardiography,* ed 6. Chicago, Year Book Medical Publishers, 1972. Used by permission.)

bundle ECGs (see Fig 4–4) show that the major delay is usually between the A and H deflection and thus occurs in the AV node itself. Conduction in the ventricle is over the normal pathways. Therefore, the form of the P, QRS, and T deflections is not affected.

Occasionally, the delay at the AV node will progressively increase from beat to beat until conduction to the ventricle is blocked. This causes the P–R interval to become longer and longer until finally a P wave occurs without a following QRS complex and T wave. By the time the SA node fires again, AV conduction has had time to recover, and the sequence starts over. This variation of a *second-degree AV block* is also known as the *Wenckebach phenomenon* or a *Mobitz type I block* (Fig 6–12,D).

A second variation of this type of AV block is the *Mobitz type II block*. In this condition, the delay at the AV node is sufficiently long that occasionally an atrial impulse fails to reach the ventricle (Fig 6–12,B). This usually occurs in a regular sequence such as 2:1, 3:2, or 4:1 (the ratio is that of atrial to ventricular beats). In this condition, the His bundle ECG usually shows a prolonged H–V interval due to involvement of the lower portion of the His bundle.

Third-degree or *complete AV block* indicates failure of any conduction between the atria and the ventricles. In this condition the SA node serves as the pacemaker for the atria, and an ectopic pacemaker serves in that capacity in the ventricle. The result is that, although P and QRS waves occur rhythmically in the ECG, there is no correlation between them. As the atrial rate usually is faster than the ventricular rate, there are more P waves than QRS complexes (Fig 6–13). Ventricular depolarization, because of its disturbed conduction, produces the characteristic wide, bizarre QRS complexes and abnormal T waves typical of an ectopic ventricular focus.

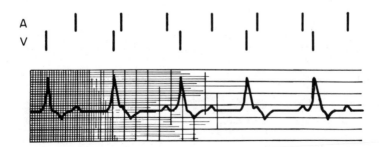

FIG 6–13.
Third-degree AV block with a ventricular pacemaker. The ECG tracing shows two independent rhythms: the atrial rate is 75 beats per minute, the ventricular rate 53 beats per minute.

BUNDLE-BRANCH BLOCK

Bundle-branch block is produced by delay or interruption of the ventricular conductive pathways below the level of the bifurcation of the common bundle. Because conduction through the atrium and AV node is normal in this condition, the P wave and P–R interval are not disturbed. However, depending somewhat on the location of the block and the conductive fibers that are interrupted, depolarization in areas of the ventricle will be delayed. In addition, the activation process will travel through the affected areas in an aberrant fashion due to the disruption of the normal conduction sequence. This causes the QRS complex to have a wide, bizarre form similar to that produced by an ectopic ventricular focus (Fig 6–14).

Localization of the block to the right or left bundle branch (or to a specific fascicle of one of the bundles such as occurs in hemiblocks) can frequently be accomplished by considering the direction of the early, middle, and late ventricular activation vectors. For example, the early ventricular forces in *right bundle-branch block* will be directed to the right side due to depolarization of the septum from the unaffected left bundle branch (Fig 6–15). During the middle part of ventricular depolarization, the average cardiac vector will point toward the left due to the normal activation of the large left ventricular muscle mass. The terminal electric forces will swing again to the right as the excitation process invades the right ventricle below

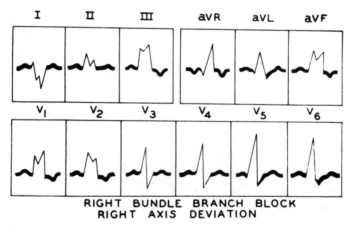

RIGHT BUNDLE BRANCH BLOCK
RIGHT AXIS DEVIATION

FIG 6–14.
Representative QRS complexes showing right bundle-branch block with right axis deviation. (From Lipman BS, Massie E, Kleiger RE: *Clinical Scalar Electrocardiography,* ed 6. Chicago, Year Book Medical Publishers, 1972. Used by permission.)

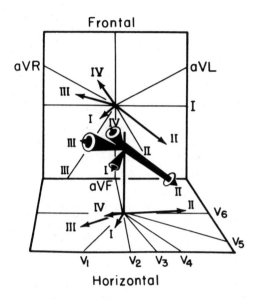

FIG 6–15.

Projections on frontal and horizontal plane of the four vectors representing phases of ventricular depolarization in a patient with right bundle-branch block. This figure shows, for example, that, in lead V_1, vector I will produce an initial upward deflection; vector II gives a downward deflection; and vectors III and IV produce tall upright R or R' waves. (From Lipman BS, Massie E, Kleiger RE: *Clinical Scalar Electrocardiography*, ed 6. Chicago, Year Book Medical Publishers, 1972. Used by permission.)

the area of the block after traveling through the slower-conducting septal myocardium. The electric forces due to the late activation of the right side of the heart will now be unopposed by simultaneous activity in the left ventricle. This leads to an unusually large late vector force directed anteriorly and to the right. This will characteristically produce a terminal tall R wave in leads that show right ventricular activity (V_1 and aV_R) and a slurred, late S wave in leads over the left ventricle (V_5, V_6, and V_L).

Interruptions of the left anterior fascicle of the left bundle branch will delay activation of the anterior ventricular septum and of the anterior and lateral wall of the left ventricle. The initial ventricular depolarization forces, as a result, will point inferiorly and to the right due to the normal activation of the remainder of the myocardium. Late activation of the ventricular muscle supplied by the blocked conductive fibers will occur by lateral spread of the depolarization process from the surrounding myocardium. This produces a terminal vector force that is directed superiorly and to the left. As a result, the typical ECG finding in cases of *left anterior hemiblock* will have QRS complexes that are at the upper limit of the normal duration or longer and show left axis deviation. Lead I will have a qR configuration and leads II, III, and aV_R will show an RS pattern.

A *left posterior hemiblock* due to interruption of the left posterior fascicle of the left bundle branch results in delayed activation of the lateral and posterior portion of the wall of the left ventricle. As a result, initial ventricular forces point superiorly and to the left, whereas the late activation vector is usually directed inferiorly and to the right. This sequence of events usually leads to an rS pattern in lead I and a qR configuration in leads II, III, and aV_F along with a mean electric axis that is shifted to the right.

Recently a third fascicle of the left bundle branch has been described that innervates primarily the interventricular septum and the base of the heart. Electrocardiographic interpretation of blockage of these fibers is more difficult and may require the use of a vectorcardiogram.

DISTURBANCES OF SERUM ELECTROLYTES

Characteristic changes in the ECG are produced by alterations in serum potassium or calcium levels. A reduction in serum potassium to 3 mEq/L or below *(hypokalemia)* results in a shortening of phase 2 and prolongation of phases 3 and 4 of the ventricular transmembrane potential. This in turn leads to flattening or reversal of the T wave. Prominent U waves frequently occur, and the Q–U interval may be prolonged. The U wave may blend with the low T wave and suggest prolongation of the Q–T interval. *Hyperkalemia* (serum potassium level of 5.5 mEq/L or higher) results in a reduction in the resting ventricular membrane potential (E_m), slower phase 0 depolarization, reduction in phase 2, and increase in rate of development of phase 3. This leads to characteristic tall, narrow T waves and prolongation of both the P–R interval and the duration of the QRS complex. Potassium concentrations in excess of 9.0 mEq/L result in the disappearance of P waves, bizarre QRS complexes, and the production of ventricular fibrillation or cardiac standstill. Low serum calcium levels *(hypocalcemia)* are associated with prolongation of the Q–T interval. This interval is reduced with high serum calcium levels *(hypercalcemia)*, which apparently results from an increase in potassium conductance of the myocardial cell membrane due to the increased Ca^{2+} level. In each case, the alteration in the Q–T interval is due to changes in the ST segment, and the T wave itself is not affected.

DISTURBANCE OF MYOCARDIAL BLOOD FLOW

The electric activity of the cardiac cell is sensitive to changes in myocardial oxygenation because of the oxidative mechanisms involved in both the maintenance of a resting membrane potential and the process of excitation (see Chapter 3). Thus, it is not surprising that changes in coronary blood flow will produce characteristic alterations in the ECG. In addition, the presence of devitalized myocardium or scar tissue will lead to ECG abnormalities particularly in the V leads recorded over the affected area. A detailed analysis of the ECG diagnosis of myocardial lesions is beyond the scope of this chapter; nevertheless, a brief summary of the changes produced by injury, ischemia, and necrosis is appropriate for this discussion.

The rate of myocardial repolarization, particularly of the epicardium, appears to be quite sensitive to mild ischemia. As a result, a small reduction in myocardial blood flow will frequently reverse the direction of the repolarization forces in the affected area. This change will result in a characteristic symmetric inversion of the T wave that will be most prominent in leads recorded from the chest near the ischemic area. (Metabolic and other factors can also affect T-wave orientation, so care must be used in interpreting such changes.) Ischemic T-wave changes can usually be reversed, with restoration of normal myocardial blood flow.

More severe levels of myocardial ischemia lead to tissue injury and interference with the membrane pumps: intracellular sodium increases, and there may be a reduction in intracellular potassium. As a consequence of these ion shifts, the resting membrane potential is reduced in the injured area. The difference in the surface electric charge between this area and the adjacent normal myocardium leads to the flow of a small electric current (the "injury" current) into the injured area (Fig 6–16, top).* Electrocardiograms recorded from a chest electrode near this injured area will show the injury current as a downward deflection of the trace, which continues throughout diastole but will disappear when the muscle is depolarized and the potential of the entire myocardium is reduced to zero. The ECG record during this period (ST segment) will return to the true "zero" baseline (Fig 6–16, bottom). This has the appearance of being an elevated ST segment, as the displacement of the diastolic baseline usually is not apparent. An ischemic inversion of the T wave is usually present due to tissue hypoxia at the margin of the injured area.

---

*This area has the potential to develop into a pacemaker and may lead to ectopic rhythms.

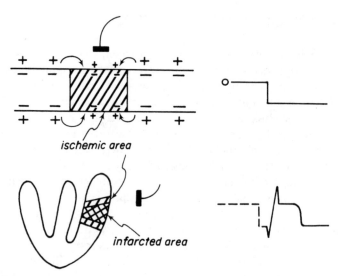

FIG 6–16.
Top left, diagram of a section of resting myocardium showing flow of current into ischemic area from surrounding normal muscles. *Top right,* downward deflection produced in an ECG when connected to an electrode near the ischemic area. *Bottom left,* effect on a typical ECG of "injury" current produced by zone of ischemia that surrounds infarcted area. *Bottom right, dashed* portion of the record shows zero potential position and effect of connecting the electrode. See text for further discussion.

Myocardial infarction produces an area of necrotic tissue that is no longer electrically active. In this sense, it acts as a window and permits body surface electrodes to pick up the negativity of the ventricular cavity early in the depolarization process. As a result, abnormal Q waves are present in the ECG record from such leads. Following recovery from the acute effects of a myocardial infarction, the injury and ischemia pattern regress and often disappear, leaving only the Q waves.

SUMMARY

The physiologic principles developed in Chapter 5 provide the framework for the discussion in this chapter of clinical cardiac arrhythmias. Disturbances in cardiac rhythm due to ectopic or reentry mechanisms and AV block are discussed and related to the changes produced in the electrocardiogram. In addition, the important diagnostic changes produced in the ECG by electrolyte abnormalities, myocardial ischemia, and infarction are summarized.

BIBLIOGRAPHY

Cranefield PF: *The Conduction of the Cardiac Impulse.* Mt Kisco, NY, Futura Publishing Co, 1975.

Damato AN, et al: A study of heart block in man using His bundle recordings. *Circulation* 1969; 39:297.

Goldman MJ: *Principles of Clinical Electrocardiology*, ed 12. Los Altos, California, Lange Medical Publishers, 1986.

Hecht HH, Kossmann CE: Idioventricular and intraventricular conduction: Revised nomenclature and concepts. *Am J Cardiol* 1973; 31:232.

Jose AD: Effect of combined sympathetic and parasympathetic blockage on heart rate and cardiac function in man. *Am J Cardiol* 1966; 18:476.

Lazzara R, Scherlag BJ: Generation of arrhythmias in myocardial ischemia and infarction. *Am J Cardiol* 1988; 61:20A.

Lewis, T, Drury AN, Iliescu CC: A demonstration of circus movements in clinical fibrillation of the auricles. *Heart* 1921; 8:361.

Lipman BS, Dunn M, Massie E: *Clinical Electrocardiography*, ed 7. Chicago, Year Book Medical Publishers, 1984.

Printzmetal M, et al: *The Auricular Arrhythmias.* Springfield, Ill, Charles C Thomas, Publishers, 1952.

Rosen K (ed): Cardiac electrophysiology symposium. *Arch Intern Med* 1975; 135:387.

Surawicz B: Ventricular fibrillation. *Am J Cardiol* 1971; 28:268.

Uhley HN: Some controversy regarding the peripheral distribution of the conduction system. *Am J Cardiol* 1972; 30:919.

Witt, AL, Rosen MR, Hoffman BF: Electrophysiology and pharmacology of cardiac arrhythmias: II. Relationship of normal and abnormal electrical activity of cardiac fibers to the genesis of arrhythmias. *Am Heart J* 1974; 88:664.

Chapter 7 _____

The Output of the Heart and Its Control

_____

The pump function of the heart is regulated so closely that under normal circumstances cardiac output is maintained equal to the perfusion needs of the tissues over a wide range of physiologic conditions. This control is accomplished by an interacting series of mechanisms of different sensitivity and response time. Ultimately, the action of the heart represents a composite of the effect of each control system. In this chapter, methods of measuring cardiac output are considered; then the major regulatory mechanisms are examined individually; and finally their collective action in the control of cardiac output is summarized.

GENERAL CONSIDERATIONS

Cardiac output is the quantity of blood moved per minute by the heart from the great veins to the aorta. It is also called the *minute volume* and is the product of the volume ejected by the heart with each beat (the *stroke volume*) and the heart rate. It is frequently more meaningful to relate the cardiac output to the size of the individual than to use its absolute value. For this reason, cardiac output is frequently expressed as the *cardiac index*. This is the cardiac output, in liters per minute, divided by the body surface area in square meters. Typical values for a normal adult in the supine position are shown in Table 7–1.

TABLE 7–1.

Typical Cardiovascular Data for the Normal Supine Adult

Heart rate (beats/min)	70.0	Pressures (mm Hg)	
Cardiac output (L/min)	5.6	Right atrial	
Stroke volume (ml/beat)	80.0	Mean	4.0
Cardiac index (L/min/sq m)	3.2	Range	1–6
Stroke index (ml/beat/sq m)	45.7	Right ventricular	
Left ventricular end-systolic volume (ml)	65.0	Systolic	24.0
		End-diastolic	4.0
Left ventricular end-diastolic volume (ml)	145.0	Left atrial	
		Mean	8.0
		Range	2–12
		Left ventricular	
		Systolic	130.0
		End-diastolic	7.0

TABLE 7–2

Changes in Heart Rate, Stroke Volume, Average Ejection Velocity, and Cardiac Output in Man During Rest and Exercise

Status	Heart Rate (Beats/Min)	Duration of Systole* (sec)	Stroke Volume (ml)	Average Ejection Velocity (ml/sec)	Cardiac Output (L/min)
Rest	60	0.370	92	248.6	5.52
Exercise	90	0.302	97	321.2	8.72
Mild	100	0.286	109	381.1	10.90
Moderate	120	0.261	112	429.1	13.74
Heavy	154	0.230	125	543.5	19.25
Maximal	187	0.209	127	607.6	23.74

*From Bazett's formula discussed in *Heart* 1920; 7:353.

Cardiac output in the same individual may vary from a value during quiet standing that is 25% to 30% below the resting supine level to a three-fold or fourfold increase above the rest level with extreme exercise (Table 7–2). More modest increases in cardiac output are produced by anxiety or excitement or by physiologic activities such as eating, defecation, or childbirth.

MEASUREMENT OF CARDIAC OUTPUT

Cardiac output can be measured in the experimental laboratory by inserting a flowmeter into or around the aorta or the pulmonary artery. These instruments operate on the principle that the movement of blood through an electromagnetic field will produce an electric potential that is oriented at right angles to the direction of flow and is proportional to the velocity. The vessel wall is constricted to a fixed cross section by the probe. This permits velocity to be converted into volume flow by use of the relationship

$$\dot{Q} = vA \tag{7-1}$$

where $\dot{Q}$ is the volume flow (milliliters per second), v is the velocity (centimeters per second), and A is the cross-sectional area of the vessel (square centimeters). The electromagnetic technique has the disadvantage of requiring placement of the probe either by cardiac catheterization or surgical exposure of the vessel.

Ultrasonic techniques for flow measurement utilize the shift in frequency of a sound reflected from the moving blood that is proportional to the velocity of the blood flow (Doppler effect). The ultrasonic transducer can be placed on the surface of the body, and it is not necessary to expose the blood vessel. With clinical ultrasound equipment (see Chapter 4), the difference between the frequency of the outgoing signal and the sound reflected from the moving column of blood produces a signal within the audible range. This signal can be monitored directly, or it can be displayed in graphic form.

The ultrasonic Doppler technique can be used to measure blood flow velocity in the heart and great vessels as well as in peripheral arteries or veins. However, when used to quantitate blood flow, the angle of the ultrasonic beam and the size of the blood vessel become critical. In addition, variations in flow velocity across the diameter of the vessel, along with differences in aortic size, have presented problems.

The first major clinical procedures for measurement of cardiac output make use of either the Fick principle or the Stewart-Hamilton indicator-dilution technique. In 1870, Adolf Fick, the German biophysicist also known for his law of diffusion, proposed a procedure for measuring the quantity of blood that flows through the lungs. Under steady-state conditions, this value is the same as the cardiac output. The volume of blood passing through the lungs can be calculated from the volume of oxygen absorbed by the pulmonary blood per minute and the amount of oxygen taken up in the lungs by each unit of blood (Fig 7–1).

In actual practice, oxygen consumption was determined by collecting the patient's expired air. A sample of arterial blood was obtained from a peripheral artery, and a mixed venous blood sample was obtained from the pulmonary artery using right heart catheterization. The amount of oxygen picked up by each 100-ml unit of blood as it passes through the lungs was estimated from the difference in the oxygen content of the arterial and ve-

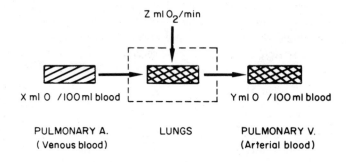

FIG 7–1.
Diagram illustrating use of Fick's principle for measuring cardiac output *(C.O.)*. Each 100-ml unit of blood is visualized as containing X ml of oxygen in the pulmonary artery and Y ml of oxygen in the pulmonary veins. Z ml of oxygen is absorbed from the lungs per minute.

nous blood samples (A_{O_2} – V_{O_2}). Cardiac output (C.O.) was then calculated from these data as follows:

$$C.O.\ (ml/min) = \frac{\text{oxygen consumption (ml } O_2/min)}{A_{O_2} - V_{O_2}\ (ml\ O_2/100\ ml\ blood)} \times 100$$

Fick's procedure gives the average cardiac output for the period needed to determine oxygen consumption and secure blood samples. It will have meaning only if the subject is in a steady state and cardiac output does not undergo marked changes during this period. The stroke volume was determined by dividing the cardiac output by the average heart rate.

Fick's principle utilized in cardiac output determinations is also used in a number of physiologic measurements such as the measurement of liver and kidney blood flow; however, its use for routine clinical cardiac output measurement has now been largely replaced by other methods.

The indicator-dilution method for measuring cardiac output was first suggested in 1898 by the American physiologist G. N. Stewart and subsequently modified by W. F. Hamilton and other investigators. In this procedure a known quantity of an indicator* is injected rapidly as a bolus into

---

*Originally saline was used; however, a nontoxic dye such as indocyanine green that attaches to the plasma proteins and thus is retained in the vascular system is now usually employed as the indicator. This dye has the advantage that its concentration in arterial blood can be determined by photodensitometry.

the venous circulation or directly into the ventricle via an intracardiac catheter. The indicator quickly mixes with the cardiac contents, and during the next few beats the entire blood-indicator mixture is then pumped out of the heart into the circulation. The concentration of indicator in the proximal circulation during this period of washout is determined by continuously sampling from the femoral or radial artery. Under these conditions, the concentration of indicator increases to a peak and then falls exponentially with time as it moves on into the circulation (Fig 7–2). If the average concentration of indicator is determined for the entire period of time that it appears in the proximal arterial circulation, the volume of blood that would be required to dilute the injected indicator to that concentration can be determined. This calculated volume will then represent the total cardiac output for the period of time required to wash the indicator out of the heart. These calculations are shown in Figure 7–2.

In theory, the indicator-dilution procedure should give an accurate measurement of cardiac output during the few beats required for its determination. However, the complexities of the cardiovascular system introduce a number of difficulties. First, recirculation of indicator through the heart begins before the first pass has been completely washed out of the

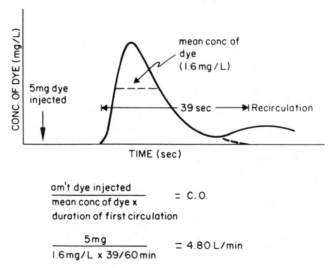

$$\frac{am't\ dye\ injected}{mean\ conc\ of\ dye\ \times\ duration\ of\ first\ circulation} = C.O.$$

$$\frac{5mg}{1.6mg/L \times 39/60\ min} = 4.80\ L/min$$

FIG 7–2.
Time plot of the concentration of dye in the aorta following injection of a 5-mg bolus into the heart. The expected time of disappearance of the dye without recirculation is obtained by extrapolation. Average concentration of dye in the aorta during the first circulation is shown. This is determined from the area under the concentration curve, as determined for the first pass. Calculations are shown for determining cardiac output (C.O.) from the above indicator-dilution data.

aorta. This occurs because of the short circulation time through such pathways as the coronary circulation. As a result, the concentration of indicator in the proximal circulation does not reach zero but instead shows a secondary increase. To overcome this difficulty, it is necessary to estimate the time required to clear the aorta if recirculation did not occur. This is accomplished by extrapolating the exponential part of the fall in the concentration of indicator to zero concentration. The result of such an extrapolation is shown in Figure 7–2. Second, the assumption that complete mixing of the indicator occurs within the heart probably is not justified. In addition, streamlined flow in the aorta may pose sampling problems. However, despite these difficulties, this method of measuring cardiac output has proved useful for clinical studies.

The indicator-dilution method has recently been applied to the measurement of cardiac output in critically ill patients by using a *thermal-dilution* modification. With this technique, a catheter with a temperature-sensitive element at the end and a side opening a few centimeters from the tip is floated into the pulmonary artery after insertion into a peripheral vein. Cold glucose solution is rapidly injected into the right atrium via the side opening, and the time course of the temperature change in pulmonary artery blood is recorded. Cardiac output is determined by substituting the temperature information for the indicator concentration in the indicator-dilution calculation.

Noninvasive procedures for the measurement of cardiac output in addition to the Doppler technique discussed above have recently been developed. These include (1) the use of echocardiographic techniques for the measurement of end-diastolic and end-systolic ventricular volume with calculation of stroke volume (see Chapter 3), and (2) gated radionuclide imaging. In this latter procedure, a suitable isotope such as sodium pertechnetate Tc 99m is injected intravenously, and its concentration in the various chambers of the heart is detected by an external scintillation camera. The number of counts corrected for background radiation over the left ventricle determined at peak systole and during diastole can then be used to calculate the stroke volume and ejection fraction (see below). Other procedures for estimating cardiac output have been suggested. They include analysis of the changes in the aortic pressure pulse and the use of ballistocardiography or impedance cardiography. The first procedure makes use of the magnitude of the pressure pulse as a function of the stroke volume and the physical properties of the arterial reservoir. The second technique relates the counterthrust given to the body as a result of the ejection of blood by the heart to the size of the stroke volume, and the third utilizes alterations in the electrical impedance of the thorax due to changing volume of blood in the heart. At present, these methods do not appear sufficiently reliable for general use.

REGULATION OF CARDIAC OUTPUT

The major factors that regulate cardiac pump function are (1) preload, (2) afterload, (3) heart rate and rhythm, and (4) myocardial contractility. Each factor is, in turn, modified by physiologic events so that in the normal individual their combined effect is to maintain cardiac output at an optimal level. These mechanisms can be subdivided into a primary and secondary group. The first acts rapidly and constitutes the major mechanism for the acute regulation of cardiac output. The secondary mechanisms operate more slowly and are involved in the long-term modification of cardiac function.

PRIMARY CONTROL OF CARDIAC OUTPUT

Preload.—The contractile force developed by a muscle fiber is related to its initial length (see Chapter 3). It is customary to express this length-tension relationship for the isolated papillary muscle by plotting the sarcomere length against the developed isometric tension (or the contraction work) (see Fig 3–16). These parameters are, at best, difficult to estimate in the intact beating heart. In the late 1890s, Otto Frank, a German physiologist, attempted to circumvent these difficulties by an ingenious series of experiments that set the stage for much of our current thinking about the control of cardiac output. He recorded phasic ventricular pressures from an isolated beating frog heart in which the aorta had been occluded. Contraction in this model was nearly isometric throughout systole as ventricular emptying was prevented. Contraction force under these circumstances was expressed entirely as pressure, as energy was not utilized for muscle shortening or conversion into kinetic energy (Fig 7–3, left). The volume of blood in the ventricle was increased between each beat. This caused ventricular end-diastolic pressure to increase according to the diastolic elastic characteristics of the ventricle. As end-diastolic volume increased, systolic pressure and the maximum rate of pressure development (dP/dT) also increased up to a maximum value. When end-diastolic volume was increased beyond this point, systolic pressure and the rate of pressure development were reduced.

The systolic pressure generated by such isometric contractions plotted against ventricular end-diastolic volume (see Fig 7–3, right) represents the relationship between maximal contraction force and ventricular volume. The significance of this relationship will be described later in this section as part of the discussion of ventricular afterload.

Replotting the difference between systolic and diastolic pressure (the contraction or developed pressure) shown in Fig 7–3 permits construction

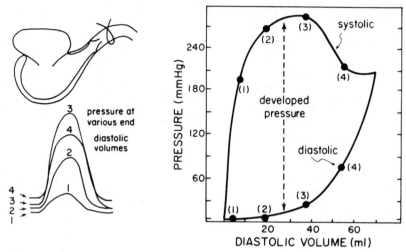

FIG 7–3.
Left, series of isometric ventricular pressure curves as recorded by Otto Frank from the frog heart at different end-diastolic volume levels. (See text for discussion.) *Right,* plot of ventricular end-diastolic pressure and peak systolic pressure against the end-diastolic volume. Numbers refer to pressure curves shown on the *left.*

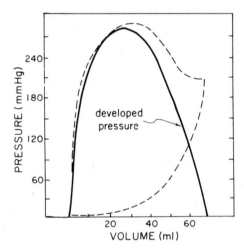

FIG 7–4.
Replotting of difference between systolic and diastolic pressures shown in Figure 7–3 (indicated here by *dashed lines*) against the ventricular end-diastolic volume.

of a ventricular volume-developed tension diagram (Fig 7–4) similar to the length-tension relationship of an isolated muscle. This similarity becomes even greater if one assumes that the volume of the ventricle has a fixed relationship to the length of the ventricular muscle fibers. This is, of course, not a simple relationship or even a linear one and can be changed by factors that affect ventricular distensibility. Nevertheless, it does permit, as a first approximation, the length-tension principle to be applied to the intact heart.

Frank-Starling Relationship.—In 1914, Ernest Starling, the English physiologist, extended the work of Frank to the mammalian heart. He and co-workers developed an experimental preparation using the anesthetized dog (Fig 7–5) in which heart rate, venous pressure, venous return, and arterial resistance were controlled, and arterial pressure, ventricular vol-

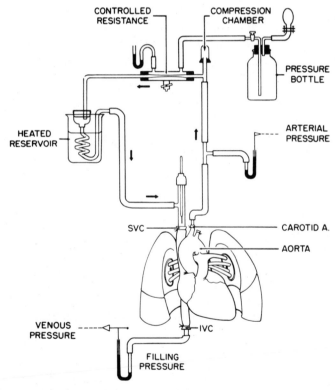

FIG 7–5.
Schematic diagram of a Starling heart-lung preparation. SVC = superior vena cava; IVC = inferior vena cava.

ume, and cardiac output could be measured. This *heart-lung preparation* isolated the heart from the remainder of the circulation by supplying inflow to the right atrium from an external reservoir and diverting left ventricular output via an arterial cannula back to the same venous reservoir. Normal blood gas concentrations were maintained by artificially ventilating the lungs, and myocardial circulation was supplied from the proximal aorta by the coronary circulation. This early ancestor of the heart transplant procedure permitted the cardiac output to be related to ventricular volume over a range of different arterial resistances and venous pressure levels. When the energy output of such a heart (measured as cardiac output) was plotted against ventricular diastolic size (as estimated by the mean venous pressure), the resulting "Starling curve" (Fig 7–6) followed the same general pattern as a length-tension plot described by Frank for the frog heart.

At this point it should be clear that the Frank-Starling relationship for cardiac muscle is in essence the same as the Blix length-tension relationship of skeletal muscle (see Chapter 3); that is, the total work output of the ventricle is related to the presystolic length of the individual muscle fibers. The principle of the Blix-Frank-Starling relationship is frequently loosely

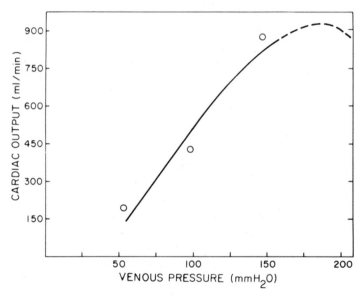

FIG 7–6.
Schematic representation of a "Starling curve" showing energy output of the heart-lung preparation measured as cardiac output, plotted against ventricular diastolic size as reflected by the venous pressure level. (Modified from Patterson SW, Piper H, Starling EH: *J Physiol,* 1914; 48:465.)

stated by relating a number of cardiac parameters that reflect changes in myocardial sarcomere length and contractile energy output. For example, stroke volume, stroke work, or even systolic pressure can be plotted on the ordinate of the Starling diagram for the heart and related to the end-diastolic volume, ventricular end-diastolic pressure, or even mean venous pressure on the abscissa. This latter parameter is an index of the preload described in Chapter 3, as it determines the initial length of the myocardial fibers prior to contraction. Although these terms cannot be used interchangeably with contraction work or sarcomere length with any precision, their use has permitted elucidation of the way the heart adjusts its output so that it "pumps what it gets."

The ability of the heart to acutely keep the stroke volume equal to venous return can be illustrated by the use of a Frank-Starling cardiac length-tension curve. At the initial operating point (Fig 7–7,D), the average end-diastolic length of the myocardium is sufficient to give a normal stroke output. If venous return is now suddenly increased and there is no change in heart rate, ventricular volume at the end of diastole also will be larger. This, in turn, will increase the myocardial fiber length and move the operating point on the length-tension curve. The result will be that the next cardiac contraction is more vigorous, and stroke volume will increase to match the extra venous return. In a similar manner, a reduction in venous inflow will cause the operating point to move down on the cardiac length-tension curve so that again cardiac output will equal venous return.

This mechanism will maintain cardiac output equal to input even in the face of an acute increase in output resistance (i.e., increased afterload; see next section) as, for example, produced by a sudden elevation in aortic pressure. In that case, the ventricular contraction that was determined by the previous end-diastolic volume will now be insufficient to empty the heart to the same degree. This will result in a larger than usual volume of blood remaining in the ventricle at the end of systole. During the next diastole, normal venous return will then be added to this remainder, and the size of the heart at the onset of the next beat will be increased. As a consequence, the operating point of the heart will "move up" on the length-tension curve. Stroke work will be increased so that cardiac output will equal venous return despite the increased resistance to ejection. This equilibrium is, however, achieved at the cost of a larger ventricular size. A similar series of events will adjust the stroke volume after a change in venous return.

This regulatory function of the Frank-Starling mechanism has been called *heterometric regulation* (i.e., hetero = altered; metric = length) as it is achieved by altering the myocardial fiber length. This mechanism is probably largely responsible for balancing the output of the right and left

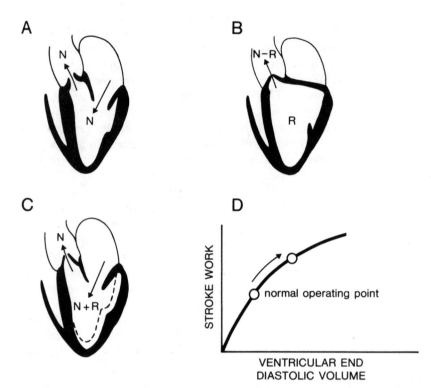

FIG 7–7.
Schematic diagram illustrating the mechanism of heterometric regulation. **A,** control.
The normal return *(N)* to the ventricle during diastole results in the same volume being
ejected during systole. **B,** a sudden increase in output resistance at the end of diastole
results in the stroke volume being less than N; N − R is ejected, and *R* (remainder of
the stroke volume) remains in the ventricle. **C,** during the next beat, the normal venous
return *(N)* is added to the volume remaining from the last beat *(R)*. This increased diastolic volume *(N + R)* causes the next ventricular contraction to be more forceful. This
returns stroke volume equal to venous return. **D,** the above sequence of events causes
the cardiac operating point to move on the cardiac function curve (Starling curve)
from its normal operating point to a larger end-diastolic volume and increased stroke
work.

ventricles because over a period of time any sustained difference in the
output of the two sides of the heart will either overfill or empty the pulmonary vascular system. In the first situation, the higher pulmonary blood
pressure will increase left ventricular filling and cause its output to rise. A
reduction in pulmonary pressure will have the opposite effect and reduce
left ventricular filling. In either instance, the output of the ventricles will
be equalized. In this way, right ventricular output tends to determine cardiac output.

Afterload.—The afterload, as described in Chapter 3, is the tension developed by a muscle before it can begin to shorten. In the same way, the cardiac afterload is the force required to begin ventricular ejection. For the left ventricle, opposition to ejection includes (1) aortic pressure, (2) the flow resistance offered by the aortic valve orifice, (3) the distensibility and capacitance of the vascular system, (4) peripheral vascular resistance, and (5) reflected pressure waves in the aorta. Because of the pulsatile nature of cardiac ejection, the opposition to ventricular ejection provided by the circulatory system is best quantitated in terms of the arterial input impedance (see Chapter 10); however, arterial blood pressure is sometimes used as an index of this parameter.

In addition to the circulatory factors that must be overcome before myocardium shortening begins, cardiac size also plays a role in determining the afterload. Myocardial force is related to both ventricular pressure and the chamber radius. This relationship is discussed in the next chapter (the law of Laplace). However, it is sufficient here to point out that to maintain the same ventricular pressure in a dilated heart, myocardial wall tension is increased over that produced in a small heart. Thus, cardiac afterload is directly related to cardiac chamber size.

In summary, cardiac afterload, which unless specified for the right ventricle, is the left ventricular myocardial force necessary to overcome opposition to ventricular ejection. In the clinical setting, as a rough index, it is frequently related to aortic pressure.

It may be helpful here to point out that with a fixed preload, an increase in afterload results in a greater proportion of the contraction effort being used to generate pressure, and consequently, the stroke volume is reduced. This relationship between afterload and cardiac stroke volume will be discussed in the next section.

Contractility.—Cardiac output is determined not only by the preload and afterload but is also directly affected by the level of what is called *contractility.* This is a poorly defined term (see Chapter 3) that describes the relative ability of the myocardium to develop contractile force. The level of contractility, as described below, is probably related both to the concentration of intracellular calcium and the number of active force-generating sites. The importance of this factor in the regulation of cardiac output was recognized when it was found that under some circumstances, heterometric regulation of cardiac output does not appear to operate. For example, the increase in myocardial contractility produced by stimulation of the sympathetic supply to the left ventricle can lead to an increase in stroke work without a change in ventricular diastolic pressure. In addition, the puzzling observation that the heart size of world-class athlete may become smaller during exercise at a time when cardiac output is elevated is clearly at variance with the "Starling" heterometric regulatory mechanism. These findings were pursued by S. J. Sarnoff and associates at the National Institutes of Health during the 1950s. They showed, in a classic series of experiments, that the Frank-Starling relationship for the myocardium was not fixed, but rather, the curve could be moved to the right or left depending on the degree of autonomic nervous system stimulation (see Chapter 3 and Fig 3–22).

Sarnoff plotted left ventricular work (stroke volume × mean aortic pressure) against mean left atrial pressure or ventricular end-diastolic pressure producing a *cardiac function curve*. He also showed that each ventricle can be represented by a family of these curves (Fig 7–8). Furthermore, the heart is able to move its performance characteristics from one curve to another depending on the balance of the autonomic input to the heart. This shows that the intrinsic length-tension relationship of the myocardium is subjected to modification just as the ability of the heart to generate its own contraction is modulated by reflexes from the central nervous system. Sarnoff suggested the name *homeometric regulation** for this ability to change contraction vigor without altering the initial myocardial length (i.e., homeo = same; metric = length). Positive inotropic actions cause the cardiac function curve to shift to the left; deleterious influences, such as decreased coronary perfusion or myocardial disease, will depress myocardial function and cause the curve to move to the right.

The mechanism for the *positive inotropic* effect of sympathetic stimulation on cardiac function (i.e., the increase in the force and vigor of contraction) is not completely settled. However, a number of the steps have been established. For example, it is known that the neurotransmitter, norepinephrine, liberated at the sympathetic neuromuscular endings, binds to β-adrenergic myocardial membrane receptors. As discussed in Chapter 8, activation of these receptors, operating via the second messenger cyclic 3′, 5′ (cAMP), AMP stimulates glycogenolysis and facilitates the uptake of calcium by the sarcoplasmic reticulum. This latter action may explain the accelerated relaxation that occurs with sympathetic stimulation. In addition, cAMP induces a cascade of biochemical reactions that lead to phosphorylation of the voltage-dependent calcium-channel proteins. With phosphorylation, these channels have an increased ability to open during membrane depolarization. This permits a greater influx of calcium into the cell during the action potential and a greater statistical chance for cross-bridge formation and development of tension. During excitation, cAMP also acts to

---

*Originally used to describe the small increase in contractility at constant fiber length that followed an acute change in afterload (the "Anrep Effect"). Through common usage the term *homeometric regulation* has now been extended to include any change in myocardial contractility without change in muscle length.

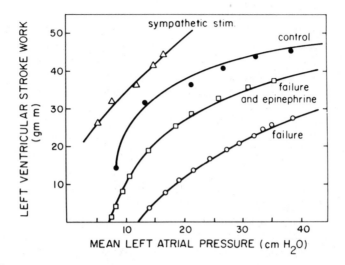

FIG 7–8.

Composite diagram of ventricular function curves obtained in the open-chest dog preparation showing family of curves representing the relationship between mean left atrial pressure and left ventricular stroke work. From top: (1) effect of stimulation of the isolated left stellate ganglion, (2) control curve, (3) effect of myocardial failure plus epinephrine, (4) myocardial failure. (Modified from Sarnoff SJ: *Physiol Rev* 1955; 35:107, and Sarnoff SJ, et al: *Circ Res* 1960; 8:1108.

mobilize intracellular calcium from intracellular stores. The result is that intracellular and carbohydrate energy are made available to facilitate excitation-contraction coupling and the development of myocardial tension.

Heart Rate.—Sympathetic stimulation, in addition to its effect on cardiac contractility, has a *positive chronotropic* effect, i.e., it acts to increase the heart rate (see Chapter 3). This can also have an important effect on cardiac output; however, the mechanism is somewhat complex. At heart rates within the normal range of 60 to 90 beats per minute, the reciprocal relationship between rate and the time that is available between beats for ventricular filling tends, in the absence of an increase in venous return, to reduce ventricular end-diastolic volume (the preload) and keep the product of rate and stroke volume (the cardiac output) nearly constant. When cardiac rate is increased into the tachycardia range (i.e., above 100 beats per minute), the greater contraction frequency itself has a positive inotropic effect. This *staircase phenomenon* (or, as it is sometimes called, *treppe*) is apparently related to a small imbalance between the flux of Ca^{2+} into and out of the cardiac cell at fast heart rates. This is thought to increase the intracellular Ca^{2+} sufficiently during contraction to facilitate greater cross-bridge formation. In addition, the sympathetic stimulation that produced the tachycardia also causes an increase in myocardial contractility. The result is that with tachycardia the duration of systole is reduced, the peak ejection velocity is increased, and the stroke volume is maintained at about the pre-tachycardia level despite a lower preload. Cardiac output is the stroke volume multiplied by the heart rate. Therefore, increasing the heart rates up to 150 to 160 beats per minute will produce a progressive increase in cardiac output (see Table 7–2).

It is of clinical interest that in contrast to a normal tachycardia, an ectopic or reciprocating reentry tachycardia (see Chapter 6) is frequently accompanied by a decrease rather than an increase in cardiac output. This occurs because the rapid heart rate in these patients is usually not initiated or accompanied by an increase in sympathetic discharge; thus, myocardial contractility is not increased to the same extent as with a sinus mechanism. The result is that these patients may develop dizziness or syncope because of the reduced cardiac output.

The normal effect of heart rate as a determinant of cardiac output operates in a different fashion outside of its physiologic range; for example, a rapid tachycardia (more than 170 beats per minute) or a very slow rate (fewer than 40 beats per minute) will result in a marked reduction in the minute output of the heart. With rapid heart rates, the time available for cardiac filling is so abbreviated that it infringes on the phase of rapid ventricular filling (see Fig 4–12). When this occurs, ventricular end-diastolic volume (and therefore the stroke volume) is materially reduced. Under these circumstances the small ejection volume more than offsets the effect of the rapid heart rate, and the output per minute (cardiac output) falls. This mechanism underlies the acute symptoms of inadequate cardiac output that may occur with a very rapid tachycardia. In contrast, a bradycardia prolongs the period of ventricular filling; however, as the major inflow occurs early in diastole, it provides for only a small increase in end-diastolic volume. As a result, at very slow rates the stroke volume is not increased sufficiently to compensate for the reduction in number of beats per minute, and cardiac output falls markedly. This reduction may also produce symptoms and require treatment such as insertion of a pacemaker or use of a sympathomimetic drug to increase the heart rate.

The interrelationship between the chronotropic and homeometric effect of sympathetic stimulation on cardiac performance has been documented by Robert F. Rushmer and co-workers at the University of Washington. They studied the effect of position and exercise on cardiac output of unanesthetized dogs that had had flow probes, dimensional gauges, and pressure sensors previously connected. In these animals the sympathetic stimulation produced by changing their position from the supine to upright or

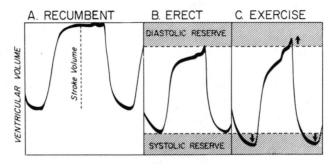

FIG 7–9.
Schematic plot of the change in ventricular volume during the cardiac cycle showing effect of posture and exercise. In the supine position *(A)*, the diastolic volume is near maximal, and the stroke volume is large. On standing *(B)*, diastolic ventricular volume and stroke volume are reduced. During exercise *(C)*, the increase in stroke volume is attained by either greater diastolic filling, more complete systolic ejection, or both. (From Rushmer RF: *Cardiovascular Dynamics*, ed 3. Philadelphia, WB Saunders Co, 1970. Used by permission.)

by starting them running on a treadmill caused an immediate increase in heart rate and a reduction in both the systolic and diastolic dimensions of the heart (Fig 7–9). Stroke volume remained the same or increased slightly, whereas cardiac output showed a considerable increase. The metabolic advantage of this smaller heart size will be discussed in the next chapter.

Atrial Reflexes.—Sarnoff and co-workers, in a separate series of experiments, showed that the vigor of atrial contraction can be controlled by the level of arterial blood pressure through a baroreceptor reflex (see Chapter 10). This mechanism permits a fine control of ventricular end-diastolic volume (preload) on nearly a beat-by-beat basis. A slight drop in arterial pressure, for example, is sensed by stretch receptors in the carotid sinus area. This leads to reflex sympathetic stimulation and a more vigorous atrial contraction. As a consequence, the contribution made by the atrium to ventricular filling is increased (see Chapter 4). Ventricular end-diastolic pressure is increased and, due to heterometric regulation, ventricular contraction becomes stronger, stroke volume is increased, and blood pressure is returned to its normal level.

PRELOAD, AFTERLOAD, AND CARDIAC STROKE VOLUME

Ventricular Pressure-Volume Relationship

The interaction between preload, afterload, and myocardial contractility can now be related to cardiac pump activity by considering it in conjunction with the ventricular pressure-volume (P-V) relationship. The significance of the early observation of Otto Frank that when cardiac ejection was prevented, peak isovolumic ventricular pressure increased as diastolic volume increased (see Fig 7–3) was not fully appreciated until Suga, Sagawa, and others showed in the 1970s that the peak left ventricular pressure-volume relationship is essentially linear over the physiologic range of ventricular volume (Fig 7–10). Furthermore, as discussed below, the upper left-hand corner of the P-V loop of an ejecting beat lies near this end-systolic pressure-volume line (Fig 7–11).

It is helpful in discussing this latter finding to first consider the relationship between ventricular pressure and volume during a normal ejecting beat (the P-V loop). Initial myocardial contraction force, as set by its level of contractility, is determined by the preload, i.e., left ventricular end-diastolic volume (LVEDV) (*A* in Fig 7–11). The contraction energy is first utilized to increase ventricular pressure to the level of aortic diastolic pressure without change in volume as the aortic and mitral valves are closed (*A–B* in Fig 7–11). When left ventricular pressure exceeds aortic pressure, the aortic valve opens. Myocardial fibers can then shorten as blood is ejected through the open aortic valve into the aorta, and ventricular volume decreases. After the contraction reaches its peak and the myocardial fibers

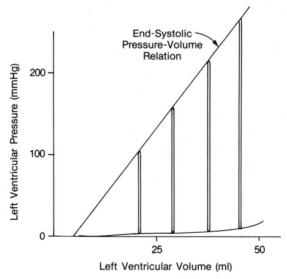

FIG 7–10.
Left ventricular pressure-volume loops generated by isovolumic (i.e., nonejecting) beats at various volumes. The peak pressure generated by each beat falls along a straight line, the end-systolic pressure-volume relation.

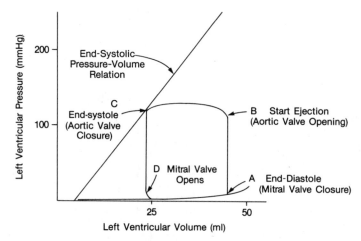

FIG 7–11.
A representative left ventricular pressure-volume loop produced by a normal contraction *(ABCD)*. The upper left-hand corner of the loop *(C)* lies near the end-systolic pressure-volume relation determined from isovolumic beats. See text for further discussion.

begin to relax, the ventricular pressure begins to fall below aortic pressure. The aortic valve then closes as soon as the forward momentum of the blood leaving the heart is no longer able to maintain cardiac ejection (*C* in Fig 7–11). Ventricular pressure then declines rapidly as the ventricle relaxes (*C* and *D* in Fig 7–11). With opening of the mitral valve, left ventricular filling begins (*D–A* in Fig 7–11), and the ventricular pressure-volume loop is completed.

The upper left-hand corner of the pressure-volume loops of variably loaded beats, as noted above, falls along the nearly linear end-systolic pressure-volume relationship (Figs 7–11 and 7–12). The slope of this line has units of pressure per volume and denotes the maximum stiffness or *elastance* of the ventricle during systole.

The end-systolic elastance is insensitive to changes in preload or afterload (see Fig 7–12); however, the maximal elastance increases or decreases with like changes in myocardial contractility (Fig 7–13). For this reason, ventricular end-systolic elastance appears to be a useful measure of myocardial contractility.

The pressure-volume diagram provides a convenient method to illustrate the effect of changing preload or afterload on ventricular performance. An increase in afterload results in a greater proportion of the contraction energy being utilized to develop pressure (Fig 7–14) so that less energy is available for myocardial shortening. As a result, stroke volume is reduced (*B'-C'*). With a larger preload without change in afterload, the left ventricle

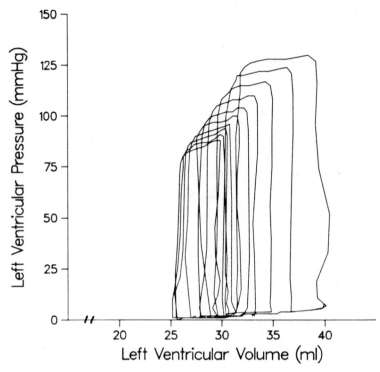

FIG 7–12.
A series of ventricular pressure-volume loops recorded in the conscious dog following partial occlusion of the venae cavae. Each beat starts at a different preload. Ejection stops when ventricular pressure reaches the end-systolic volume pressure line. (From Little WC: *Circ Res* 1985; 56:808. Used by permission of the American Heart Association.)

starts from a larger end-diastolic volume but empties to the same end-systolic size *(C);* thus, the stroke volume is increased.

In the previous illustrations, each variable is altered one at a time for illustrative purposes while the remainder are unchanged. When the circulation is stressed, it is usual for each variable, i.e., contractility, preload, and afterload, to change. For example, preload and afterload may be increased with both exercise and heart failure, but myocardial contractility (and cardiac output) is increased in the former and reduced in the latter disturbance.

Ejection Fraction

The ventricles do not empty completely during ejection, but as indicated in Table 7–1, a considerable volume of blood (the *end-systolic volume*)

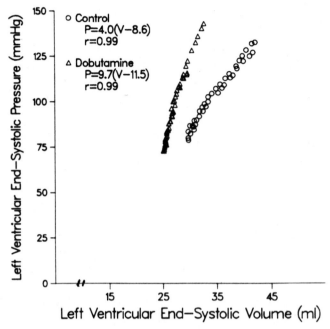

FIG 7–13.
Left ventricular end-systolic pressure-volume relationships in a conscious dog during control conditions and after an increase in myocardial contractility produced by infusion of dobutamine. The relationship is linear, but the slope increases after dobutamine. (From Little WC: *Circ Res* 1985; 56:808. Used by permission of the American Heart Association.)

remains in the heart at the end of systole. Thus, for the left side of the heart,

$$LVEDV = SV + LVESV$$

where LVEDV is left ventricular end-diastolic volume, LVESV is left ventricular end-systolic volume, and SV is stroke volume. The end-systolic volume serves as a reserve that can be drawn on by an increase in myocardial contractility to acutely increase SV.

It is clinically useful to relate SV to LVEDV by calculation of the *ejection fraction* (EF) as follows:

$$EF = \frac{SV}{LVEDV}$$

The normal *EF* in man is 0.50 to 0.75. This ratio serves as a measure of left ventricular pump function as it is affected by heterometric (preload)

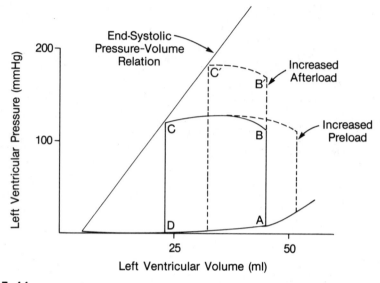

FIG 7–14.
Effect of increased preload and increased afterload on the normal pressure-volume loop *(ABCD)* defined in Figure 7–12. See text for discussion.

forces, homeometric (contractility) forces, output resistance (afterload), and, to some extent, heart rate. This value is usually determined in man from echocardiographic or angiocardiographic (roentgenographic or radionuclide) studies. An EF below 0.50 at rest or failure of EF to increase with exercise or inotropic stimulation is a sign of significant left ventricular impairment.

Cardiac Reserve

One of the advantages of the Frank-Starling diagram, as modified by Sarnoff (see Fig 7–8), is that it permits a graphic appreciation of the concept of cardiac reserve. For example, when the response to an increase in venous return is plotted on such a curve, the operating point will be moved at least transiently to a higher position. As a result of the larger volume, cardiac output will be increased, and the heart will have used some of its ability to respond to an increased myocardial fiber length. The closer the operating point on the cardiac function curve to the point of maximum response, the less cardiac reserve remains for preload regulation.

A diseased heart has a depressed cardiac function curve. This heart must then use some of its reserve to maintain its normal pump function. As a result, there is a reduced reserve available to meet emergencies. A patient with reduced reserve could, for example, be symptom free at rest but might develop difficulties at normal levels of activity.

This concept can be expanded to include the extrinsic cardiac control mechanisms. The steps theoretically taken by a heart suddenly subjected to a reduction in myocardial contractility are shown in Figure 7–15. Stroke volume is initially depressed (*A* to *B*). Compensation then results in a return of the stroke volume to the normal range (*B* to *C*) at the expense of preload reserve. As a result of the simultaneous sympathetic stimulation, or perhaps the administration of a positive inotropic drug, the cardiac function curve is then further shifted to the left. The heart is then able to produce the normal stroke output at a smaller size (*C* to *E*). This has the advantage of minimizing the reduction in cardiac reserve. It also reduces the mechanical and metabolic disadvantage of a large heart. This latter point is discussed in Chapter 8.

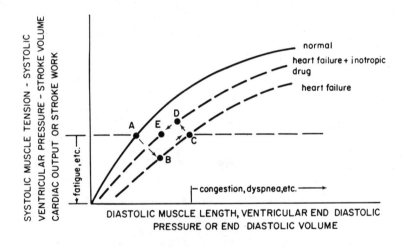

A to B   initial decrease in contractility

B to C   use of Frank-Starling compensation

C to D   increase in contractility due to use of a positive inotropic drug

D to E   drug permitted reduction in the use of the Frank-Starling compensation

FIG 7–15.
Diagrammatic representation of compensatory steps used to maintain cardiac output after an acute decrease in myocardial contractility. See text for discussion. (Redrawn from Spann JF Jr, Mason DT, Zelis RF: *Mod Concepts Cardiovasc Dis* 1970; 39:79.)

SECONDARY CONTROL OF CARDIAC OUTPUT

The primary role of ventricular end-diastolic volume in the heterometric regulation of cardiac output was pointed out earlier in this chapter. The magnitude of ventricular filling is determined, in part, by the size of the blood volume and the vascular capacitance and indirectly by the extracellular fluid volume as these compartments are in dynamic equilibrium with each other. This relationship between fluid volume and output of the heart permits the control mechanisms that regulate the hydration of the body to have a secondary effect on the level of cardiac output. These mechanisms are relatively slow; their response time is measured in terms of hours or days; nevertheless, they play an important role in the long-term regulation of cardiac action.

Vascular Reflexes.—The right and left atria have a rich supply of subendocardial unencapsulated nerve endings (Fig 7–16). These endings have been divided into two functional groups: A receptors that are sensitive to atrial pressure and B receptors that respond to changes in atrial volume.

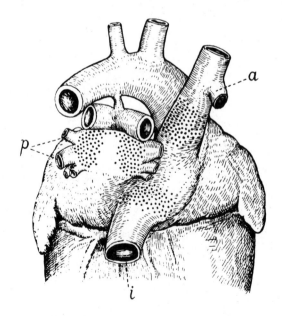

FIG 7–16.
Posterior view of heart of a kitten showing location and approximate extent of receptor areas of the veins as they join the atria *(dotted areas)*; *a* = azygos vein; *i* = inferior vena cava; *p* = pulmonary vein. (From Nonidez JF: *Am J Anat* 1937; 61:203. Used by permission.)

The latter receptors normally fire at the peak of the atrial V wave when atrial volume is greatest. These receptors also can be stimulated experimentally by inflation of an intra-atrial balloon and by the increases in atrial volume brought about by negative-pressure breathing.

Afferent impulses from the atrial receptors travel to the medulla with the vagi and end near the fibers from the carotid and aortic baroreceptors (see Chapter 10). Internuncial fibers pass to the hypothalamus and synapse with neurosecretory cells in the supraoptic area. These connections are inhibitory in nature and prevent secretion of the *antidiuretic hormone* (ADH), *vasopressin*. This substance enhances renal reabsorption of water from tubular urine by increasing the permeability of the distal tubules and collecting ducts. As a result of this negative feedback loop (Fig 7–17), a decrease in atrial volume, such as may occur following a hemorrhage, will increase the circulating level of ADH, limit the loss of water by producing a concentrated urine, and tend to return extracellular volume to normal. The cardiovascular response to a hemorrhage is discussed more fully in Chapter 15.

In the presence of a prolonged elevation of atrial volume, as may occur, for example, in congestive heart failure, adaptation to the atrial stimulus appears to occur, and blood levels of ADH may return to the normal range.

An additional cardiac reflex has been described that originates with the atrial mechanoreceptors. In 1915, the English physiologist F. A. Bainbridge suggested on the basis of infusion studies that an increase in venous return to the heart will produce a reflex tachycardia. This offered a partial explanation for the increase in heart rate that occurs with exercise. Unfortunately, the evidence for this reflex is controversial. It now appears that the *Bainbridge effect*—there is some question if it is a true reflex—depends on the resting heart rate. If it is less than 110 beats per minute, an increase in venous return will result in an increase in heart rate, whereas in a resting heart rate of over 110 beats per minute, the response will be cardiac slowing.

Hormonal Effects.—In addition to the action of ADH discussed above, there are other hormonal pathways that affect cardiac function via the extracellular volume. The first has its receptor mechanism in the kidney. A decrease in either the mean blood pressure, the pulse pressure in the afferent arteriole of the renal nephron (Fig 7–18), or a reduction in plasma sodium stimulates specific *juxtaglomerular cells* in the vessel wall to secrete a proteolytic enzyme called *renin*.* This renal hormone, acting through a

---

*The macula densa and the polkissen, the other cells of the juxtaglomerular complex, are not directly involved in the reflexes discussed here. Their role in the regulation of extracellular volume is beyond the scope of this chapter.

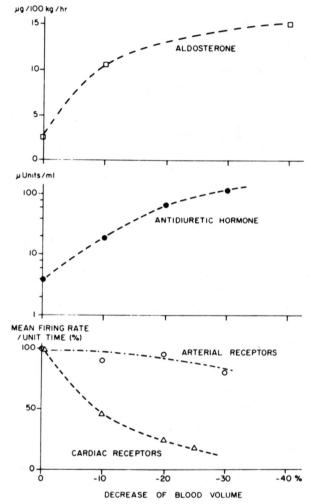

FIG 7–17.
Data showing effect of graded hemorrhage in the experimental animal on aldosterone levels, antidiuretic hormone, mean firing rate of arterial baroreceptors, and atrial mechanoreceptors. (From Gauer OH, Henry JP, Behn C: *Am Rev Physiol* 1970; 32:547. Used by permission.)

series of intravascular events, results in formation of the polypeptide *angiotensin II* (Fig 7–19).

In addition to being a potent vasopressor agent, angiotensin II serves as a powerful stimulus for the production and release of the mineralocorticoid *aldosterone* from the zona glomerulosa of the adrenal cortex. Aldoste-

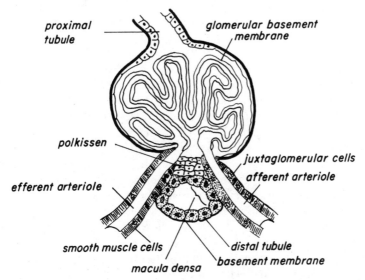

FIG 7–18.
Schematic diagram of the juxtaglomerular complex showing the relationship of the juxtaglomerular cells in the wall of the afferent arteriole to the macula densa of the distal tubule and the polkissen. (Modified from Dustan HP, Frohlich ED, Tarazi RC, in Frohlich ED [ed]: *Pathophysiology: Altered Regulatory Mechanisms in Disease.* Philadelphia, JP Lippincott Co, 1972. Used by permission.)

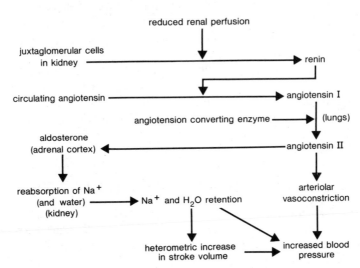

FIG 7–19.
Schematic pathways for action of the renal enzyme renin. See text for discussion.

rone has its primary site of action in the kidney where it increases the reabsorption of sodium by the distal tubules. Concomitant with this saving of sodium, there is an obligatory reabsorption of water from the tubular fluid to maintain normal osmotic relationships. Thus, the final limb of this reflex set in motion by a drop in renal blood pressure is an isotonic expansion of extracellular fluid volume.

The reflex increase in extracellular volume just described acts as a compensatory mechanism to return renal blood pressure to normal by increasing cardiac output through its effect on cardiac filling. This mechanism may be triggered by such clinical events as (1) a reduction in mean arterial pressure as, for example, might be produced by a hemorrhage or a drop in cardiac output or (2) a reduction in pulse pressure due to generalized vasoconstriction of a renal artery as a result of disease processes. The later mechanism has been implicated in the etiology of renal *hypertension*.

When cardiac reserve is decreased, the various compensatory reactions available to support cardiac function may not be able to maintain the cardiac output equal to the needs of the body. In this situation, the negative feedback part of the renal reflex described above will not operate, and the extracellular volume may undergo expansion. As a result, what under more normal circumstances is a protective mechanism designed to maintain cardiac output can become a source of difficulties such as vascular congestion, edema, and problems with pulmonary function. This mechanism underlies many of the signs and symptoms of *congestive heart failure*.

In addition to the effect of angiotensin on sodium reabsorption, a vasodilator peptide extracted from atrial cells, the *atrial natriuretic factor* (hormone), has been shown to act specifically on the kidney to increase excretion of sodium. This peptide, which may be present in several forms, is secreted when the extracellular fluid volume is expanded probably as a result of stretch of the atrial wall. It lowers the blood pressure by reducing the responsiveness of vascular smooth muscle to vasoactive substances. It also acts to reduce the secretion of renin and vasopressin. A similar peptide has recently been identified in neurons in the brain; however, its function is still unclear.

Interrelation Between Venous Return and Cardiac Output

So far the intrinsic and extrinsic factors that regulate cardiac output have been considered one at a time. In the intact individual, each of these control mechanisms operates concurrently and is interrelated in a complex fashion. Since the cardiovascular system is a closed loop, both cardiac output and venous return are dynamically coupled. As a result, a variation in the level of either variable will cause the other to change. Because of this interdependence, circuit analysis can be used to describe the outcome.

Arthur C. Guyton of the University of Mississippi has provided the experimental and conceptual basis for the following analysis. He and his co-workers divided the circulation into two major units. The first segment is the heart pump and its associated pulmonary system. The second is the peripheral circulation. Guyton suggested a graphic procedure for relating the functional characteristics of each segment in a single diagram. This diagram has two parts: (1) a *cardiac function curve* similar to that proposed by Sarnoff except that left ventricular output is related to right atrial pressure, and (2) a *systemic function curve* that relates venous return to the same right atrial pressure. As a convenience, this common parameter is plotted on the abscissa since this variable is interdependent and operates simultaneously in both systems. A Guyton cardiovascular function diagram is shown in Figure 7–20. A normal systemic and cardiac function curve indicated by the solid lines and the effect of exercise on these relationships is shown by

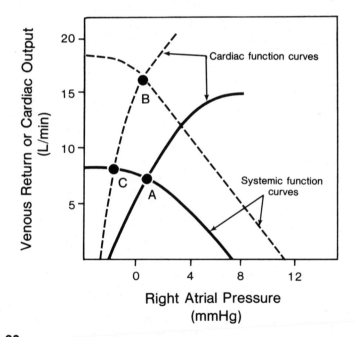

FIG 7–20.
A Guyton cardiovascular function diagram. The *solid lines* show a normal cardiac function curve relating cardiac output to right atrial pressure and a normal systemic function curve relating venous return to right atrial pressure. The result of exercise is indicated by the *dashed lines*. See text for further explanation.

the dashed lines. Before proceeding further with an analysis of this diagram, each of the function curves will be examined in detail.

Systemic Function Curves

Mean Systemic Pressure.—Normal blood volume is larger than the filling volume of the vascular system. As a result, if the circulation is suddenly stopped and fluid is prevented from entering or leaving, blood will distribute itself throughout the system according to the distensibility characteristics of each segment and a common static pressure will develop due to elastic recoil of the vessel walls. This pressure is the *mean systemic pressure.* Its magnitude is a function of the lumped volume elastic characteristics of the system, the vascular filling volume (i.e., the capacity of the undistended vascular system), and the blood volume. Guyton has suggested that the mean systemic pressure is the same as the *average pressure* that exists near the venous end of the systemic capillaries when the circulation is intact. This pressure varies from about 3.5 to 14 mm Hg and is about 7 mm Hg under normal conditions.

Factors Affecting Venous Return.—Right atrial pressure normally is lower than mean systemic pressure (or mean capillary pressure) so that a gradient, which has been termed the *vis a tergo* (push from behind), is present between the capillaries and the heart. This gradient supplies the force to move blood through the veins, and within physiologic limits venous return is linearly related to its magnitude. In the framework of this discussion, it should be clear that venous return will stop in the absence of any compensatory mechanisms if right atrial pressure is raised to the level of mean systemic pressure. This point is indicated in Figure 7–17 by the systemic function curves intercepting the right atrial pressure axis at zero venous return.

If right atrial pressure falls below atmospheric, the negative pressure in the great veins causes them to collapse as they leave the chest. This obstruction prevents venous return from significantly increasing further if right atrial pressure falls to subatmospheric levels. As a result, the systemic function curve reaches its peak at zero right atrial pressure and remains essentially at this level with lower atrial pressures.

Factors that modify mean systemic filling pressure will shift the systemic function curve. Increased sympathetic activity, for example, causes the smooth muscle in both arterioles and venous capacitance vessels to contract. This causes (1) a reduction in size of the vascular compartment and (2) a decrease in distensibility of the vessel walls. As a result, the vascular system becomes tighter, mean systemic filling pressure is increased, and the systemic function curve is shifted upward and to the right. An example of this shift is shown in Figure 7–17 where the systemic function curve indicated by the dashed lines shows the effect of sympathetic stimulation combined with the increase in venous return due to exercise. In a similar manner, changes in the systemic filling pressure due to alterations in blood volume or changes in the slope of the curve due to variations in systemic vascular resistance will cause the systemic function curve to assume different configurations.

Cardiac Function Curve

As indicated earlier, the cardiac function curve is similar to the Starling relationship between atrial pressure and cardiac output. As experimentally determined in intact animals, it is somewhat more S-shaped, it has a less prominent peak, and the terminal downslope is minimal or does not occur. Under the influence of sympathetic stimulation or other positive inotropic intervention, the curve is moved to the left and becomes steeper (see Chapter 3). This positive inotropic response is shown in Figure 7–17 by the shift of the curve to the left. Negative inotropic interventions such as myocardial disease, valvular lesions, or hypoxia that decrease myocardial function shift the curve to the right, and it becomes less steep.

Analysis of the Guyton Diagram

Under steady-state conditions, venous return and cardiac output are equal. If the myocardium has adequate reserve and can respond to an increase in venous flow, venous return becomes the limiting factor and thus can be viewed as the regulator of cardiac output. However, if cardiac reserve is exceeded, the pump function of the heart becomes the limiting factor. In this case, the heart is unable to pump what it receives, venous pressure increases, cardiac output falls, and the heart is said to have "failed."

The complicated relationship among venous return, atrial pressure, and cardiac output, as well as their ability to maintain a steady-state relationship despite perturbations to the system, is illustrated by the complementary quality of the systemic and cardiac function curves. Under normal conditions an intervention such as, for example, a sudden temporary increase in venous return will increase right atrial pressure and cardiac output. At the same time, the increase in right atrial pressure will reduce the pressure gradient between the capillaries and the heart. Loss of the normal vis a tergo will then have the negative feedback effect of reducing venous return. This action will, in time, (1) limit the original increase in cardiac output and (2) tend to return the system to its steady-state position. However, as explained below, if the increase in venous return is maintained, the systemic function curve will be rotated upward and to the right, and the increase in cardiac output will be sustained.

The Guyton diagram shows this relationship graphically; that is, the parameters that regulate venous return and cardiac output can be simultaneously resolved at only one right atrial pressure. This steady-state point is indicated by the intersection of the systemic and cardiac function curves. Thus, a sudden perturbation may temporarily change this operating point; however, such a change will be transitory, and the system will gradually return toward its equilibrium position. However, if the perturbation is accompanied by a change in one or both of the function curves, either directly or as a compensatory reaction to the intervention, the equilibrium point will stabilize at the intersection of the new curves.

The series of events just described can be illustrated by considering the effects of exercise on cardiac function (see Chapter 15 for a fuller discussion of this subject). As suggested above, both the systemic and cardiac function curves will be altered. The positive inotropic effect of the increased sympathetic stimulation that accompanies physical exercise will cause the cardiac function curve to move to the left and become steeper. At the same time, the increased sympathetic discharge will reduce vascular compliance and increase the mean circulatory filling pressure. This combined with the increase in venous return due to muscular activity will shift the systemic function curve to the left. The result is that the steady-state relationship between these two function curves will move (from *A* to *B* in Fig 7–17), and cardiac output will be materially increased. It is interesting that cardiac size (i.e., right atrial pressure) will remain essentially unchanged.

This analysis also indicates the importance of venous return to the cardiovascular adaptations to exercise. If the systemic function curve was unaltered, the increase in cardiac contractility alone would result in the operating point moving only from *A* to *C*, and cardiac output would not increase significantly.

SUMMARY

A number of techniques are available for measuring cardiac output. These include electromagnetic flow probes, indicator-dilution techniques, ultrasound (Doppler), or isotope procedures as well as blood gas determinations using the Fick Principle. Cardiac output can be acutely modulated by altering the preload (Starling's law), afterload, heart rate, and level of myocardial contractility. The ventricular pressure-volume diagram and end-systolic pressure-volume relationships have recently provided new insight into myocardial performance and pump function. The secondary control of cardiac output includes vascular reflexes and their regulation of body fluid levels through endocrine, renal, vascular, and other organ systems. The interaction between venous return and cardiac output operates in a closed loop. This complex relationship can be illustrated by plotting cardiac and systemic function curves on a Guyton diagram. Stable changes in this relationship can be accomplished only by altering either or both the cardiac and systemic function curves.

BIBLIOGRAPHY

Antani JA, Wayne HH, Kuzman WJ: Ejection phases indexes by invasive and noninvasive methods. *Am J Cardiol* 1979; 43:239.

Aviado DM, Schmidt CF: Reflexes from stretch receptors in blood vessels, heart and lungs. *Physiol Rev* 1955; 35:247.

Bodenheimer MM, Banka VS, Helfant RH: Nuclear cardiology: I. Radionuclide angiographic assessment of left ventricular contraction: Uses, limitations and future directions. *Am J Cardiol* 1980; 45:661.

Braunwald E, Ross J Jr: Control of cardiac performance, in Bern RM, Spirelakis N, Geiger SR (eds): *Handbook of Physiology, Section 2: The Cardiovascular System*, vol 1. Bethesda, American Physiological Society, 1979.

Fick A: Ueber die Messung des Blutquantums in der Herzventrikeln. S.B. *Phys-Med Ges Wurzburg*, July 9, 1870.

Frank D: On the dynamics of cardiac muscle, Chapman CB, Wasserman E (trans from *Z Biol* 1895, 32:370. *Am Heart J* 1959; 58:467.

Glower DD, Rankin JS, et al: Linearity of the Frank-Starling relationship in the intact heart: The concept of preload recruitable stroke volume. *Circulation* 1985; 71:994.

Guyton AC: Determination of cardiac output by equating venous return curves with cardiac response curves. *Physiol Rev* 1955; 35:123.

Guyton AC: Venous return, in Hamilton WF, Dow P (eds): *Handbook of Physiology: Circulation*, Section 2, vol II. Washington, DC, American Physiological Society, 1963.

Guyton AC, Jones CE, Coleman TG: *Circulatory Physiology: Cardiac Output and Its Regulation*. Philadelphia, WB Saunders Co, 1973.

Hamilton WF, Remington JW: The measurement of the stroke volume from the pressure pulse. *Am J Physiol* 1947; 148:14.

Little RC, Downes TR: Atrial transport and its importance to cardiovascular function. *Cardiologic Consultant* 1987 (summer); 8:1.

Little RC, Little WC: Cardiac preload, afterload and heart failure. *Arch Intern Med* 1982; 142:819.

Little WC: The left ventricular dP/dt_{max}-end-diastolic volume relation in closed-chest dogs. *Circ Res* 1985; 56:808.

Mason DT: Afterload reduction and cardiac performance. *Am J Med* 1978; 65:115.

Moore JW, et al: Studies on the circulation: II. Cardiac output determinations: Comparison of the injection method with the Fick procedure. *Am J Physiol* 1929; 89:331.

Patterson SW, Piper H, Starling EH: The regulation of the heart beat. *J Physiol* 1914; 48:465.

Porter R, Fitzsimons DW (eds): *The Physiological Basis of Starling's Law*, a CIBA Foundation Symposium. Amsterdam, Associated Scientific Publishers, 1974.

Powers ER, Foster JR, Powell WJ Jr: Interaction of interval-force relationship with aortic pressure and stroke volume. *Am J Physiol* 1976; 230:893.

Reuter H: Modulation of ion channels by phosphorylation and second messengers. *News in Physiol Sci* 1987; 2:168.

Rushmer RF, Smith OA, Franklin D: Mechanisms of cardiac control in exercise. *Circ Res* 1959; 7:602.

Sagawa K: The end-systolic pressure-volume relation of the ventricles: Definition, modification and clinical use. *Circulation* 1981; 63:1223.

Sarnoff SJ, Berglund B: Ventricular function: I. Starling's law of the heart studied by means of simultaneous right and left ventricular function curves in the dog. *Circulation* 1954; 9:706.

Sarnoff SJ, et al: Regulation of ventricular contraction by the carotid sinus: Its effect on atrial and ventricular dynamics. *Circ Res* 1960; 8:1123.

Shippley RE, Gregg DE: The cardiac response to stimulations of the stellate ganglia and cardiac nerves. *Am J Physiol* 1945; 143:396.

Starr I, et al: Studies on the estimation of cardiac output in man, and of abnormalities in cardiac function, from the heart's recoil and the blood impacts. The ballistocardiogram. *Am J Physiol* 1939; 127:1.

Stewart GN: Researches on the circulation time and on the influences which affect it. IV. The output of the heart. *J Physiol* 1897; 22:159.

Suga H, Kitabatake A, Sagawa K: End-systolic pressure determines stroke-volume from fixed end-diastolic volume in the isolated canine left ventricle under a constant contractile state. *Circ Res* 1979; 44:238.

Weber KT, Janicki JS: The dynamics of ventricular contraction: Force, length and shortening. *Fed Proc* 1980; 39:188.

Chapter 8 _____

Energetics of the Heart

_____

The heart converts metabolic energy into the pressure and kinetic force necessary to maintain blood pressure and provide circulation of blood to tissues. This activity is carried out in a series of steps that include (1) conversion of substrate energy into myocardial wall tension by means of oxidative metabolism and action of the cardiac contractile machinery, (2) transference of myocardial wall tension into intracardiac pressure, and (3) utilization of these forces to produce ejection of the stroke volume into the circulation.

The energy consumption of the heart and the efficiency with which it is converted to useful work is influenced by (1) the type of load, (2) the geometry of the ventricles, (3) the level of myocardial contractility, and (4) the heart rate.

CARDIAC METABOLISM

In contrast to skeletal muscle, which obtains its energy for contraction almost exclusively from the metabolism of glucose or glycogen, the heart can utilize a wide variety of substrates in addition to glucose to support its activity. These energy sources include esterified and nonesterified fatty acids, lactate, ketone bodies, and, to a lesser extent, amino acids. Under normal conditions, the myocardium appears to preferentially utilize the substrate that is present in the largest concentration. Following a carbohydrate meal, for example, the heart uses glucose and pyruvate as its primary source of energy. However, in the postabsorptive state, the myocardium switches to the metabolism of fatty acids and ketones. When presented with blood containing a normal mixture of metabolic materials, the heart will utilize almost equal amounts of glucose and lactate; however, these materials will contribute only one third of the total energy needs of the heart, and the remainder will come from noncarbohydrate sources (Table 8–1).

If the arterial concentration of glucose is above 3.33 mmol/L (60 mg/dl), glucose enters the myocardial cell by facilitated diffusion. The rate of this transfer is increased by insulin, anoxia, and high levels of cardiac work. Once inside the cell, glucose undergoes phosphorylation to glucose-6-phosphate (G-6-P) and is then either converted to glycogen via the uridine diphosphoglucose system or enters the glycolytic energy pathway through conversion to fructose-6-diphosphate (Fig 8–1).

Myocardial glycogen serves primarily as a reserve store of substrate. It can, however, be mobilized as a result of sympathetic stimulation. The catecholamines liberated by sympathetic endings bind to myocardial receptors of the adenylate cyclase system. This, in turn, leads to the formation of cyclic 3′,5′-AMP (cAMP) within the cell and activation of phosphorylase *b* into the active *a* form, which then catalyzes the breakdown of glycogen.

The second step in the Embden-Meyerhof pathway where fructose-6-phosphate is converted to fructose-1,6-diphosphate is an important control point for regulation of cardiac metabolism. The activity of phosphofructokinase, which catalyzes this reaction, is inhibited by ATP and citrate. As these are the end products of the glycolytic and Krebs cycle, this mechanism permits a negative feedback control of the entire metabolic pathway.

TABLE 8–1.

Relative Contribution (%) of Various Substrates to Total Uptake of Oxygen by the Heart*†

Carbohydrate	
Glucose	17.90
Lactate	16.46
Pyruvate	0.54
Total	**34.90**
Noncarbohydrate	
Fatty acids	67.0
Amino acids	5.3
Ketones	4.3
Total	**76.6**

*Total equals more than 100% due to storage or conversion of substrate into other forms.
†Data from Bing RJ: *Circulation* 1955; 12:635.

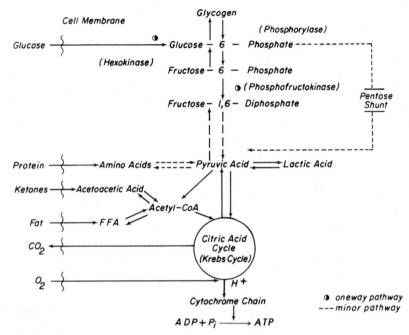

FIG 8–1.
Outline of myocardial metabolism showing major steps and principal enzymes in the glycolytic pathways. ADP = adenosine diphosphate; CoA = coenzyme A; FFA = free fatty acids.

The significance of this regulation is enhanced by the fact that production of pyruvate from G-6-P via the pentose (hexose monophosphate) shunt is usually not important in the myocardium. It is also significant that the activity of phosphofructokinase is stimulated by cAMP and by high levels of inorganic phosphate. This provides an important means of increasing production of metabolic substrate when ATP stores are reduced by hydrolysis or when metabolic activity is stimulated by the sympathetic nervous system.

Free fatty acids (FFA), triglycerides, and ketone bodies enter the myocardium passively, provided their concentration in the blood is above a threshold level (for FFA this value is about 0.35mM). Uptake of these substances is not affected by insulin or other substances. Once inside the cardiac cell, FFA are bound to intracellular protein but after activation can be converted to tissue lipids or enter the citrate cycle in the mitochondria in the form of acetyl coenzyme A. Endogenous lipid is usually not employed as an energy source, and the myocardium apparently preferentially uses carbohydrate. Although the myocardium is also able to use acetoacetate and β-hydroxybutyrate as energy sources, there is no evidence that these are used as a major source of energy.

Under normal conditions of oxygen availability, the energy contained in pyruvate enters the citric acid cycle in the mitochondria and is transformed by oxidative phosphorylation into the high-energy bonds of adenosine triphosphate (ATP) by way of the electron chain mechanism of the flavoprotein-cytochrome system. When oxygen is limited, pyruvate is able to act as a hydrogen acceptor and is converted to lactic acid rather than entering the citrate cycle. This allows hydrogen to be transferred from the hydrogenated coenzyme, nicotinamide adenine dinucleotide ($NADH_2$) with the re-formation of NAD. This permits it to continue to serve as an electron carrier in the synthesis of ATP. This mechanism is limited in the myocardium and, as discussed below, is not able by itself to maintain myocardial activity for any length of time.

During cardiac contraction, the adenosine triphosphatase (ATPase) of the actomyosin cross bridges results in hydrolysis of ATP with formation of adenosine diphosphate (ADP) and inorganic phosphate along with the liberation of energy (see Chapter 3). The ADP is then promptly converted back to ATP by energy from the Krebs cycle. Creatine phosphate (CP) acts as a reservoir of energy in the form of phosphate bonds that can be called on to regenerate ATP (Fig 8–2). Recent studies have shown that formation of CP from ATP and creatine is catalyzed in the mitochondria by the enzyme creatine phosphokinase. The high-energy CP diffuses to the myosin-actin interface where it is hydrolyzed. The phosphate can then be utilized to reconstitute ATP from ADP, and the creatine is free to return to the mitochondria. In this way, CP serves as a shuttle to bring mitochondrial energy to the contractile proteins.

The metabolic pathways just described are designed for aerobic metabolism. Under normal conditions, these systems provide adequate energy for ATP regeneration, and the heart does not incur an oxygen debt. However, if the supply of oxygen is reduced, the metabolic activities of the mitochondria are inhibited. As a result, as discussed above, they do not metabolize pyruvate at the normal rate, and lactate accumulates in the circulation. In addition, hypoxia, probably acting via sympathetic stimulation and formation of cAMP, stimulates glycogenolysis, glycolysis, and the uptake of glucose by the cardiac cells. The excess pyruvate produced by this activity then appears as the metabolite lactic acid. Finally, the supplies of CP are degraded to provide energy for ATP regeneration. As a result, the level of myocardial inorganic phosphate is increased. Under these conditions, the heart can incur a small oxygen debt. However, it should be emphasized that because the ability of the heart to provide energy from

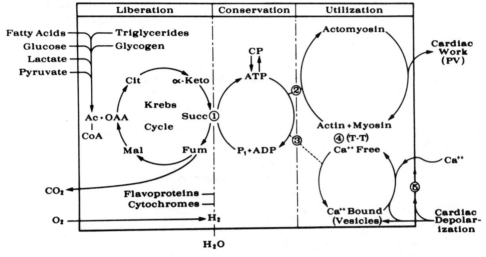

FIG 8–2.
Metabolic pathways involved in energetics of the heart. Points primarily affected by anoxia include (1) oxidative phosphorylation, (2) actomyosin ATPase, (3) reticulum calcium pump, (4) troponin-tropomyosin-calcium system; and (5) cell membrane ion pumps. (Modified from Olson RE, Dhala NS, Sun CN: *Cardiology* 1971; 56:114. Used by permission.)

anaerobic sources is severely limited, the myocardium cannot operate without oxygen for any appreciable period of time. Thus, the availability of oxygen becomes the limiting step in the metabolism of the heart.

In view of the importance of the aerobic pathways to myocardial metabolism, it should not be surprising that cardiac muscle cells have a greater number of mitochondria than have other types of muscle. In addition, the heart contains a high concentration of the hematin compound, myoglobin (1.5% to 2% by weight in myocardium vs. 0.1% to 0.2% in white skeletal muscle fibers). This protein is localized in close association with the mitochondria. It accepts oxygen from hemoglobin and stores it for release to the cytochrome oxidase system when myocardial oxygen tension is reduced. In this respect, the metabolism of the myocardium is similar to that of red skeletal muscle in that both are designed for a constant work load over an extended period without the necessity for rest periods. This is in contrast to white skeletal muscle, which is organized for short bursts of intense work and the accumulation of a considerable oxygen debt. This latter event requires a period of rest while the debt is repaid largely by oxidation of the lactic acid produced during the period of muscle activity. In view of these functional differences, it should not be surprising that white skeletal muscle has a much larger store of CP and the enzyme systems involved with anaerobic glycolysis than do red skeletal muscle and the myocardium, which have a richer store of oxidative enzymes.

CARDIAC CONTRACTION AND MYOCARDIAL WALL TENSION

The first step in the conversion of the energy contained in ATP into the forces that maintain the circulation is carried out by the contractile machinery of the myocardium. Activation of these elements causes them to shorten against the recoil of the muscle series elastic units (see Chapter 3) and to produce a longitudinally oriented tension (stress) within the muscle fibers. This tension causes the myofibrils that encircle the ventricle (see Fig 2–10) to press on the blood inside, just as a stretched rubber band placed around a paper tube tends to occlude the lumen. This compression of the ventricular contents results in the development of an outward force, the ventricular pressure. With opening of the aortic and pulmonary valves, the ventricular myocardium is able to shorten and add additional force to the system in the form of kinetic energy as blood is ejected into the circulation. The magnitude of this transfer of metabolic energy to ventricular pressure and flow is subject to modification by the control mechanisms (see Chapter 7) that regulate the force and vigor of ventricular contraction.

Law of Laplace

The interdependence of myocardial wall tension, ventricular pressure, and cardiac size has important implications for the way the heart responds to stress. This relationship was worked out for a thin-walled soap bubble in 1820 by the Marquis de Laplace. Expressed for a sphere, this relationship is given by

$$T_w = P \cdot r/2 \qquad (8-1)$$

where T_w (tension, wall) is the tangential hoop tension (longitudinal tension) that is expressed per length of the circumference, P is the internal pressure, and r is the radius (Fig 8–3,A). The myocardial hoop tension (T_w) is oriented so that it will pull open a slit place in its wall (Fig 8–3,B). The total longitudinal tension acting on this slit is the hoop tension (equation 8–1) times the length of the opening. If the slit is extended so that it circles the sphere, the total tension developed in the ventricular wall (TW)

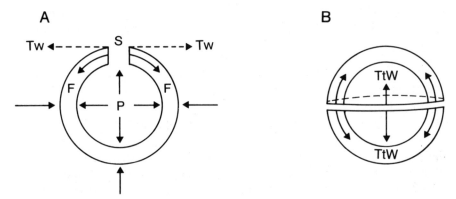

FIG 8–3.
Wall tension (*tw*) is the force *(F)* developed in the myocardium that would pull apart the small slit *(S)* shown in the cross section of the heart **(A)**. Total wall tension (T_{tw}) is the force that would tend to pull both halves of the heart apart if the slit were extended around the heart to form a circumference **(B)**. This T_{tw} can be normalized for ventricular thickness and expressed as wall stress. P = internal pressure. See text for further discussion.

is the hoop tension times the circumference of the sphere. For a thin-walled vessel this is given by

$$T_{tw} = \frac{P \cdot r}{2} \times 2\,\pi r = P \cdot \pi r^2 \tag{8–2}$$

While the heart is not a perfect sphere, the *law of Laplace* can be applied in an approximate manner if one assumes that the left ventricle is spheroid* and the muscle fibers are homogenously oriented in a circumferential manner. This relationship can then be modified for the heart with its thicker wall by normalizing the total hoop tension described in equation 8–2 for the average thickness of the myocardium as follows:

$$\sigma = P \cdot \pi r^2/h \tag{8–3}$$

where h is the average wall thickness, and σ is the normalized total wall tension or wall stress, (i.e., the tension per unit of cross-sectional of the ventricle).

---

*Other more complicated geometric forms such as an ellipsoid of revolution have been proposed. See the article by Mirsky listed in the bibliography for details.

The ability of the heart to convert myocardial tension into ventricular pressure is also dependent on cardiac size. This can be illustrated by rearranging equation 8–3 as follows:

$$P = \frac{\sigma \cdot h}{\pi r^2} \tag{8–4}$$

This relationship shows that a larger normalized total wall tension or stress (σ) will be required to develop the same ventricular pressure (P) when the heart has a greater volume (i.e., the value of r is increased). This prediction is confirmed by the finding that the metabolic energy expenditure, as measured by the myocardial oxygen consumption, is greater for the same ventricular pressure when generated by a dilated heart than when it is developed by a small heart.

This relationship also illustrates the compensatory effect of cardiac hypertrophy where the increase in muscle thickness (h) permits a lower wall stress for the same developed pressure (see discussion below).

TOTAL WALL TENSION-VOLUME DIAGRAM

It is useful to consider the relationship between total wall tension and chamber volume. In this analysis, a spherical thin-walled ventricle with a constant level of contractility will be discussed first before the effect of cardiac dilation, increase in cardiac preload, and myocardial hypertrophy are considered.

Instantaneous total wall tension (equation 8–2) plotted against ventricular volume in a normal-sized ventricle is shown in Figure 8–4,A. During isovolumic contraction, ventricular pressure increases rapidly while the radius does not change. As a result, total wall tension increases. During ejection, both ventricular volume and radius decrease, but the radius decreases to a greater extent. This follows because of the third-power relationship between volume and radius (Fig 8–5). In a small heart, the reduction in radius during ejection is sufficiently large that even though ventricular pressure continues to increase, total wall tension, that is, the product of pressure and πr^2, is progressively reduced as the heart empties. During isovolumic relaxation, wall tension then falls rapidly before again increasing gradually as the ventricle fills during diastole.

This ability to reduce the level of wall tension during ejection is lost when the heart becomes dilated as may occur with heart failure (see Fig 8–4,B). In such a patient, a larger end-diastolic volume (preload) is required for the failing heart to maintain a normal stroke volume. The increased end-

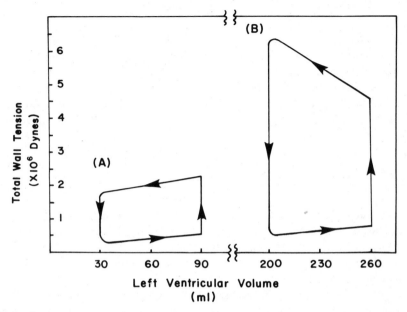

FIG 8–4.
Diagrammatic total wall tension volume curves for a normal-sized heart *(A)* and a dilated heart *(B)* for one cardiac cycle. The *arrows* indicate chronologic sequence. (Modified from Burch GE, Ray CT, Cronvich JA: *Circulation* 1952; 5:504.)

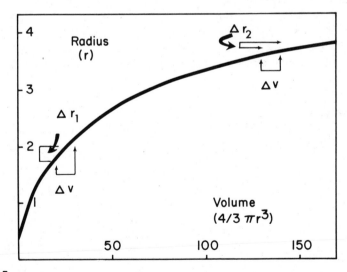

FIG 8–5.
Relationship of the volume of a sphere to its radius. This illustrates the principle that the
same change in volume (ΔV) will produce a much large change in the radius of a
normal-sized heart (Δ_{r1}) than in that of a large heart (Δ_{r2}).

diastolic size of the left ventricle also results in an increase in myocardial wall tension. Furthermore, the dilated heart operates at a mechanical disadvantage as total wall tension may *increase during ejection*. This occurs because the same stroke volume in the larger heart results in a smaller reduction in the ventricular radius than is the case with a normal-sized heart. Illustrative values of total wall tension calculated for a small and dilated heart are summarized in Table 8–2.

CARDIAC HYPERTROPHY

Prolonged cardiac dilation acts as a stimulus for nucleic acid and protein synthesis and invariably leads to cardiac fiber hypertrophy. This may take one of two forms depending on the initiating stress. A *concentric* type of hypertrophy results when the heart is subjected to a prolonged pressure load such as produced by arterial hypertension or obstruction to cardiac ejection by a stenotic aortic valve. In this condition, muscle mass increases without significant change in the size of the ventricular cavity. In contrast, a chronic volume overload, as produced by an intracardiac shunt or an insufficient (leaking) cardiac valve, produces an *eccentric* type of hypertrophy. In this condition, the ventricular wall becomes moderately thicker, but the major increase in cardiac size is due to dilation of the ventricular cavity.

The functional importance of cardiac hypertrophy is somewhat different depending on its etiology. Concentric hypertrophy due to a pressure load permits systolic tension to be distributed over a larger muscle mass so

TABLE 8–2.

Effect of Heart Size on Total Wall Tension Developed at Beginning and Peak of Ventricular Ejection

Pressure	Start of Ejection (9,331 pascals [70 mm Hg])	Peak of Ejection (15,996 pascals [120 mm Hg])
Small Heart		
Volume	9×10^{-5} cu m (90 ml)	3×10^{-5} cu m (30 ml)
Radius	0.028 m (2.8 cm)	0.019 m (1.9 cm)
Wall thickness	0.010 m (1 cm)	0.010 m (1 cm)
Total wall force	2,298 newtons	1,814 newtons
Dilated Heart		
Volume	2.6×10^{-4} cu m (260 ml)	2.0×10^{-4} cu m (200 ml)
Radius	0.039 m (3.9 cm)	0.036 m (3.6 cm)
Wall thickness	0.010 m (1 cm)	0.010 m (1 cm)
Total wall force	4,458 newtons	6,512 newtons

that normalized wall tension or stress (increase in h in equation 8–3) frequently remains in the normal range. As discussed in the next section, this will minimize the need for increased myocardial oxygen supply and permit relatively normal cardiac function.

Chamber dilation due to a chronic volume overload permits the heart to support the increased stroke volume by operating at an increased sarcomere length (the Frank-Starling mechanism). However, because of the law of Laplace (see Fig 8–4), the larger ventricle is at a mechanical disadvantage and must develop a greater wall tension to maintain the normal stroke volume. The increase in wall thickness in eccentric hypertrophy compensates for this increased wall tension and returns wall stress back toward normal (see equation 8–3). Progression of the hypertrophic response to myocardial stress may eventually result in insufficient coronary blood flow to maintain the increased muscle mass, and myocardial hypoxia may occur. Furthermore, long-standing hypertrophy may damage the myocardium, decreasing its contractile ability, and in some cases lead to cardiac failure.

CARDIAC WORK

Work, in the terminology of physics, describes the energy transfer when a mass is moved or a volume is displaced. When applied to the heart, the concept of work has taken a somewhat broader definition. In a general sense, cardiac work is used to describe the myocardial transfer of energy from its metabolic substrate to the pressure and kinetic energy of the blood in the vascular system. In this process, several types of work are described. For example, the *pressure-volume or external mechanical work* of the heart describes the energy utilized in the ejection of the stroke volume against aortic or pulmonary pressure. *Total cardiac work* is related to the energy used by the heart and is inferred from the metabolic oxygen demands. This parameter includes the internal as well as the external work. The *internal cardiac work* describes the energy dissipated in the form of heat or that utilized to open and close valve cusps as well as to carry out the normal basal tissue activities.

Pressure-Volume Diagram

The external work of the left ventricle can be illustrated graphically by relating instantaneous ventricular volume and pressure during the cardiac cycle. The area of the diagram produced for a single cardiac cycle is the pressure-volume or external mechanical work. In Figure 8–6 (see also Fig 7–10), the diagram shows that during the isovolumic phase of ventricular contraction, pressure increases, but cardiac volume remains constant. During the period of cardiac ejection, ventricular volume decreases rapidly, whereas the pressure continues to increase. With closure of the aortic valve, ventricular pressure falls rapidly during the period of isovolumic relaxation without change in ventricular volume. Finally, as the heart fills during diastole, there is a large increase in ventricular volume, with only a small increase in pressure. The area bounded by this loop (*ABCDA* in Fig 8–6) represents the net pressure-volume work. This area is the product of ventricular pressure and the stroke volume over the period of systole, i.e.,

$$W_{(t)} = \int_{V_o}^{V_i} P_v \cdot dV \qquad (8-5)$$

where W is the work, V_o is end-ventricular diastolic volume, V_i is end-ventricular systolic volume, P_v is ventricular pressure, and V is ventricular volume.

The shaded area under the diastolic portion of the loop shown in Figure 8–6 represents the work expended by venous return in stretching the

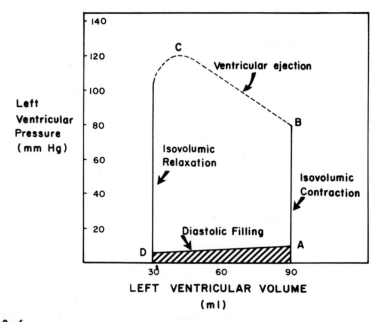

FIG 8–6.
Schematic diagram of the relationship between left ventricular pressure and volume for one cardiac cycle. The area *ABCDA* represents net pressure-volume work. See text for further discussion.

ventricular wall during the period of filling between beats. This energy is returned to the system during systole so that the total work is represented by the sum of the two areas.

Aortic pressure is frequently used instead of ventricular pressure to calculate left ventricular work. This pressure differs from left ventricular pressure in that some of its energy has been converted to kinetic or flow energy. Therefore, when aortic pressure is used, it must be corrected by the addition of a kinetic energy term. The equation becomes

$$W = \int_{V_o}^{V_i} P_a \cdot dV + \int_{V_o}^{V_i} \frac{1}{2} \rho v^2 dv \qquad (8\text{--}6)$$

where P_a is aortic pressure, ρ is the density of the blood, and v is the velocity of flow. During conditions of high-velocity flow, such as may occur with extreme levels of exercise or in other states where a large cardiac output is achieved, the kinetic energy term in the above equation may become significant; however, it is frequently disregarded because, under rest conditions, it accounts for only about 5% of the cardiac work.

Pressure and Volume Work

Cardiac work can be further classified according to the major load presented to the heart. For example, if the heart pumps a normal stroke volume against a higher than normal arterial pressure (increased afterload), the area added to the pressure-volume diagram will represent additional *"pressure" work* (Fig 8–7,A). In this case, the higher pressure will require a larger static effort on the part of the heart to raise and hold ventricular pressure equal to this increased load. By the same reasoning, if the heart moves a larger than normal stroke volume against the same arterial pressure, the extra work will represent added volume or dynamic work, and the fraction of the total work that is devoted to static work will decrease.

Myocardial Oxygen Consumption

The cost of cardiac activity, as discussed above, is met by the oxidative metabolism of energy sources. As a result, the utilization of oxygen by the myocardium can serve as a measure of its energy expenditure and total work. Oxygen utilization is usually expressed as milliliters of oxygen per minute per 100 gm of left ventricle ($m\dot{V}_{O_2}$). This is determined from the coronary blood flow and the arteriovenous oxygen difference across the left ventricle, as determined by sampling from the arterial system and the coronary sinus.

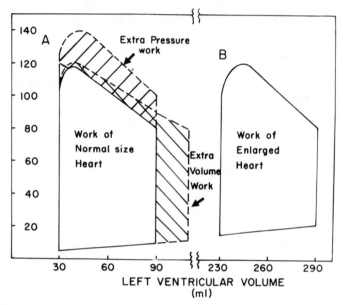

FIG 8–7.

A, schematic diagram illustrating the extra pressure work required to eject the normal stroke volume against a high systemic pressure and the extra volume work required to eject a large stroke volume against the normal arterial pressure. *B,* the work diagram for an enlarged heart ejecting the normal stroke volume against the same arterial pressure on the ordinate.

The basal metabolic needs of the myocardium without regard to the contraction process are about 2 ml/minute/100 gm or about 20% of the oxygen needs of the normal beating heart under basal conditions. An additional 0.04 ml of O_2 per minute per 100 gm is utilized as a direct consequence of cardiac electric activity. The remainder of the 8 to 15 ml or more of O_2 per minute per 100 gm consumed by the beating heart represents the energy used in pumping blood to the tissues.

It should be apparent from the above discussion why attempts to correlate $m\dot{V}_{O_2}$ with cardiac work have met with difficulties. It has been known, for example, since early work with the Starling heart-lung preparation, that pressure work was more costly in terms of oxygen consumption than the same volume work, due to the large amount of energy-consuming static work associated with the development of a high arterial pressure. In addition, because of the effect of heart size on the relationship between wall tension and ventricular pressure, work carried out in a dilated heart will require more oxygen than the same amount and kind of work performed by a normal-sized heart (Fig 8–8).

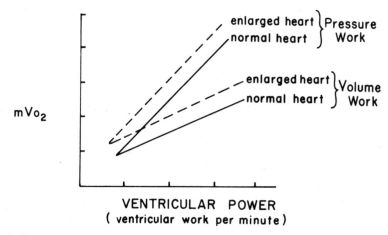

FIG 8–8.
Diagrammatic representation of myocardial oxygen consumption for the different levels of cardiac work performed as pressure or volume work in a normal or enlarged heart. Work is expressed as the cardiac pressure-volume work per minute, or myocardial power. (Based on data from Sarnoff S, et al: *Am J Physiol* 1958; 129:148; Rodbard SC, et al: *Am Heart J* 1959; 57:348, and Simann J: *Cardiovasc Res* 1974; 8:534.)

Efforts have been made to find other parameters of cardiac function that correlated better with $m\dot{V}_{O_2}$ than mechanical work. Attention was focused on the static work of the heart, and attempts were made to incorporate the duration of this effort as well as its magnitude. This led to the use of the area under the systolic portion of the ventricular pressure pulse as a *tension-time index*. This parameter (mean systolic pressure × the duration of systole × the heart rate) correlated well with $m\dot{V}_{O_2}$ provided there were no changes in myocardial contractility or heart size.

The peak total wall tension (T_{tw}) or the area under the T_{tw}-volume diagram* (see Fig 8–4) may be a more useful definitive determinant of myocardial energy utilization than is the tension-time index. In addition, $m\dot{V}_{O_2}$ is also modified by the level of myocardial contractility. For example, sympathetic stimulation or administration of positive inotropic drugs, such as digitalis or norepinephrine, increases both the rate of contractile energy utilization (V_{max}) and the number of force-generating sites (see Chapter 3). Thus, an increase in myocardial contractility will result in the expenditure of larger amounts of metabolic energy and thereby increase $m\dot{V}_{O_2}$. Finally, an elevation in the heart rate, in addition to its positive inotropic effect on the myocardium (see Chapter 3), also adds to the meta-

*Wall stress (σ) (equation 8–3) can be substituted for T_{tw}.

bolic needs for oxygen because of the increased number of cardiac contractions per minute (Fig 8–9).

The left ventricular pressure-volume diagram has recently provided a satisfactory method for quantitating the oxygen cost of cardiac work. As discussed in Chapter 7, the upper left-hand corner of the systolic ventricular pressure-volume loop lies on the end-systolic pressure-volume line while the slope of this relationship is determined by the contractile state of the myocardium (see Fig 7–12). The area of the pressure-volume loop represents external left ventricular mechanical stroke work (Fig 8–10). The remaining triangular area between the end-systolic and end-diastolic pressure-volume relationship has been related to the potential mechanical ventricular work that could have been performed if the systolic pressure was sufficiently low. Suga and co-workers have recently demonstrated that myocardial oxygen consumption is directly related to the sum of the potential and external stroke work.

This concept offers an explanation for the observation discussed earlier that the oxygen cost of pressure work is greater than that of volume work. As illustrated in Figure 8–11, the ventricle that ejects a small volume at high pressure (i.e., that performs mostly pressure work) has a greater area

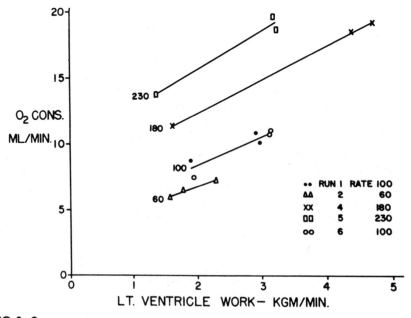

FIG 8–9.
Relationship between myocardial oxygen consumption and left ventricular work in the same dog heart at various heart rates. (From Berglund E, et al: *Acta Physiol Scand* 1958; 42:185. Used by permission.)

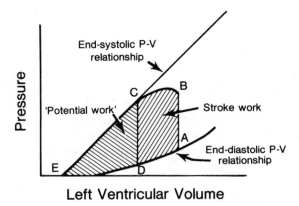

FIG 8–10.
Schematic illustration of left ventricular systolic pressure-volume *(P-V)* area. The pressure-volume loop area *ABCD* represents external stroke work, and the triangular area *DCE* represents end-systolic "potential" work. (Based on data of Suga H, Hisano R, Goto Y, et al: *Circ Res* 1983; 53:306.)

of "potential" work than the ventricle that ejects a large stroke volume at low pressure. In this illustration the external mechanical stroke work produced is the same for both ventricles, but the total of the potential and actual work and the oxygen consumption is greater for the ventricle that is pressure loaded.

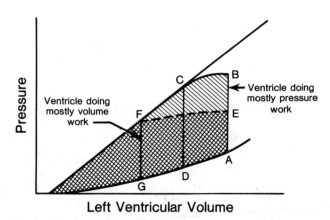

FIG 8–11.
Schematic diagram of two pressure-volume loops that represent the same external mechanical work. Loop *ABCD* represents predominantly pressure work and loop *AEFG* predominantly volume work. The *double-hatched* area shows the total external and potential work accomplished by the *AEFG* loop, and the total *single- and double-hatched* area shows the total external and potential work for the *ABCD* loop.

Summary

Metabolic energy is transferred to myocardial wall tension through the action of the contractile elements as modulated by their initial length and level of contractility. Wall tension is, in turn, converted into intracardiac pressure. The efficiency of this conversion is inversely related to the volume of the heart. The energy in the form of ventricular pressure is then utilized along with the energy added by contractile element shortening to eject the stroke volume into the circulation. The proportion of each of these energy sources utilized by the heart depends on the type of load.

CARDIAC EFFICIENCY

The mechanical efficiency of a machine is defined as the ratio of the useful work produced to the total energy expended. For the heart, this can be expressed as the ratio of external work to total work. In the beating heart, energy utilization is related to oxygen consumption. Therefore, in calculating the efficiency of the heart, $m\dot{V}_{O_2}$, along with the appropriate energy equivalent of 1 ml of oxygen, can be used for the energy term. To obtain net cardiac efficiency, oxygen consumption of the resting heart (non-beating) is subtracted from the total oxygen consumption. The work expression used in the numerator is calculated from the area of the pressure-volume diagram for the left ventricle times the heart rate. The equation becomes

$$\% \text{ net efficiency} = \frac{100 \times \text{cardiac work (kg-m/minute)}}{(m\dot{V}_{O_2 \text{ total}} - m\dot{V}_{O_2 \text{ resting}}) \times (2 \text{ kg-m/ml } O_2)} \qquad (8\text{--}8)$$

where $m\dot{V}_{O_2}$ is the myocardial oxygen consumption per minute, kg-m/minute means kilogram-meters per minute and kg-m/ml O_2 means kilogram-meters per milliliter of oxygen. When calculated in this fashion, the efficiency of the human left ventricle has been estimated to average about 23%.

It is of clinical interest that the efficiency with which the heart is able to respond to various work loads depends on the type of load as previously discussed. Aortic stenosis or arterial hypertension, for example, represents essentially a pressure load. With these conditions, the heart must increase the proportion of high-cost static work that goes into the total cardiac pressure-volume work. As a result, there is a disproportionate increase in the denominator of the efficiency equation, and cardiac efficiency is markedly reduced. In contrast, the increase in stroke volume that occurs with exercise or aortic insufficiency represents essentially a volume load for the heart. This requires only a small increase in m$\dot{V}_{O_2}$, and as a result, cardiac efficiency is not affected to the same degree as with a pressure load. In fact, under these circumstances, cardiac efficiency may be improved. This fact has led to the suggestion that moderate muscular exercise, such as provided by a golf game, is not ordinarily taxing to the heart provided the player does not become emotionally upset by missing a putt or having a poor drive. In that circumstance, an elevation in blood pressure will add considerably to the work of the heart and markedly reduce its efficiency.

A modest increase in heart rate will result in a corresponding increase in cardiac output. The greater output is achieved, in this case, at the cost of a decrease in efficiency because of (1) the increased metabolic energy that will be utilized due to the greater contractility associated with the faster rate and (2) the increase in internal work associated with the larger number of contractions per unit time. Similarly, the decreased efficiency of the failing heart is made worse when it is combined with the tachycardia that often accompanies heart failure.

SUMMARY

The heart requires a continuous supply of oxygen but can utilize a variety of substrates in addition to glucose as an energy source. The myocardial contractile machinery converts the energy of ATP into cardiac wall tension (stress). This ventricular force is interrelated to its internal pressure and heart size through the law of Laplace. As a result, a small heart can reduce ventricular wall tension during the period of ejection, while wall tension increases during the same period in a dilated heart. Cardiac hypertrophy has the compensatory effect of permitting a lower wall stress (wall tension per unit of myocardium) for the same developed pressure.

Cardiac work can be divided into internal and external (mechanical) work. Cardiac work used to produce pressure (pressure work) requires more oxygen than the same work utilized to move volume (volume work). Cardiac oxygen utilization and cardiac efficiency is related to the geometry of the ventricle, the level of myocardial contractility, the ratio of pressure to volume work, and the heart rate.

BIBLIOGRAPHY

Bing RJ: Cardiac metabolism. *Physiol Rev* 1965; 45:171.
Braunwald E: Control of myocardial oxygen consumption: Physiologic and clinical considerations. *Am J Cardiol* 1971; 27:416.

Bugaisky L, Zak R: Biological mechanisms of hypertrophy, in Fozzard HA, Habel E, Jennings RB, et al (eds): *The Heart and Cardiovascular System: Scientific Foundations*. New York, Raven Press, 1986, pp 1491–1506.

Burch GE, Ray CT, Cronvich JA: Certain mechanical peculiarities of the human cardiac pump in normal and diseased states. *Circulation* 1952; 5:504.

Burton AC: The importance of the size and shape of the heart. *Am Heart J* 1957; 54:801.

Katz AM: Contractile proteins of the heart. *Physiol Rev* 1970; 50:63.

Khalofbeigui F, Suga H, Sagawa K: Left ventricular systole pressure-volume area correlates with oxygen consumption. *Am J Physiol* 1979; 237:566.

McClellan G, Weisberg A, Winegrad S: Energy transport from mitochrondria to myofibril by a creatine phosphate shuttle in cardiac cells. *Am J Physiol* 1983; 245:C423.

Mirsky I: Elastic properties of the myocardium. A quantitative approach with physiological and clinical application, in Bern RM, Sperelakis N, Geiger SR (eds): *Handbook of Physiology, Section 2: The Cardiovascular System*, vol 1. Bethesda, American Physiological Society, 1979, pp 497–532.

Opie LH: Metabolism of the heart in health and disease. *Am Heart J* 1968; 76:685.

Rodbard SC, et al: Myocardial tension and oxygen uptake. *Circ Res* 1964; 14:139.

Sandler H, Dodge HT: Left ventricular tension and stress in man. *Circ Res* 1963; 13:91.

Schlant RC: Metabolism of the heart, in Hurst JW, Logue RB (eds): *The Heart*, ed 3. New York, McGraw-Hill Book Co, 1974.

Sonnenblick EH, et al: Velocity of contraction as a determinant of myocardial oxygen consumption. *Am J Physiol* 1965; 209:919.

Suga H: Total mechanical energy of a ventricle model and cardiac oxygen consumption. *Am J Physiol* 1979; 236:H498.

Suga H, Hisano R, Goto Y, et al: Effect of positive inotropic agents on the relationship between oxygen consumption and systolic pressure volume area in canine left ventricle. *Circ Res* 1983; 53:306.

Tarazi RC: The progression from hypertrophy to heart failure. *Hosp Prac [off]* 1983; 18:101.

Weber KT, Janicki JS: Myocardial oxygen consumption: The role of wall force and shortening. *Am J Physiol* 1977; 233:H421.

Weber KT, Janicki JS, et al: The contractile behavior of the heart and its functional coupling to the circulation. *Prog Cardiovasc Dis* 1982; 14:375.

Wiggers CJ: *Circulatory Dynamics*. New York, Grune & Stratton, 1952.

Wildenthal K, et al (eds): *Regulation of Cardiac Metabolism*. Dallas, American Heart Association, 1976.

Chapter 9 _____

Hemodynamics

Flow through the vascular system of the body is influenced by the unique characteristics of both the blood and the vascular system. These properties are summarized in this chapter and related to the physiology of the circulation. In a general sense, the forces that govern the movement of blood in the body are the same as those that apply to the flow of water in the plumbing system of a building. For this reason, the steady flow of fluid through a series of different-sized pipes will be considered first. The relationships developed for this simplified model will then be applied in an approximate manner to the circulation. Finally, the more complicated pulsatile flow of blood in the arteries will be discussed.

RHEOLOGY OF BLOOD

Streamlined Flow

Under normal circumstances, both the movement of water in a plumbing system and the flow of blood in the body are *streamlined*. In this type of flow, the cohesive attraction between fluid and vessels keeps the molecules of liquid that are in contact with the wall from moving. The next thin layer of fluid toward the center of the vessel slides past the stationary layer and so on until, at the center, the fluid moves at its fastest velocity (Fig 9–1). With this type of laminar flow, resistance results from friction between the concentric fluid layers and not from interactions between the fluid and wall of the tube.

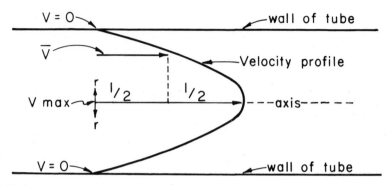

FIG 9–1.
Diagram of steady laminar flow of a Newtonian fluid in a rigid tube. The velocity profile increases parabolically with decreasing radical distance. The average velocity ($\bar{V}$) is half the maximal velocity (V_{max}) at the center of the tube. (Modified from McDonald DA: *Blood Flow in Arteries,* ed 2. Baltimore, Williams & Wilkins Co, 1974.)

Viscosity

During laminar flow, the friction between fluid layers sliding past each other tends to impede their movement. The *coefficient of viscosity* is defined as the ratio of the energy loss due to this internal resistance (shear stress) to the relative velocity of adjacent fluid layers (shear rate). In practical terms, an increase in the resistance between fluid layers will result in a relatively smaller change in the velocity gradient across the face of the vessel. As a result, the value of their ratio increases and the coefficient of viscosity becomes larger. For this reason, the viscosity coefficient of molasses, for example, is greater than the coefficient of a slippery solution such as water.

Viscosity is measured in newtons times seconds per square meter (in the centimeter-gram-second [CGS] system the unit is the *poise*, where 1 poise equals 1 dyne · second/sq cm). It is difficult to measure viscosity directly, and it is often easier in dynamic studies to use the *viscosity ratio* or *relative viscosity*. This dimensionless ratio relates the viscosity of the test fluid to that of water. It usually is obtained by comparing the flow rate of the two solutions under the same conditions of temperature, pressure head, and size of tube. The relative viscosity of plasma is about 1.8, whereas whole blood normally has a value of 3 to 4.

Technically, blood is a non-newtonian fluid because, like other suspensions of colloidal particles, its viscosity increases when the flow becomes very slow (Fig 9–2). This property, known as *anomalous viscosity*, usually is not of importance in the body. However, when cardiac output is markedly reduced, as in cardiovascular shock, venous flow may be slowed

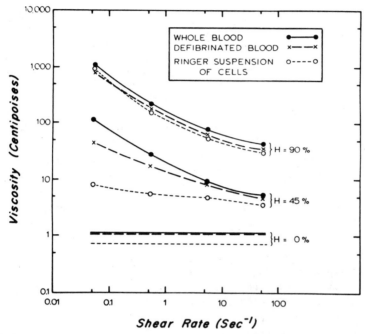

FIG 9–2.

Relationship between logarithm of viscosity and logarithm of flow rate for blood, defibrinated blood, and Ringer's suspension of cells at hematocrit reading (H) of 90%, 45%, and 0%. (Modified from Chien S, et al: *J Appl Physiol* 1966; 21:81.)

to the point that increased viscosity becomes an important factor in determining the movement of blood through those vessels.

In addition to flow-dependent changes, the viscosity of blood moving in a small vessel is related to the diameter of the tube. This is known as the *Fabraeus-Lindqvist effect*. An explanation for this phenomenon is suggested by the process of *axial streaming*. In this condition, erythrocytes become concentrated at the center of the vessel during laminar flow. This accumulation results from the rapid rate of change in the velocity profile near the wall. This velocity gradient pulls the long axis of the erythrocytes parallel to the direction of flow and forces the cell toward the center of the tube where the flow is more stable (Fig 9–3). This process leaves a relatively cell-free sleeve of plasma near the wall and may lead to *plasma skimming*. In this condition, the red cell concentration may be markedly reduced in the small side vessels that are filled from the plasma layer at the edge of the axial stream.

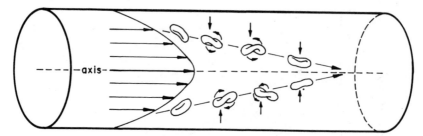

FIG 9–3.
Illustration of rotational effect of velocity profile on erythrocytes that tends to line the cells with the axial flow and concentrate them at the center of the tube.

Significant axial streaming will not occur in vessels larger than 1 mm in diameter because in these tubes the velocity profile changes more slowly and the concentrating force is insufficient to offset the dispersing effect of cell collisions.

The relatively cell-free marginal zone associated with axial streaming becomes proportionally larger as the lumen of the tube is decreased. As a result, the viscosity of the blood appears to be reduced. The Fahraeus-Lindqvist effect may play a role in decreasing resistance to the flow of blood in the arterioles and venules (see below). However, this phenomenon does not occur in capillaries because the red blood cells (RBCs) squeeze through the lumen one at a time. This action tends to isolate the plasma into separate units between the cells and prevents continuity of plasma flow.

The viscosity of blood is also affected by changes in its cellular composition. At normal or low hematocrit* levels, changes in the size of the cell fraction result in a nearly proportional change in viscosity (Fig 9–4). However, if the hematocrit level is elevated above the normal value of 40% to 45%, blood viscosity undergoes a proportionally larger change with further increase in the cell fraction.

In clinical conditions in which the hematocrit level is elevated, as in dehydration, cyanotic congenital heart disease, or polycythemia (increase in total number of RBCs), the increased viscosity of the blood may be sufficient to increase cardiac work. This factor may become of significance in patients with long-standing pulmonary emphysema or other chronic lung diseases who have *cor pulmonale* (failure of the right heart due to a combination of chronic high pulmonary vascular resistance and anoxia). In contrast, patients with anemia may find the associated reduction in blood vis-

---

*The hematocrit is the fraction of the blood volume occupied by cells. It is measured by centrifuging a sample of blood and expressing the volume of packed cells as a percentage of the total volume.

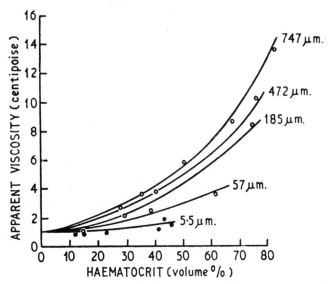

FIG 9–4.
Blood viscosity plotted against hematocrit level of blood flowing in glass tubes of various diameters. Because of the Fahraeus-Lindqvist effect, the viscosity approaches that of plasma for very small tubes despite high hematocrit levels. (From Burton AC, in Wolstenholme GEW, Knight J [eds]: *Circulatory and Respiratory Mass Transport,* Ciba Foundation Symposium. Boston, Little, Brown & Co, 1969. Used by permission.)

cosity due to the lower number of red blood cells to be helpful by increasing blood flow to the tissues.

BIOPHYSICAL FACTORS THAT REGULATE BULK FLOW

The relationship between pressure head, size of the tube, and steady flow in a small rigid tube was independently described in the middle of the last century by the German engineer G. Hagen and the French physician Jean Poiseuille. This relationship, as formulated by others, has become the *Hagen-Poiseuille law*. It is stated

$$\dot{Q} = \frac{\Delta P \pi r^4}{8 l \eta} \qquad (9\text{–}1)$$

where $\dot{Q}$ is the volume flow per unit time, ΔP is the pressure head, r is the radius, l is the length of the tube, and η is the viscosity of the fluid.

Although this relationship holds only for the steady streamlined flow of a Newtonian fluid, its application to the circulation permits a qualitative understanding of the flow of blood and other fluids in the body. For example, equation 12–1, presented in Chapter 12 that describes the bulk flow through the capillary wall, becomes the *Hagen-Poiseuille equation* when the bulk flow constant (K_B) is written in its expanded form as

$$K_B = \frac{\pi r^4}{8l\eta} \qquad (9\text{–}2)$$

The Swiss physicist Daniel Bernoulli established in 1738 that the energy of fluid moving in a pipe or of blood flowing in a vessel can exist in three forms: (1) *pressure*—usually measured as the lateral pressure exerted at right angles to the direction of flow and representing potential energy at the point of measurement that is available for conversion to kinetic energy or for utilization to overcome resistance; (2) *gravitational energy*—the potential energy of the fluid that exists because of its position or level; and (3) *kinetic energy*—the energy contained in the moving mass of fluid.

These three forms of energy are interchangeable. For example, if the flow in a tube is stopped by closing a faucet at the lower end (Fig 9–5), all of the fluid energy in the tube, neglecting gravitational factors, will exist in the form of pressure. If the faucet is opened, the amount of pressure

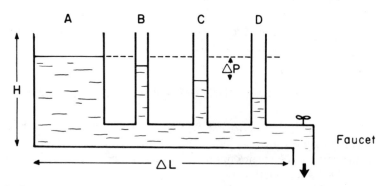

FIG 9–5.
Schema showing flow of a Newtonian fluid from a reservoir *(A)* through a horizontal tube. When the faucet is closed, lateral pressure in the horizontal tube (as shown by height of the liquid in the side tubes *B, C,* and *D)* will be equal to pressure of the fluid in the reservoir *(H)*. When the faucet is open, pressure is converted to kinetic energy, and the lateral pressure along the horizontal tube will fall. The pressure gradient *ΔP/ΔL* between the reservoir and side tube *C* is shown.

energy that is converted to kinetic energy will depend on the rate of flow in the tube. As a result, if the flow is fast, less potential pressure energy is left and the lateral pressure will drop rapidly along the length of the tube. If the flow rate in the horizontal tube remains constant so that there is no change in the kinetic energy between its ends, the drop in pressure over the length of the tube will represent the energy lost overcoming friction. This drop in pressure can be expressed by rearranging the Hagen-Poiseuille equation as follows:

$$\Delta P = \frac{8l\eta\dot{Q}}{\pi r^4} \tag{9-3}$$

Resistance

Resistance can be defined by means of *Ohm's law*. When applied to a dc electrical circuit, this law states

$$\text{current (I)} = \frac{\text{electromotive force (E)}}{\text{resistance (R)}}$$

Ohm's law can be applied to steady nonturbulent flow of fluid in a tube with a constant radius as follows:

$$\dot{Q} = \frac{\text{pressure head } (\Delta P)}{\text{resistance (R)}}$$

Rearranging provides:

$$R = \frac{\Delta P}{\dot{Q}}$$

From equation 9-1

$$R = \frac{8l\eta}{\pi r^4} \tag{9-4}$$

This provides a definition of resistance that is a function of the size of the tube and the viscosity of the fluid.

In a tube of varying diameter, the velocity of flow at any point along the tube is inversely related to the cross-sectional area of the tube and directly related to the volume flow through the tube. This is shown by:

$$v = \frac{\dot{Q}}{\pi r^2}$$ (9–5)

where v is the velocity of flow, and r is the radius of the tube. Rearranged, the relationship becomes

$$\dot{Q} = v \pi r^2$$

Substituting into equation 9–3 and rearranging provides

$$v = \frac{\Delta P}{R \pi r^2}$$ (9–6)

These manipulations show that the loss of pressure (ΔP) due to the constant flow of fluid in a tube is directly related to the resistance offered by the tube. The physiologic importance is that a great deal of energy is required to overcome resistance for rapid flow through a narrow tube.

General Rules for Steady Streamlined Flow of Newtonian Fluid

The biophysical factors just discussed that govern the steady flow of fluid through a series of tubes such as the vascular system can be summarized in three general rules:

1. Flow is directly related to the pressure and fourth power of the radius and is inversely related to length of tube and viscosity of fluid.
2. Resistance to flow is proportional to both length of tube and viscosity of fluid and is inversely related to the fourth power of the radius.
3. When volume flow is constant, velocity is inversely related to the cross-sectional area of the flow path.

Total Peripheral Resistance

The concept of vascular resistance developed for steady flow through a single vessel is frequently extended in a qualitative manner to the entire circulation. This is accomplished by ignoring the pulsatile nature of blood flow in the arterial segment and using cardiac output and arterial pressure minus mean right atrial pressure, respectively, as the flow and pressure variables. Total peripheral resistance (TPR) is determined as follows:

$$\text{TPR} = \frac{\text{mean arterial pressure} - \text{mean right atrial pressure (mm Hg)}}{\text{cardiac output (ml/minute)}}$$

This computation is sometimes simplified by considering mean right atrial pressure to be zero. Total peripheral resistance (TPR) is usually expressed in empirical peripheral resistance units of mm Hg per ml per minute. Total peripheral resistance determined in this way can only be an approximation since blood flow is pulsatile in the arterial portion of the circulation and the pressure-flow relation for this part of the circulation, as discussed below, should be quantitated in terms of fluid impedance. Nevertheless, calculation of TPR is useful as a way of clinically estimating changes in arteriolar resistance.

PRESSURE-MEAN FLOW RELATIONSHIPS IN THE VASCULAR SYSTEM

The Hagen-Poiseuille relationship that describes the steady flow of fluid in a single tube is modified in the body by the parallel arrangement of the circulation (see Fig 2–17). Under steady-state conditions, there is continuity of flow so that the same volume of blood per minute moves through each anatomical subdivision. This geometric organization is illustrated in the simplified schema shown in Figure 9–6. As arterial flow is pulsatile, this discussion must be applied to that portion of the circulation only in an approximate manner. Oscillatory flow in these larger vessels will be discussed below.

In the model shown in Figure 9–6, flow starts from a single relatively large aorta and proceeds through a series of branching, essentially parallel, vessels until it reaches the arterioles. Each arteriole supplies a capillary network made up of very narrow tubes. Again, the essentially parallel arrangement is maintained. Flow from each capillary bed is collected and returned to the vena cava via a coalescing series of progressively widening veins.

The number of arteries increases, and their individual diameters become smaller as flow proceeds toward the capillary bed. These dimensional changes are roughly proportional so that the total cross-sectional area only increases slowly through the arterial portion of the circulation. At the level of arteriole, the total cross-sectional area of all the parallel vessels has been estimated to range from 12 to 125 times that of the aorta. While this appears to be a sizable increase, in relationship to the very large increase in total

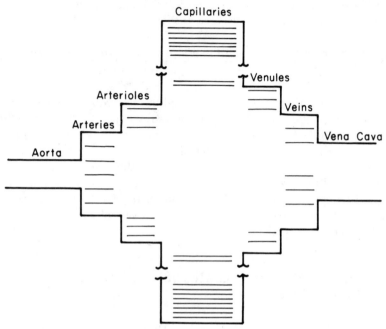

FIG 9–6.
Schema of vascular system showing total cross-sectional area of various subdivisions.

cross-sectional area that occurs in the capillaries, it can be considered to be only moderate. As a result, the flow velocity (equation 9–6) remains relatively rapid through the entire arterial system (Fig 9–7). As described above, considerable energy must be expended to maintain the relatively rapid flow through the small-diameter, high-resistance arterioles; this loss of energy is reflected in a major drop in blood pressure in this segment.

In the capillaries, the total cross-sectional area increases 700 to 800 times, and the vascular stream widens into a large lake. Due to the reciprocal relationship described earlier between velocity and total cross-sectional area, capillary flow becomes very slow. This permits ample time for capillary exchange, and it allows blood to flow through the small capillaries with minimal loss of energy even though the resistance of the individual capillary vessel is high.

The essentially parallel arrangement of the vessels in each capillary network also permits the high total flow resistance of that unit to be lower than might be predicted from the small size of the individual vessels. This can be shown by a simple example. Three parallel capillaries are assigned the resistance values of 5, 10, and 20 units, respectively. Addition of par-

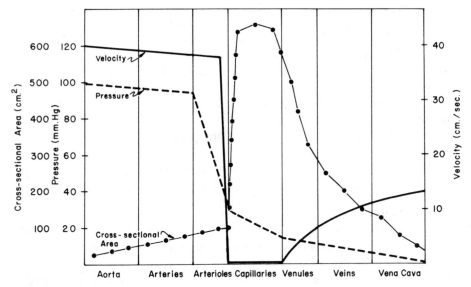

FIG 9–7.

Graph showing changes in cross-sectional area of the vascular bed, average velocity of flow, and mean pressure in various segments of the circulation.

allel flow resistances uses the same reciprocal arrangement as employed in adding parallel electric resistances. Thus, resistance of this unit is determined by the following equation:

$$\frac{1}{R_t} = \frac{1}{R_1} + \frac{1}{R_2} + \frac{1}{R_3} \qquad (9–7)$$

in which R_1, R_2, and R_3 are the individual resistance values. In this illustration, the total resistance (R_t) becomes

$$R_t = \frac{1}{1/5 + 1/10 + 1/20}$$
$$= 2.85$$

Because of this reciprocal relationship, the resistance of the total unit, as shown in this example, is less than any of the individual resistance values. This relationship has physiologic importance. Despite their individual narrow caliber, the large number of short parallel vessels in any capillary bed provides an aggregate resistance that is relatively low. This, plus the slow velocity of flow in each individual vessel, requires only a small pressure drop across the vascular segment to maintain capillary perfusion.

The coalescence of the venous system toward the vena cava permits the total vascular cross-sectional area to be reduced, whereas the diameter of individual veins is increased. As a consequence, when the blood approaches the vena cava, the velocity increases moderately. However, the total cross-sectional area of each segment of the venous system never decreases to the level of the corresponding part of the arterial system, and the velocity of venous flow remains relatively slow. As a result, the energy loss in this segment of the circulation is low, and the pressure declines only moderately.

To summarize, in the model of the circulation, there is a small drop in pressure between the aorta and small arteries because of their low resistance. The large pressure loss in the arterioles is caused by their small individual radius and relatively fast velocity of flow. The pressure drop over the capillary bed is relatively small because of the relatively low total resistance due to their parallel arrangement and the slow flow in that area. There is a smaller loss of pressure in the venous system than on the arterial side of the circulation because of its large cross-sectional area and slower velocity of flow.

Turbulent Flow

When the velocity exceeds a critical level for the size of the vessel and physical characteristics of the contents, the silent movement of one fluid layer past the next changes and the flow becomes *turbulent*. The flow develops swirls and vortices and becomes noisy (Fig 9–8). The English engineer Osborne Reynolds showed in 1883 that the point at which turbulence begins can be predicted from the following relationship:

$$R_e = \frac{Vd\rho}{\eta} \tag{9-8}$$

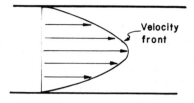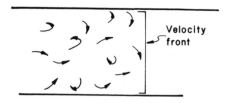

FIG 9–8.
Left, diagram showing laminar flow with its parabolic velocity front. *Right,* turbulent flow with swirls and vortices. This type of flow has a square velocity front.

R_e is the dimensionless term, the *Reynolds number*, V is the average linear velocity, d is the diameter of the tube, ρ is the density, and η is the viscosity of the fluid. When the Reynold's number of blood exceeds about 2,000, turbulence occurs.*

Under normal body conditions, turbulence is most apt to develop at the aortic or pulmonic valve orifice during cardiac ejection because of the fast flow velocity in this area and the relatively small size of these openings. This tendency for turbulent flow is important for proper positioning of the aortic valve cusps (see Chapter 2). The role of turbulence in the production of murmurs is discussed below.

When turbulent flow is fully developed, the velocity profile changes from the parabolic shape of laminar flow and becomes rectangular. Now, all fluid molecules travel at about the same linear speed in relation to the vessel wall. Extra energy is, however, utilized to maintain the eddy currents in their random motion. As a result, the relationship between the pressure head and blood flow no longer follows the linear Hagen-Poiseuille relationship (described above) for laminar flow, and instead, the flow becomes proportional to the square root of the driving pressure (Fig 9–9).

The fact that turbulent flow requires the expenditure of more energy than does streamlined flow has clinical significance. With aortic stenosis, for example, the increased cardiac afterload due to the resistance of the small valve orifice and the additional energy required by the turbulent flow in the area of the stenotic valve will require the heart to expend extra energy to eject its normal stroke volume.

Cardiovascular Sounds

Characteristic sounds, usually called murmurs or bruits, are heard over a blood vessel in which the flow is turbulent. For years it was thought that these sounds resulted from the oscillatory nature of the transfer between pressure and kinetic flow energy in the turbulent eddy currents. Although this vibratory action undoubtedly plays a role, engineering studies suggest that the level of energy produced by turbulence alone is insufficient to account for audible sound and other mechanisms must also be involved.

In addition to producing random turbulence, narrowing of the lumen of a blood vessel also will tend to produce a fluctuating vortex trail in the flow below the lesion. In this way the obstruction will act like an aeolian wind harp (Fig 9–10). It is interesting that in these Aegean instruments the round strings do not vibrate; rather, the wind traveling past each string

*If the radius of the vessel is used instead of the diameter in calculating the Reynold's number, the critical value will be 1,000.

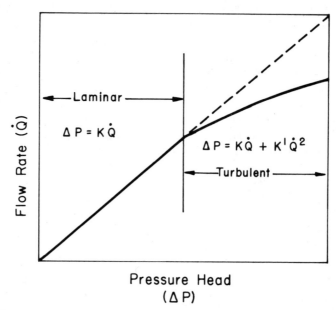

FIG 9–9.
Pressure-flow curve for streamlined and turbulent flow of a Newtonian fluid. With turbulent flow, energy is expended in eddy formation so that a greater driving force is required for the same bulk flow rate. Slope of the F-P curve changes when the flow becomes turbulent and begins to decrease progressively with increasing flow. This indicates a progressive decrease in flow conductance (increase in resistance).

produces an alternating wake as it is shed from one side and then the other. This trail flutters back and forth like a flag waving in a strong breeze. This wake then produces a series of vortices to form a van Karman trail in the stream below the string. The rate at which these vortices are produced by a wind harp determines the fundamental frequency of the tone produced. In the vascular system, such a vortex trail soon degenerates below the ob-

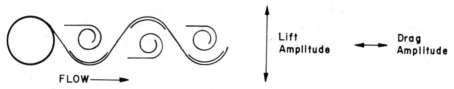

FIG 9–10.
Diagrammatic representation of the alternating wake beyond the string of an aeolian harp. The direction and relative strength of both lift and drag fluctuations are shown. (Modified from Bruns DL: *Am J Med* 1959; 27:360.)

struction into a turbulent jet. However, the combination of the aeolian mechanism, the turbulent jet, and the general turbulence produced in the vascular system by the obstruction apparently releases sufficient energy below the obstruction at right angles to the vascular flow to set the vessel wall in vibration and to produce an audible sound or murmur that may be heard with a stethoscope over the vessel.

The characteristic sound of murmurs produced by obstruction to the flow of blood in the vascular system varies from a semipure tone (musical murmur) to a more random type of noise without obvious harmonics (blowing or noisy murmur). The specific type depends on the dominant production factor. The aeolian mechanism is more apt to produce a musical murmur, whereas the random motion resulting from eddy currents and turbulence is more likely to produce sound vibrations without a dominant frequency.

PULSATILE FLOW IN ARTERIES

Vascular Impedance

The relationship between pressure and flow in the arterial segment of the circulation is more complicated than indicated by the analysis of steady-state flow just presented. The pulsatile nature of arterial pressure and flow combined with the elastic properties of the vessels, viscosity and inertial nature of blood, and the variable capacity and geometry of the vascular system introduce phase relationships between pressure and flow that are similar to the relationship between voltage and current in an ac electric circuit. This follows because in a sinusoidally oscillating system containing both capacitance, resistive, and inductive elements, peak pressure and flow are separated (the phase angle) because of the alternating storage and discharge of the capacitance. Mathematically, these factors can be combined into a single vector force, the *impedance*. This complex mathematical quantity is more appropriate for the study of arterial circulatory dynamics than the resistance value used in the discussion of mean flow.

Analysis of arterial input impedance is further complicated by the nonsymmetric form of the arterial pressure and flow pulse. These fluctuations may, however, be mathematically divided by harmonic or *Fourier analysis* into a mean value, a fundamental sine wave, and a series of harmonic waves, each with a different amplitude and phase angle. When these waves are placed in the proper juxtaposition, i.e., with the proper phase angle, and are mathematically added, they will reconstitute the original wave form (Fig 9–11). Analysis of cardiovascular pulses usually requires only a set of four or five harmonics to provide a reasonable degree of accuracy as

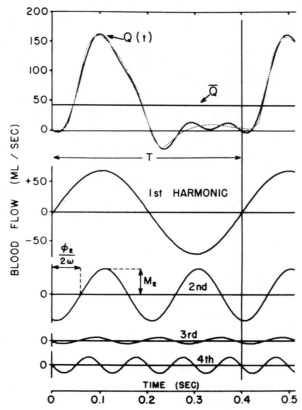

FIG 9–11.
Example of a Fourier analysis of a blood flow pulse from the pulmonary artery. The original pulse is shown at the top *(dotted line)* along with the pulse *(solid line)* reconstituted from the four harmonics shown below. (From Bergel DH, Milnor WR: *Circ Res* 1965; 16:401. Used by permission.)

the fundamental and first harmonics account for nearly 80% of the pulse form.

Like electrical impedance, vascular impedance* has two parts: (1) a modulus that represents the ratio of the peak amplitude of a sinusoidal pressure oscillation to the sinusoidal flow oscillation and (2) a phase angle that indicates the time difference between the sinusoidal pressure and flow (Fig 9–12). It is important to recognize, however, that in the calculation of electrical impedance, only one sine wave frequency (for example, 60 cps)

---

*The impedance vector is determined mathematically in the complex plane as the ratio of capacitance and resistive factors.

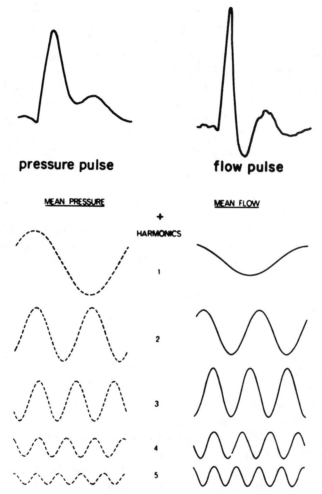

pressure pulse   **flow pulse**

MEAN PRESSURE   MEAN FLOW

\+

HARMONICS

1

2

3

4

5

FIG 9–12.
Determination of vascular impedance. Pressure and flow pulses are each resolved into a mean value and a series of harmonic sine waves. (Modified from O'Rourke MF, Taylor MG: *Circ Res* 1966; 18:126. Used by permission.)

is usually involved. Under this condition, a single impedance modulus and phase angle will reflect the complex interaction of the resistance and reactance parameters of the system. In contrast, the more complicated arterial pulse as described above contains a number of individual sinusoidal pressure and flow oscillations. Thus vascular impedance cannot be accurately described by a single modulus or phase angle; rather, the circulatory pressure and flow pulse must first be converted into its sinusoidal components and the impedance expressed as a series or spectrum of individual moduli and phase angles over the range of harmonic frequencies used in the analysis (Fig 9–13). Nevertheless, an average impedance value is sometimes used in describing the impedance characteristics of a vascular bed.

Analysis of impedance data obtained from the vascular system is complicated and still open to some question. Nevertheless, this procedure has provided a powerful analytic method for understanding the dynamics of the circulation. Some of the implications of this mathematical treatment of pressure and flow data are summarized below. Interested readers are referred to specific sources listed in the bibliography for more detailed information.

The impedance modulus for a vascular bed during a state of continuous flow (i.e., at an oscillation frequency of zero) is the resistance for the unit, as described previously in the discussion of nonpulsatile flow. When oscillatory flow is present, inertial, elastic, and capacitance properties of the system act to impede the movement of blood. These factors combine to give a characteristic impedance profile for the vascular bed under study. This value is called the *input impedance* when it also includes the opposition to flow produced by reflected pressure waves. This aspect is discussed further below.

CONTOUR OF THE ARTERIAL PULSE

Generation of the aortic pulse by action of the heart was described in Chapter 4. The rapid increase in proximal aortic pressure produced by left ventricular ejection (the arterial pulse) propagates toward the periphery in the same manner as a pressure pulse in an elastic tube. The physical characteristics of the arterial system cause the form of this pulse to change as it progresses through the large and small arteries toward the capillary bed (Fig 9–14). The upstroke becomes steeper, and the pulse wave becomes more triangular. At the periphery, the sharp systolic peak is followed by a prominent dicrotic oscillation. Systolic pressure increases as the pulse travels away from the heart, whereas diastolic and mean pressure decrease slightly. By the time the pulse reaches the lower femoral artery, the pulse pressure may have increased as much as 50%. This phenomenon underlies the fact that systolic blood pressure is normally 20 to 30 mm Hg higher in the legs than in the arms. The *incisura*, which marks closure of the aortic valve, is prominent in recordings from the aortic arch. It becomes slurred and is lost in the distal arteries. In addition, a secondary positive wave occurs immediately after the incisura in the aortic arch. The foot of this

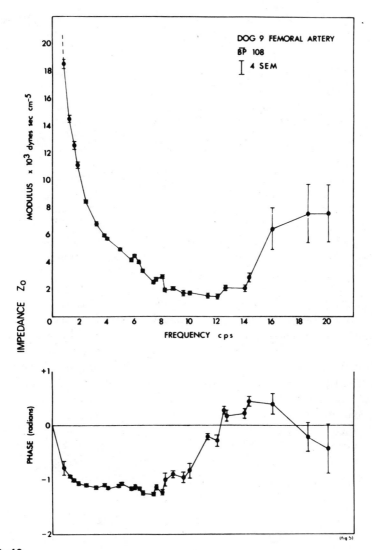

FIG 9–13.
Graph of vascular impedance of the dog femoral artery showing the modulus *(top)* and the phase *(bottom)*. Data from 57 pulses obtained during control conditions at various heart rates. (From O'Rourke MF, Taylor MG: *Circ Res* 1966; 18:126. Used by permission.)

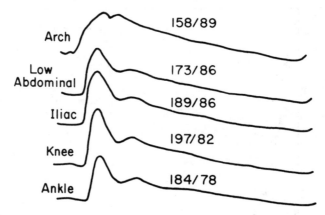

Arch 158/89
Low Abdominal 173/86
Iliac 189/86
Knee 197/82
Ankle 184/78

FIG 9–14.
Pressure pulses recorded from various locations in aorta and femoral artery. (Modified from Remington JW, O'Brien LJ: *Am J Physiol* 1970; 218:437.)

secondary wave is defined by the *dicrotic notch*. This reflected or dicrotic wave occurs progressively later in more distal parts of the arterial system.

The mechanism responsible for changes in the arterial pulse has been elucidated by recent studies of pulse wave reflection in both elastic tubes and arteries by McDonald, O'Rourke, Murgo, and others. Although physiologists differ as to the details, it is now generally recognized that some of the energy imparted to the blood by ventricular contraction is reflected back toward the heart from various sites in the circulation. These backward pressure waves merge with the forward moving wave to produce the characteristic form of the arterial pulse. The high-frequency vibrations produced during aortic valve closure are quickly damped by the viscous and inertial properties of blood and the vascular wall. These rapid components are lost, and the pulse assumes a rounder, smoother shape (see Fig 9–14) by the time it reaches the carotid or femoral arteries.

Pulse Wave Reflections

In the iliac artery of the dog, summation of the forward pulse wave and the reflected wave from nearby sites in the leg takes place while arterial pressure is still maximal. As a result, the pulse wave is amplified, systolic pressure is increased, and the form of the pulse becomes peaked. Passage of this reflected wave back toward the heart (Fig 9–15), along with reflected waves from other sites in the circulation, leads to a diastolic pressure wave following the incisura in the proximal aorta. At the same time, passage of the primary pulse wave into the lower legs results in a second reflection

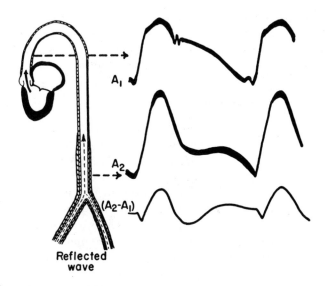

FIG 9–15

Drawing showing distortion produced in arterial pulse wave as it travels away from the heart. The primary pulse contour A_1 is shown as recorded from the arch of the aorta; A_2 is the pulse recorded from the distal aorta. The difference between these pulses $(A_2 - A_1)$ is the reflected pulse wave that travels toward the heart from the arterioles. (Modified from Rushmer RF: *Cardiovascular Dynamics*, ed 3. Philadelphia, WB Saunders Co, 1970. Used by permission.)

from sites in the foot that provides further systolic amplification at the knee and a prominent diastolic wave in the iliac artery.

Despite the increase in the peak systolic pressure as the pulse moves away from the heart, blood flows from the central to the peripheral arteries. Pressure energy is lost overcoming resistance so that mean arterial pressure falls almost linearly with distance from the larger to smaller vessels. Superimposed on this pressure drop are the oscillations due to changes in systolic and, to some extent, diastolic pressure. Forward flow, however, is maintained by the mean pressure gradient directed toward the periphery.

Wave Reflection and Abnormal Pulse Contour

Arterial distensibility is reduced with age or the occurrence of arteriosclerosis. Pulse wave velocity is increased in such patients. As a result, the early return of the reflected waves from the periphery can lead to disappearance of the diastolic wave, a late systolic peak in the pulse, and increase in the pulse pressure. This is discussed further in Chapter 10. In contrast, in patients with hypovolemic shock (see Chapter 15), the high level of arteriolar vasoconstriction causes increased peripheral pulse reflections while the low blood pressure causes a slower pulse wave velocity. This can result in a further reduction in the pulse pressure and the presence of a prominent diastolic wave in the peripheral pulse.

Source of Reflected Waves

A pressure wave reflected from a point downstream from the site of measurement will oppose the forward movement of fluid, thus adding to the impedance of the system. Based on studies of reflected waves in electric transmission lines and elastic tubes, the effect of the reflected wave on the impedance modulus will be minimal at a distance that is one quarter of a wavelength away from the reflection site and will be maximal at a distance of one-half wavelength. The length of a traveling wave is the velocity divided by the frequency. As a consequence, determination of the minimal modulus of impedance over a spectrum of frequencies will permit an estimation of the distance between the site of reflection and measurement.

Additional information regarding reflected waves can be obtained from changes in the impedance phase angle. In an ideal elastic system filled with a nonviscous fluid and with total reflection at one end (i.e., a closed-end tube), pressure and flow are 90 degrees out of phase at the point of reflection. This relationship changes 180 degrees at the node of the wave, and flow now leads pressure. In such an ideal system, the impedance phase angle will change from -90 degrees to $+90$ degrees at a distance that is one-quarter wavelength from the reflection site. In the vascular system, the magnitude of this phase shift will depend on, among other things, the amount of the wave energy that is reflected. The change in phase angle may, however, be used to indicate the proportion of the incident wave that is reflected.*

The input impedance modulus for the femoral artery of the dog shown in Figure 9–13 reached minimal value, and the phase angle reversed at a frequency of 12 cps. It is interesting that, despite the complicated geometry of the femoral arterial bed, these data suggest that the femoral arterial system behaves as if there is only one reflecting site located a short distance below the knee. It is probable that this site represents a composite effect of a number of reflected waves, and the indicated reflection is from a virtual rather than an actual site.

The changes in vascular impedance, just described for the femoral bed, are minimized or abolished by intra-arterial injection of acetylcholine

---

*A reflection coefficient can be calculated from the characteristic input impedance and the impedance of the system below the reflection site.

(which produces vasodilation of the small arteries and arterioles) and are increased by injection of the vasoconstrictor norepinephrine. These changes suggest that the small arteries, and particularly the arterioles, are the major sources of the reflected waves.

In addition to supplying information about reflection sites, the vascular impedance profile furnishes data on the energy cost of moving blood through the circulation. Figure 9–16 shows a spectrum of the modulus of impedance for the aorta. Impedance is quite high at zero frequency (the resistance) but falls rapidly as the frequency increases and then remains essentially constant above a frequency of 2 cps. This suggests that the impedance presented to the forward flow of blood by the circulation is reduced as the heart rate increases up to about 120 beats per minute. Furthermore, the impedance at heart rates above this value remains much lower than would be predicted by the resistance value calculated for mean flow.

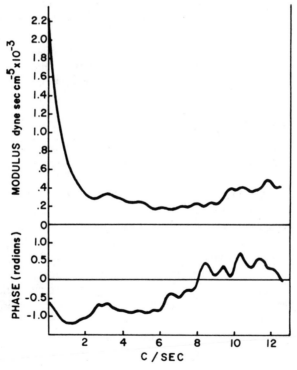

FIG 9–16.
Aortic impedance showing modulus and phase. (Redrawn from Taylor MG: *Circ Res* 1966; 19:585. Used by permission.)

PULSATILE WORK

The energy cost for the movement of blood through the arterial system can be divided into two components: (1) the steady-state work used largely to overcome arteriolar resistance and (2) pulsatile work dissipated in the rise and fall of the arterial pulse. Because of the low-input impedance of the arterial system at normal heart rates (see Fig 9–13), the latter value is estimated to be only 5% to 15% of total left ventricular work. In the presence of hypertension or large-vessel arteriosclerosis, more energy is used in generating arterial pulsations so that in these disease states the pulsatile work may be appreciably increased.

SUMMARY

Blood is a suspension of colloidal particles that undergoes a change in viscosity when its flow is slow (anomalous viscosity) or travels through a small diameter vessel (Fahraeus-Lindqvist effect). Under normal conditions, steady blood flow in vessels is streamlined and related to the pressure head, size of the vessel, and the blood viscosity (Hagen-Poiseuille law). The resistance of the vessel for such flow is the pressure head divided by the volume flow. When applied to the entire circulation, that relationship determines the total peripheral resistance.

The major loss of circulatory pressure occurs in the arterioles due to their high resistance to flow (small diameter and fast flow). Capillary flow is slow due to its large total cross-sectional area. The pressure drop in these vessels is low due to the slow flow and their parallel arrangement. The pressure loss in the venous system is less than in the corresponding arterial segment due to its larger cross-sectional area and slower flow.

Turbulent flow is noisy and requires more energy than streamlined flow. Turbulence and a fluctuating wake are involved in the production of cardiovascular sounds. Analysis of the pulsatile blood flow in the large arteries makes use of the complex quantity, impedance, rather than resistance as used for steady flow. The contour of the arterial pulse generated by cardiac ejection is modified as it travels toward the periphery by reflected pressure waves. The upstroke becomes steeper, systolic pressure increases, and the pulse becomes more triangular in shape.

BIBLIOGRAPHY

Attinger EO (ed): *Pulsatile Blood Flow.* New York, McGraw-Hill Book Co, 1964.

Avolio AP, et al: A comparative study of pulsatile arterial hemodynamics in rabbits and guinea pigs. *Am J Physiol* 1976; 230:868.

Bruns DL: A general theory of the cause of murmurs in the cardiovascular system. *Am J Med* 1959; 27:360.

Byliss LE: Rheology of blood and lymph, in Frey-Wyssling A (ed): *Deformation and Flow in Biological Systems.* Amsterdam, Elsevier North-Holland Publishing Co, 1952.

Finkelstein SM, Collins VR: Vascular hemodynamic impedance measurement. *Prog Cardiovasc Dis* 1982; 24:401.

Fishman AP, Richards DW (eds): *Circulation of the Blood: Men and Ideas.* New York, Oxford University Press, 1964.

Gow BS: Circulatory correlates: Vascular impedance, resistance, and capacity, in Bohr D, Somlyo AP, Sparks HV, Jr (eds): *Handbook of Physiology, Section 2: The Cardiovascular System,* vol 2. Bethesda, American Physiological Society, 1980, pp 353–408.

Henry JP, Meehan JP: *The Circulation: An Integrated Physiologic Study.* Chicago, Year Book Medical Publishers, 1971.

McDonald DA: *Blood Flow in Arteries,* ed 2. Baltimore, Williams & Wilkins Co, 1974.

Milnor WR: Pulsatile blood flow. *N Engl J Med* 1972; 287:27.

Milnor WR: *Hemodynamics.* Baltimore, Williams & Wilkins Co, 1982.

Murgo JP, et al: Aortic input impedance in normal man: Relationship to pressure wave forms. *Circulation* 1980; 62:105.

Murgo JP, et al: Manipulation of ascending aortic pressure and flow wave reflections with the valsalva manoeuver: Relationship to input impedance. *Circulation* 1981; 63:122.

O'Rourke MF: Vascular impedance. A call for standardization, in Kenner T, Busse R, and High-fer-Szalky H (eds): *Cardiovascular System Dynamics: Models and Measurement.* Plenum Publishing Corp, 1982.

O'Rourke MF, Taylor MG: Vascular impedance of the femoral bed. *Circ Res* 1966; 18:126.

O'Rourke MF, Yaginuma T: Wave reflections and the arterial pulse. *Arch Intern Med* 1984; 144:366.

Rothe CF, *Measurement of Circulatory Capacitance and Resistance.* Ireland, Elsevier Scientific Publisher, Ltd, 1983.

Saari JT, Stinnet HO: Diameter versus number in diameter of vessel resistance. *The Physiologist* 1981; 24:51.

Sacks AH, Tickner EG, MacDonald IB: Criteria for the onset of vascular murmurs. *Circ Res* 1971; 24:249.

Chapter 10 _____

Measurement and Regulation of Arterial Blood Pressure

_____

Arterial pressure is closely regulated to maintain tissue perfusion during a wide variety of physiologic conditions. As a result, substantial changes in body position and level of muscular activity, as well as alterations in circulating blood volume, are tolerated without causing a significant deviation in blood pressure. This control is supplied by a combination of two mechanisms: (1) a system of rapidly acting vascular reflexes and (2) a group of slower mechanisms that adjust the fluid volume of the body and indirectly affect arterial pressure. The slower-acting control systems play an important role in long-term regulation of cardiac output. These were discussed in Chapter 7. The acute mechanisms that operate to maintain normal blood pressure will be summarized in this section.

Alterations in cardiac output and peripheral resistance produce characteristic changes in the pressure relationships of the arterial pulse. These relationships can supply insight into the activity of the blood pressure control mechanisms during health and disease. They are important clinically and will be discussed in this section.

ARTERIAL BLOOD PRESSURE

Definition of Terms

The basic form of the arterial pressure pulse and its modification as it propagates over the arterial tree were discussed in previous chapters. The highest pressure, at the peak of the pulse wave, is the *systolic pressure* and the lowest pressure, at the end of the diastole, is the *diastolic pressure*. The difference between systolic and diastolic pressure is the *pulse pressure*. This latter term sometimes leads to confusion. Pulse pressure, for example, should be clearly differentiated from the term "pressure pulse" used to describe the form of the phasic pressure in an artery or heart chamber during the cardiac cycle. (See Chapter 4.)

Mean pressure is the average pressure during the cardiac cycle. Because of the shape of the pressure pulse, mean blood pressure is a geometric mean that takes into consideration both the magnitude and the time the pressure is exerted (Fig 10–1). Calculation of the true mean pressure requires integration of the pressure pulse. However, this value can be approximated for central arterial pressure by using the following formula:

$$\text{mean pressure} = \text{diastolic pressure} + \tfrac{1}{3} \text{ pulse pressure}$$

Because of the change in form of the arterial pressure pulse as it travels away from the heart, the above relationship for mean pressure does not apply in the smaller peripheral arteries where systolic pressure is frequently higher but lasts for a much shorter time than in the proximal aorta.

Measurement of Arterial Blood Pressure

Human blood pressure can be determined directly by introducing a needle or catheter into an accessible artery and connecting it to a pressure measuring device; however, it is usually estimated indirectly with the aid of a special blood pressure cuff and sphygmomanometer or pressure gauge. Direct blood pressure measurement usually is restricted to research studies or diagnostic tests carried out in the cardiovascular catheterization laboratory and generally is not required for ordinary clinical use.

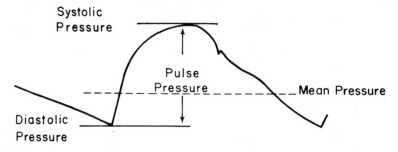

FIG 10–1.
Schematic arterial pressure pulse labeled to show pressure values usually measured for physiologic studies.

Indirect estimation of blood pressure is accomplished by balancing the pressure in an inflatable arm bag or cuff against the blood pressure in the brachial artery (Fig 10–2). When the pressure in the arm cuff is higher than brachial systolic pressure, the vessel is occluded by compression action of the cuff, and blood flow is interrupted. As the pressure in the cuff is reduced by permitting the air to gradually escape, the cuff pressure becomes lower than peak arterial systolic pressure, and the artery is forced open for a short period at the peak of the pressure pulse. Under these circumstances blood escapes through the area of constriction during the interval that arterial pressure is higher than cuff pressure. The duration of this flow will become longer as cuff pressure approaches arterial diastolic pressure, and when cuff pressure falls below the diastolic pressure level, blood flow will continue in an uninterrupted manner throughout the cardiac cycle.

Auscultation over the brachial artery below the inflated cuff as the pressure is reduced will detect characteristic sounds (Korotkoff sounds) when cuff pressure begins to fall below arterial systolic pressure. This is due to the turbulent flow of blood through the partially constricted artery

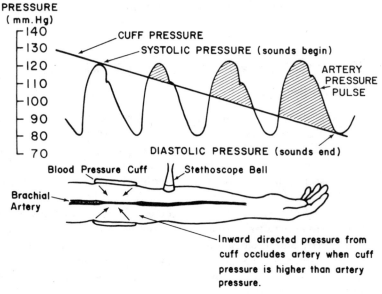

FIG 10–2.
Inflation of blood pressure cuff with a pressure above arterial occludes the brachial artery. As cuff pressure falls, the artery opens for that portion of the pulse that arterial pressure exceeds cuff pressure *(shaded area).* Turbulent forward flow of blood during this interval produces sounds below the cuff. The turbulence is decreased; thus the sounds disappear when cuff pressure is lower than diastolic arterial pressure. (Adapted from Rushmer RF: *Cardiovascular Dynamics,* ed 3. Philadelphia, WB Saunders Co, 1970.)

under the blood pressure cuff. A faint radial pulse also may be palpated at this time. The sounds heard over the artery change in character from a sharp tapping sound to a loud murmur-like noise as cuff pressure is further reduced. When cuff pressure approaches diastolic pressure, the sounds first become muffled as flow becomes more streamlined and then disappear as the cuff pressure falls below the diastolic level as the obstruction to flow is removed. The cuff pressure, when the first sound is detected, is considered to be the systolic pressure, and the pressure in the cuff at the point of complete cessation of sound is considered to be an index of diastolic pressure. In children, the diastolic pressure correlates best with the pressure at which the sounds become muffled. Under some conditions, Korotkoff sounds may continue until the bag is deflated. In this case, the point of muffling may be used to indicate diastolic pressure.

The indirect method of estimating arterial pressure at best tends to underestimate systolic pressure by 4 to 5 mm Hg and to overestimate diastolic pressure by approximately the same value, so there is an overall error of about 8 to 10 mm Hg. Despite these problems, the indirect measurement of arterial pressure is the standard in clinical practice and performs well, particularly if several consecutive determinations are made to detect obvious errors.

FACTORS THAT CONTROL MEAN BLOOD PRESSURE

General Principles

Mean blood pressure, as the average pressure during the cardiac cycle, is a calculated value that does not exist except as an instantaneous measurement during the rise and fall of the pulse. Nevertheless, it is an important physiologic parameter that avoids the complexities of pulsatile pressure changes. Its use permits the following simplified analysis of reflex control of mean arterial pressure.*

Reference has been made earlier to the elastic nature of the windkessel vessels that permit them to serve as distensible reservoirs. These vessels are always distended, and their walls are under tension. As a result, factors that increase or decrease arterial volume cause similar directional change in arterial pressure. By the same token, changes in arterial pressure result in similar changes in arterial volume. It should be emphasized that, because of the shape of the volume elastic curve of the arterial system (see Fig 10–11), these directional changes are not necessarily linearly related to each other.

The circulation is a closed system. Assuming a constant total blood

*The hemodynamic relationships summarized in Chapter 9 should be kept in mind.

volume, the fraction of this volume that is contained in the arterial reservoir during the steady state will be determined by the balance between cardiac output (input) and overall capillary flow (outflow). The effect of alterations in this balance between input and outflow on mean arterial pressure can be analyzed in a qualitative manner by considering the effect of changes in each of these variables independently while keeping the remainder constant.

Effect of Changes in Cardiac Output.—The minute output of the heart can be changed by alterations in heart rate, by cardiac stroke volume, or by changes in both of these parameters (see Chapter 7). Singly or together, these variables constitute the *central factors* that regulate arterial pressure. An increase in cardiac minute volume or cardiac output without change in peripheral resistance will upset the steady state between arterial input and outflow, and for at least a short interval, input into the arterial system will exceed runoff. As a result, both arterial volume and mean pressure will increase (Fig 10–3). However, the higher arterial pressure will then lead to

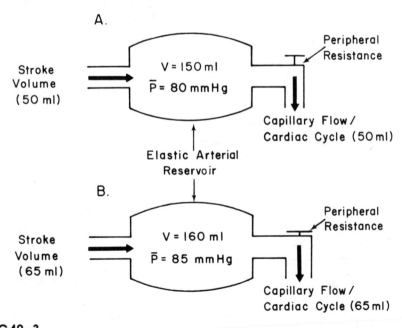

FIG 10–3.
Diagram of arterial system as elastic reservoir. **A,** steady state in which input from the heart is equal to capillary flow. Blood in the reservoir is under pressure from elastic recoil of its wall. **B,** new equilibrium point after an increase in cardiac output without change in peripheral resistance. Capillary flow again equals cardiac output. Volume and pressure of blood in reservoir are increased. (Volume *(V)* and mean pressure *(P̄)* values are arbitrary and used only as an example.)

an increase in flow through the arterioles. When this peripheral runoff comes into dynamic equilibrium with cardiac output so that one equals the other, mean arterial volume and pressure will stabilize and be maintained at its higher level. In a similar fashion, a decrease in the cardiac output will result in an immediate drop in mean blood pressure and capillary flow. Under these circumstances, arterial pressure will then stabilize at a lower level when peripheral runoff is reduced to the point that it again equals cardiac output.

Effect of Peripheral Resistance.—Mean blood pressure also can be changed by modifying the tone of the circular smooth muscle in the wall of the arterioles. This "stopcock" control of arterial runoff produced by changes in peripheral resistance constitutes the *peripheral factor* in blood pressure regulation. An increase in peripheral resistance due to generalized arteriolar constriction will temporarily reduce the runoff from the arterial reservoir. If cardiac output remains constant, this imbalance between input into the circulation and output through the capillary bed will result in an increase in both arterial volume and mean arterial pressure (Fig 10–4). The higher arterial pressure will then cause capillary flow to increase back toward control levels despite the high arteriolar resistance. Under these circumstances, mean arterial pressure will stabilize at its new higher level when capillary flow is again equal to cardiac output. The reverse of this mechanism will cause a fall in mean arterial pressure when peripheral resistance is decreased. In this situation, dilation of the resistance vessels will result in a drop in arterial volume and mean pressure, while capillary flow will increase transiently before returning to equal cardiac output.

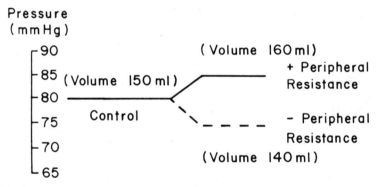

FIG 10–4.
Illustrative change in mean arterial pressure and arterial volume due to change in peripheral resistance with cardiac output kept constant. (Volume measurements are arbitrary.)

TABLE 10–1.

Factors That Affect Mean Arterial Pressure
and Capillary Flow

Factor	Mean Pressure	Capillary Flow
Peripheral resistance*		
Increased	↑	↓ than control
Decreased	↓	↑ than control
Heart rate†		
Increased	↑	↑
Decreased	↓	↓
Stroke volume‡		
Increased	↑	↑
Decreased	↓	↓

*Cardiac output maintained constant.
†Peripheral resistance and stroke volume constant.
‡Peripheral resistance and heart rate constant.

Alterations in mean blood pressure due to changes in peripheral resistance and cardiac output can be summarized by restatement of the definition for peripheral resistance (see Chapter 9). Mean arterial pressure is equal to the cardiac output in milliliters per minute times the peripheral resistance in millimeters of mercury per milliliter per minute. These relationships are summarized in Table 10–1.

NEURAL CONTROL OF CIRCULATION

The arterial pressure level reflects the composite activities of the cardiac pump and peripheral circulation. The nervous system plays an important role in the regulation of both components of the circulatory system and is pivotal to the maintenance of an adequate systemic perfusion pressure. It is, therefore, appropriate to include a summary of the neural regulation of the heart and blood vessels at this point in discussion of control of arterial blood pressure.

Central nervous system direction of the cardiovascular system is primarily a function of its autonomic division. Motor impulses in these fibers have their origin from cells in the brain stem. These medullary cells, in turn, receive a wide range of input from other brain centers such as the cortex, hypothalamus, and bulbar sites as well as sensory information from all parts of the body. Recent studies have emphasized, for example, the integrative function of the spinal neurons and the role of preganglionic fibers in processing these incoming signals. As a result, the older view of a discrete medullary cardiovascular center has been largely replaced by a more ubiquitous central nervous system control. This system involves a hypothalamic-medullary-spinal axis with input from many areas and with multiple integrative centers. A detailed discussion of this central control will not be attempted here; however, a brief overview will serve to emphasize the important features.

Cardiovascular "Centers"

The vascular smooth muscle in the wall of blood vessels is innervated by sympathetic nerve fibers. The resistance vessels have both α- and β-adrenergic receptors although their density and relative proportion vary in different vascular beds. As a result, not all respond to the sympathetic neurotransmitter norepinephrine with the same degree of vasoconstriction. (See Chapter 12 for discussion of sympathetic α and β receptors.) The capacitance venous vessels are less responsive to sympathetic stimulation than the arterioles, and as they have only α-adrenergic receptors, they control the volume of blood in the venous system by varying the contraction tone of the venous vascular muscle.

Systemic arterioles normally receive a continuous barrage of vasoconstrictor impulses. As a result, blocking or cutting the sympathetic supply to a vascular bed permits the smooth muscle in the wall of its arterioles to relax. This allows the vessels to be pushed open by the internal pressure, and blood flow to the area is increased. Ablation experiments show that this tonic sympathetic activity originates from diffusely scattered cells in the bulbopontine area of the brain stem. This longitudinally arranged group of interconnecting cells is sometimes called the *vasoconstrictor center* even though it does not constitute a true center in the anatomical sense.

Stimulation studies near the vasoconstrictor area suggest a second diffuse group of neurones that have *vasodilator* actions (Fig 10–5). However, these functions are so interwoven—and operate so closely with adjoining parts of the medulla that also regulate cardiac activity—that the whole area of the brain stem is probably best described as a single diffuse *cardiovascular center*. This area can then be subdivided functionally, if not anatomically, into: the *vasoconstrictor* and *vasodilator* areas already discussed and reciprocally acting *cardioexcitatory* and *cardioinhibitory* areas. These latter two areas send sympathetic (excitatory) or parasympathetic (inhibitory) fibers, respectively, to the heart and control cardiac contraction frequency by altering the periodic discharge rate of the sinoatrial (SA) node (see Chapters 3 and 6).

The tonically active vasoconstrictor (pressor) area of the brain stem normally maintains an output to the peripheral arterioles of one to two excit-

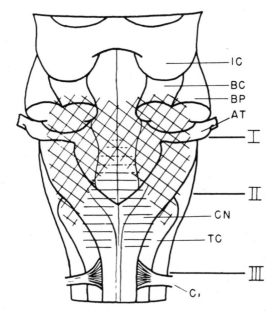

FIG 10–5.
Localization of pressor *(crosshatched)* and depressor *(horizontal lines)* areas of medulla of the cat. *IC* = inferior colliculus; *BC* = brachium conjunctivum; *BP* = brachium pontis; *AT* = auditory tubercle; *CN* = caudate nucleus; *TC* = tuberculum cinereum; *C* = first cervical nerve. (From Alexander RS: *J Neurophysiol* 1946; 9:205. Used by permission.)

atory sympathetic impulses per second. This apparently occurs because of stimulation from the reticular activating system and from other areas of the brain as well as from the direct effect of pH, partial pressure of carbon dioxide (P_{CO_2}) and partial pressure of oxygen (P_{O_2}). (A decrease in pH or P_{O_2} or an increase in P_{CO_2} frequently causes an increase in discharge.)

The basic discharge rate of the vasoconstrictor area and its stimulatory effect on the sympathetic fibers to blood vessels are also modified by efferent impulses from a large number of neural connections (Fig 10–6). The negative feedback effect of information from the aortic and carotid baroreceptors will be discussed separately below. Important modifying impulses also descend from higher brain centers via corticohypothalamic pathways to the vasomotor area in the medulla. Information carried in these fibers is involved in such diverse activities as the vascular response to anger and other emotions, the effect of stimulating thoughts on the arterial blood pressure, and the regulation of skin blood flow as part of the maintenance of body temperature. The hypothalamus and limbic system also are involved in activities with cardiovascular components such as thirst, food in-

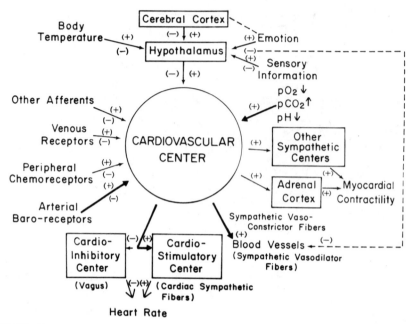

FIG 10–6.
Diagrammatic representation of cardiovascular reflexes that involve the cardiovascular center in the medulla.

take, and sexual arousal. This information is supplied to the medullary centers so that the appropriate vascular reaction will take place. In addition, input from the reticular formation brings afferent pain signals and other sensory information to the cardiovascular center. This nociceptive information, if acute, usually leads to an increase in blood pressure; however, if the pain is severe or prolonged, it may inhibit the pressor area, lead to a drop in blood pressure, and, in some instances, cause fainting.

The vasoconstrictor area has close connections with the adjoining cardioexcitatory cells in the medulla, although the functional details are not entirely clear. For example, the cardioexcitatory area is not tonically active under normal conditions. However, electric stimulation of this area may lead to an elevation of both heart rate and arterial pressure due to a generalized sympathetic discharge. The cardioexcitatory cells may also exert a reciprocal inhibition on the cardioinhibitory area and vice versa, although the excitatory area clearly is the dominant center.

In contradistinction to the pressor (vasoconstrictor) area, the vasodilator area of the medulla does not exert its effect directly on the peripheral vasculature but rather acts by sending inhibitory impulses to the preganglionic sympathetic neurons in the spinal cord. Thus, these preganglionic cells receive both excitatory impulses from the vasoconstrictor center and inhibitory impulses from the vasodilator center. In this way, activation of the vasodilator center results in blockage of excitatory impulses coming from the vasoconstrictor center and the resistance vessels passively dilate. Some additional "vasodilatory" fibers have their origin in the vasodilator area and travel via the parasympathetic system to blood vessels in the salivary glands, skin of the face and neck, gastric mucosa, and external genitalia. These fibers do not produce active dilation of the arterioles but rather achieve this function by directly inhibiting the active tone of the vascular smooth muscle or, at least in the salivary glands and the skin, by the liberation of specific vasodilatory substances (see Chapter 11). This vasodilation mechanism appears to be used primarily to increase local blood flow, and it is probably not significant in the overall regulation of arterial pressure.

Sympathetic vasodilator pathways from the hypothalamus and cerebral cortex also innervate resistance vessels of the major skeletal muscles. These fibers are not controlled by the cardiovascular center but may be selectively activated as part of a general body reaction to danger. In this situation, vasodilation of skeletal muscle arterioles will permit muscle blood flow to increase, perhaps in preparation for defensive action. As this can be prevented by blocking the neurotransmitter acetylcholine with atropine, it appears likely that both types of vasodilatory fibers are cholinergic.

Neurons from the vasodilator area of the medulla also make connections with cardiac inhibitory cells in the dorsal vagal motor nucleus. This vagal center normally is tonically active and maintains a restraining influence on the heart rate (see Chapter 3). The activity of these vagal cells, however, is not due to inherent tonic activity like the cells of the vasoconstrictor area, but instead this periodic discharge is generated reflexly by the normal input from the carotid and aortic baroreceptors that are discussed below. This stimulatory action is shown by the fact that sections of the sensory nerves from these receptors (the moderator nerves) will abolish the vagal inhibition to heart rate as effectively as will vagotomy.

Peripheral Baroreceptors and Chemoreceptors

Receptors located in the walls of the heart and in the major blood vessels supply sensory information to the cardiovascular areas of the brain (Fig 10–7). Major stretch receptors are located in the proximal aorta and in the area of the carotid sinus. (Additional receptors are found in the great veins, atria, and pulmonary artery, as well as in other areas of the cardiovascular system. The role of these low-pressure receptors in the control of cardiac

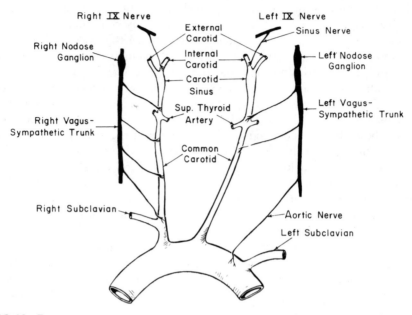

FIG 10–7.
Diagrammatic representation of major arterial baroreceptors. Major arteries and nerves are labeled.

function has been discussed in Chapter 7.) The carotid and aortic receptors are undifferentiated terminal nerve fibers, 5 μ or less in diameter, that branch extensively in the adventitial and medial layer of the vessel wall. These fibers respond to change in length by altering their rate of discharge. Although these receptors are technically *mechanoreceptors*, they usually are referred to as *baroreceptors* or *pressoreceptors* because the stimulus that leads to an increase in their length is the stretching of the arterial wall produced by an elevation in blood pressure. Each group of these receptors contains endings with a wide variation in individual sensitivity so that with increasing levels of stretch there is an increase in the number of actively firing receptors.

Fibers from the baroreceptors in the carotid sinus travel with the sinus and glossopharyngeal nerves, whereas fibers from the aortic receptors travel with the vagus nerve. In both cases, the fibers end in the vasomotor area in the medulla. Because of their role in the regulation of the circulation, these neurons have been called the *moderator* or *buffer nerves*.

The baroreceptors respond in a characteristic manner to both steady and phasic pressure changes. When exposed to static pressure, the receptors begin to fire at a low rate (i.e., 15 to 20 impulses/sec) when arterial

pressure reaches a threshold value of about 30 to 40 mm Hg. The receptors
are apparently inactive at pressure levels below this range. The relationship
between firing frequency to arterial pressure above this threshold level is S-
shaped (Fig 10–8), and the firing level stabilizes at its maximum rate (40 to
100 imp/sec) when arterial pressure reaches a level of 220 to 230 mm Hg.
The sensitivity of these receptors can be modified by drugs and by neural
input that affect the distensibility of the vessel wall. With phasic pressure
changes similar to those produced by the arterial pulse, the baroreceptors
fire more rapidly (1) with a rising pressure than with a falling pressure and
(2) with a rapid change in pressure rather than with a slow pressure change.
For this reason, the traffic in the moderator nerves coming from the baroreceptors is higher during rise of the pressure pulse than during the diastolic portion (see Fig 10–8). The sensitivity of the baroreceptors is influenced by the size of the pulse pressure so that their response at the same
level of mean blood pressure is greater with a large pulse than with a small
pulse.

Special chemoreceptors located in the carotid and aortic bodies are sensitive to decreases in both blood pH and the partial pressure of oxygen
(P_{O_2}). These organs, which are located in close proximity to the carotid
sinus and aortic arch, are very vascular and have a high metabolic rate.
The 2-mg carotid body, for example, has the highest blood flow on a
weight basis of any of the tissues (2,000 ml/100 gm/minute). Sensory nerve
fibers from these receptors make connections with both the respiratory and
cardiovascular centers. Chemoreceptor stimulation results in an increase in
pulmonary ventilation and, to a much lesser extent, in an increase in peripheral resistance. However, the direct effect of changes in the chemical
composition of the blood on the cardiovascular center is considerably more
potent than is the stimulation these changes produce in the peripheral

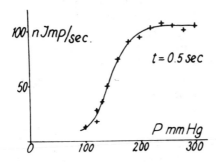

FIG 10–8.
Impulse frequency (impulses per second) of the baroreceptors in the wall of the carotid
sinus, as a function of sinus blood pressure. (From Landgren S: *Acta Physiol Scand* 1952;
26:35. Used by permission.)

chemoreceptors. The peripheral chemoreceptors adapt rather rapidly, and their input usually is not significant in cardiovascular control. During anoxia or asphyxia, however, their acute peripheral input may become important and, combined with its central effect, will lead to a powerful sympathetic outflow to the circulation.

BARORECEPTOR CONTROL OF BLOOD PRESSURE: CAROTID SINUS REFLEX

The major determinant of arterial pressure under rest conditions is arteriolar resistance; alterations in heart rate and stroke volume play an important but secondary role. This relationship changes during activities such as muscular exercise. Alterations of cardiac output then assume a more important role (see Chapter 15). However, in either case, the overall degree of arteriolar constriction is determined largely by the equilibrium achieved between the discharge rate of the pressor area of the cardiovascular center and the degree of inhibition as a result of nerve impulses coming to the brain from the baroreceptors. The effect on arterial blood pressure of removing this inhibitory contribution to the equilibrium can be shown in the experimental animal by sectioning the aortic nerve to remove impulses from the aortic baroreceptors and clamping both common carotid arteries (Fig 10–9). The drop in carotid blood pressure due to clamping of the arteries results in a loss of the normal reflex inhibition from the carotid baroreceptors. This lack of inhibition then permits the hypothalamic-medullary-spinal control axis to increase its sympathetic drive to the resistance vessels (and to a lesser extent to the SA node and the myocardium). At the same time, the lack of stimulation from the baroreceptors will result in the same cardiovascular control area no longer sending vagal impulses to the heart. The final result of this "escape" of the cardiovascular center from the inhibition produced by the baroreceptors is an immediate marked increase in blood pressure along with some increase in heart rate.

The acute negative feedback reflex that maintains blood pressure within the normal ranges depends on baroreceptor input from both carotid and aortic receptors. The carotid baroreceptors, which have been more intensely studied, appear, however, to play the dominant role in regulation of arterial pressure. For this reason, the carotid and aortic reflexes are sometimes referred to, incorrectly, as being just the *carotid sinus reflex*.

Reflex control of arterial pressure may be illustrated by following the acute mechanism triggered by a sudden drop in blood pressure (Fig 10–10). In many ways, the result is similar to the cardiovascular changes, described above, that followed clamping of the carotid arteries. If mean arte-

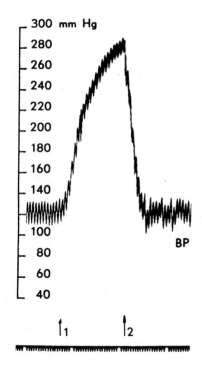

FIG 10–9.
Femoral artery pressure in the anesthetized dog. The aortic nerves have been cut. Between *1* and *2*, both common carotid arteries were clamped. The marked increase in blood pressure during this interval resulted from lack of inhibitory impulses to the cardiovascular center from the carotid sinus baroreceptor. (From Heymans C, van den Heuvel-Heyman G: *Circulation* 1951; 4:581. Used by permission.)

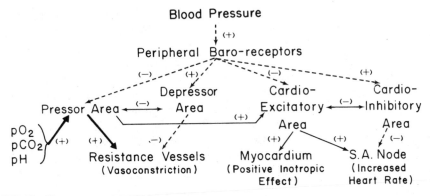

FIG 10–10.
Schematic flow chart showing the reflex regulation of mean arterial blood pressure. Effect of each input indicated by *plus* or *minus sign*. A reduction in stimulation produced by a drop in mean blood pressure is shown by *dashed arrows*; the relative degree of stimulation is indicated by width of *solid arrows*.

rial pressure falls below 70 mm Hg, the firing rate of the baroreceptors is significantly reduced. The lack of this input results in a reduction in the inhibitory output from the vasodilatory area, particularly to the preganglionic sympathetic cells in the spinal cord, so that the pressor area is able to increase its output of vasoconstrictive impulses to the blood vessels. This results in a generalized increase in peripheral resistance and reduction in venous capacitance. (The degree of arteriolar vasoconstriction will vary between different vascular beds. This aspect will be discussed in Chapter 11.) If the sympathetic discharge is sufficiently intense, it may "spread" to the heart and produce an increase in myocardial contractility. The end result of this spread is an increasing stroke volume (see Chapter 7). The concomitant decrease in moderator drive to the cardiac inhibitory center also reduces the rate of depolarization of these cells and releases the heart from its vagal inhibition. The result is that heart rate increases. If the sympathetic stimulation to the heart is intense, heart rate will be increased even further. The result of these activities is that both cardiac output and peripheral resistance are increased, and arterial pressure is returned toward normal.

The baroreceptor reflex mechanism also operates to limit a sudden elevation in arterial pressure and to return pressure to the normal range. In this situation, the higher arterial pressure results in an increase in baroreceptor input to the medulla. These inhibitory impulses reduce the tonic output of the pressor area. This occurs directly as a result of inhibitory moderator impulses and indirectly as a result of stimulation of the depressor area by the same sensory information. The increased moderator input to the cardiac depressor center also stimulates it to inhibit the cardioexcitatory center and increase vagal tone to the heart. The result is that rate is reduced and cardiac output will fall. These reactions result in vasodilation of capacitance and resistance vessels and in a decrease in cardiac minute volume with the result that blood pressure is lowered.

In summary, baroreceptor impulses via the moderator nerves *inhibit* tonically active medullary sympathetic excitatory impulses and *excite* cardiac inhibitory centers. As a result, the response to an acute increase in arterial pressure is arteriolar and venous vasodilation, slowing of the heart rate, and a drop in arterial pressure, while the response to an acute decrease in blood pressure is arteriolar and venous constriction, an increase in both the heart rate and level of myocardial contractility, and return of mean blood pressure to its normal level.

ELASTICITY OF ARTERIAL SYSTEM

Before considering the alterations in pulse pressure that accompany changes in mean arterial pressure, it will be necessary to discuss the volume-pressure properties of the windkessel vessels. As was pointed out earlier, these vessels serve as elastic reservoirs and, during systole, store a major fraction of the energy imparted to the blood by cardiac contraction before returning it to the circulation during diastole. The relationship between the volume of blood in the arterial system and internal pressure is complicated by the geometry of the vessel and the nonlinear stress-strain behavior of the vessel wall. The shape of the volume-pressure curve for the windkessel vessels, however, becomes of fundamental importance in determining the magnitude of the pulse pressure.

The static volume-pressure relationship of the human aorta for different age groups is shown in Figure 10–11. The data for these curves were obtained at autopsy by ligating all the vessels leaving the aorta and then filling the aorta with sufficient fluid to just distend its walls. A known quantity of fluid was then injected and the internal pressure determined. As the filling volume was different for each vessel studied, the injected volume was expressed as a percentage of the volume in the system just before the injection. When plotted in this manner, the volume-pressure curve approximates the in vivo elastic properties of the windkessel vessels.

The pressure-percentage volume relationship for a young individual shown in Figure 10–11 is essentially linear over the physiologic range of arterial pressure (50 to 175 mm Hg). At higher pressures, the slope of the relationship increases in a curvilinear manner that is concave toward the pressure axis. It is of interest that with increasing age, the extent of the linear portion of the curve is reduced, and the slope of the entire curve is increased. This observation is compatible with a general loss of elastic tissue and the gradual development of atherosclerotic changes in the vessel wall.

It is helpful to first consider the linear portion of the aortic pressure-volume data: The slope of this relationship is the *volume-elasticity coefficient* (E_v). It is given by

$$E_v = \frac{\Delta P}{\Delta V} \cdot V \qquad (10\text{--}1)$$

where ΔP is the change in pressure that results from a change in volume (ΔV), and V is the initial or filling volume. Thus, E_v defines the change in pressure in the system for a percentage change in its initial volume.

If V in equation 10–1 is considered to be the volume of blood in the aorta at end-diastole (V_d), the change in aortic pressure, ΔP (i.e., the pulse pressure) for a given stroke volume (ΔV) is given by rearranging equation 10–1 and substituting V_d for V as follows:

$$\Delta P = \frac{E_v \cdot \Delta V}{V_d} \qquad (10\text{--}2)$$

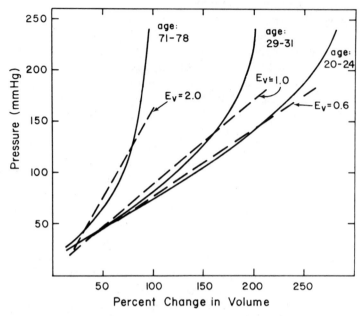

FIG 10–11.
Static volume-pressure curves of aorta determined for different age groups. Each of these curves can be approximated by a linear relationship *(dashed lines)* within the physiologic pressure range (50 to 175 mm Hg). E_v = volume elasticity. (Modified from Hallock P, Benson IC: *J Clin Invest* 1937; 16:595.)

Thus, within the linear range of the V-P relationship shown in Figure 10–11, equation 10–2 can be used to approximate, at least in a qualitative manner, the changes in pulse pressure that will accompany alterations in mean aortic pressure (Table 10–2). For example, as discussed above, an increase in peripheral resistance without change in stroke volume or heart rate in a young individual will acutely reduce arterial runoff and increase both mean blood pressure and the end-diastolic volume of blood in the aorta (V_d). Under these circumstances, as the value of E_v can be considered to be constant over any short period of time, the pulse pressure (ΔP) will be reduced. As mean arterial pressure is increased, the diastolic pressure must be increased more than the systolic pressure.

In the same manner, a sudden increase in heart rate without change in stroke volume or peripheral resistance will produce a temporary decrease in peripheral runoff due to the abbreviated diastolic time interval. Arterial volume and pressure will increase until peripheral flow again returns to control levels. Because the same stroke volume (ΔV) is now injected into a

TABLE 10–2.

Effect of Changing a Single Factor on Systolic, Diastolic, and Pulse Pressures in a Young Individual With all Other Conditions Constant

Factor	Systolic Pressure	Diastolic Pressure	Pulse Pressure	Mean Pressure
Stroke volume				
Increased	+ +	+	+	+
Decreased	– –	–	–	–
Heart rate				
Increased	+	+ +	–	+
Decreased	–	– –	+	–
Peripheral resistance				
Increased	+	+ +	–	+
Decreased	–	– –	+	–
Arterial distensibility				
Increased	–	+	–	No
Decreased	+	–	+	Change

larger aortic end-diastolic volume (V_d), the percentage change in volume and the pulse pressure (ΔP) are both reduced.

An increase in stroke volume will by itself increase both mean arterial pressure and volume. However, the rapid increase in arterial pressure during ejection will result in an increased peripheral runoff into the capillaries. The end result will be that the increased stroke volume ΔV will be proportionally greater than the increase in volume (V_d). As a result, systolic pressure increases more than diastolic, and the pulse pressure increases moderately.

The above generalizations suggest that factors that modify arterial pressure by changing peripheral arterial runoff (i.e., changes in peripheral resistance or time between beats) have their major effect on the diastolic pressure. Thus, in the clinic, special attention is given to the diastolic pressure of patients with hypertension as it may provide a measure of arteriolar resistance. Similarly, factors that primarily modify cardiac output have their major effect on systolic pressure. Thus a patient with systolic hypertension but a normal diastolic pressure is more likely to have an increased stroke volume or atherosclerotic changes in the wall of the aorta than an increase in peripheral resistance.

Unfortunately, the above "rule-of-thumb" regarding the pulse pressure is not always reliable. The effects of intervention that modify arterial pressure becomes unpredictable if they cause arterial pressure to move beyond the linear range of the volume-pressure relationship. This is most likely to occur in older individuals or patients with atherosclerosis where this portion of the relationship is abbreviated. For example, following an increase in peripheral resistance in such an individual, the value of both E_v and V_d in equation 10–2 can change so that the pulse pressure may remain the same or even increase. In addition, most physiologic interventions affect all the variables involved in the control of arterial blood pressure, and it is unusual for only a single one to be altered. Nevertheless, changes in a single factor (i.e., heart rate, stroke volume, or peripheral resistance) frequently dominate. As a result, despite these difficulties, directional changes in pulse pressure frequently can be correctly analyzed at the bedside.

SUMMARY

Regulation of arterial blood pressure is multifactorial. The circulation is a closed elastic system without empty spaces. Arterial pressure results from the interactions of cardiac stroke volume, heart rate, peripheral resistance (impedance), arterial blood volume, and the elastic properties of the arterial windkessel vessels. The steady-state arterial volume is determined, in turn, by the arterial pressure necessary to keep capillary blood flow equal to cardiac output. In addition, mean arterial pressure is maintained within normal limits by the reflex control of arteriolar resistance, heart rate, myocardial contractility and venous capacitance. These negative feedback reflex arcs receive their input from mechanical (stretch) and chemical receptors in the wall of the carotid artery and arch of the aorta plus input from other areas of the brain and vascular system. They operate via the autonomic nervous system from a cardiovascular center located in the brain stem.

The relationship between the arterial pressure and the percentage change in its volume is relatively linear over the normal range of arterial pressure. Thus, factors that modify arterial runoff have their major effect on diastolic pressure, and factors that affect cardiac output have their major effect on systolic pressure. This generalization can be used to predict the changes in the arterial pulse pressure that accompany interventions that modify arterial pressure within its normal range.

BIBLIOGRAPHY

Abrahams VC, Hilton SM, Zbrozyna AW: The role of active muscle vasodilation in the alerting state of the defense reaction. *J Physiol* 1964; 171:189.
Berne RM, Levy MN: *Cardiovascular Physiology*, ed 5. St Louis, CV Mosby Co, 1986.

Detweiler DK: Circulation, in Broebeck JR (ed): *Physiological Basis of Medical Practice*, ed 8. Baltimore, Williams & Wilkins Co, 1973.

Dobrin PB: Vascular mechanics, in *Handbook of Physiology, Section 2: The Cardiovascular System—Peripheral Circulation and Organ Blood Flow*, vol 3. Bethesda, American Physiological Society, 1983.

Donald DE, Shepherd JT: Autonomic regulation of the peripheral circulation. *Annu Rev Physiol* 1980; 42:429.

Folkow B: Range of control of the cardiovascular system by the central nervous system. *Physiol Rev* 1960; 40(suppl 4):93.

Folkow B, Neil E: *Circulation*. New York, Oxford University Press, 1971.

Hamilton WF: The patterns of the arterial pulse. *Am J Physiol* 1944; 141:235.

Hilton SM, Spyer KM: Central nervous regulation of vascular resistance. *Annu Rev Physiol* 1980; 42:399.

Korner PI: Central nervous control of autonomic cardiovascular function, in Bern RM, Sperelakis N, Geiger SR (eds): *Handbook of Physiology, Section 2: The Cardiovascular System*, vol 1. Bethesda, American Physiological Society, 1979.

O'Rourke MF, Yaginuma T: Wave reflections and the arterial pulse. *Arch Intern Med* 1984; 144:366.

Rothe CF: Reflex control of the veins and the capacitance vessels. *Physiol Rev* 1983; 63:1281.

Rushmer RF: *Cardiovascular Dynamics*, ed 4. Philadelphia, WB Saunders Co, 1976.

Sparks HV, Belloni FL: The peripheral circulation: Local regulation. *Physiol Rev* 1978; 40:67.

Steinfeld L, Alexander H, Cohen ML: Updating sphygmomanometry. *Am J Cardiol* 1974; 33:107.

Wiggers CJ: *Physiology in Health and Disease*, ed 5. Philadelphia, Lea & Febiger, 1949.

Wiggers CJ: The influence of vascular factors on mean pressure, pulse pressure and phasic peripheral flow. *Am J Physiol* 1938; 123:644.

Chapter 11 _____

Local Control of Peripheral Circulation

_____

The mechanisms that regulate arterial blood pressure and maintain an adequate pressure head for tissue perfusion have been summarized in the last chapter. This chapter will cover the control of blood flow to individual organs and vascular beds. In addition, the interactions between the control of arterial pressure and tissue flow will be discussed and related to the distribution of blood within the body.

FACTORS INVOLVED IN VASCULAR CONTROL

The control systems available to regulate tissue blood flow can be divided into two main groups: (1) those that operate remotely from the regulated vascular bed and (2) those that are confined within a single organ or tissue. Examples of the first group include the neural control exerted over the diameter of resistance vessels and the effect of circulating hormones on vascular resistance. The second group includes the effect of metabolic end products on the tone of vascular smooth muscle and the myogenic reaction of the resistance vessels themselves to varying degrees of stretch. Fundamental to both of these systems is the fact that vascular smooth muscle of the resistance vessels is normally in a state of partial contraction and thus exhibits resting "tone."

Vascular Tone

The existence of a basal level of precapillary vascular constriction after all known extravascular vasoconstrictive influences have been eliminated is demonstrated by the following comparison. Skeletal muscle blood flow, under resting conditions at an arterial pressure of 100 mm Hg, is about 3 to 5 ml/minute/100 gm of tissue. This flow will substantially increase when neuroconstrictor influences are removed by section of the sympathetic nerve supply to the muscle blood vessels. However, following this procedure, a considerable degree of vascular resistance is still present. This can be shown by the marked further increase in blood flow that follows maximal vasodilation as a result of muscle work or the use of vasodilatory drugs (Fig 11–1 and Table 11–1). Thus, it is clear that vascular tone is influenced by a complex series of factors. These mechanisms will be summarized individually.

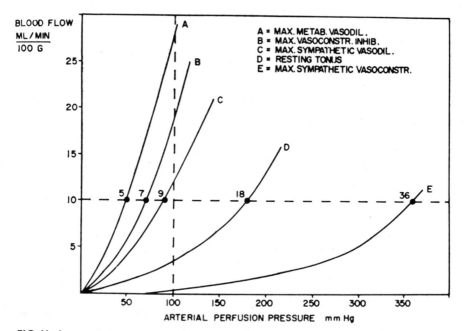

FIG 11–1.

Plot showing pressure-flow curves obtained from gracilis and gastrocnemius-plantaris muscles of the dog and cat under various conditions. The numbers indicate peripheral resistance in millimeters of mercury per milliliter per minute per 100 gm of tissue at a flow of 10 ml/minute/100 gm of tissue. (From Renkin EM, Rosell S: *Acta Physiol Scand* 1962; 54:241. Used by permission.)

TABLE 11-1.

Approximate Blood Flow and Resistance Values for Various Organs Under Normal Rest Conditions and During Maximal Vasodilation (Arterial Blood Pressure 100 mm Hg)*

Tissue	Rest		Maximal Dilation†		No. of Times Rest Resistance Increased Over Maximal Dilation Resistance
	Blood Flow (ml/min/100 gm)	Resistance (PRU$_{100}$)‡	Blood Flow (ml/min/100 gm)	Resistance (PRU$_{100}$)‡	
Skeletal muscle	2.5	40.00	60	1.66	24.0
Salivary glands	40.0	2.50	500	0.20	12.5
Gastrointestinal tract	35.0	2.85	275	0.36	7.9
Liver	29.0	3.44	176	0.56	6.1
Heart	70.0	1.42	400	0.25	5.7
Fat	8.0	12.50	30	4.54	2.8
Central nervous system	50.0	2.00	140	0.71	2.8
Skin	200.0	1.49	167	0.60	2.5
Kidney	400.0	0.25	466	0.21	1.2

*Based on data of Mellander S, Johansson B: *Pharmacol Rev* 1968; 20:117.
†Produced by vasodilatory drugs.
‡PRU$_{100}$ (peripheral resistance units) are given as millimeters of mercury per milliliter per minute per 100 gm.

Metabolic Factors.—Blood flow increases when tissues become active. For example, blood flow to muscles undergoing active exercise may increase from a basal level of 2.5 to 3 ml/minute/100 gm of muscle to as much as 60 ml/minute/100 gm. This increase is accompanied by a marked fall in vascular resistance. In addition, the functional capillary surface area of the muscle increases due to the perfusion of previously underused capillary channels.

The marked increase in vascular volume of active tissues (hyperemia) has led to the suggestion that arterioles are dilated by the metabolites or other factors that accumulate in their immediate environment as a by-product of increased tissue metabolism. Many such vasoactive substances have been implicated including adenosine triphosphate (ATP), adenosine, and other Krebs cycle intermediates, as well as various polypeptides and such substances as histamine, bradykinin, and prostaglandins (see below). The most important vasoactive metabolic substances, at least in the peripheral vascular beds, appear to be low partial pressure of oxygen (P_{O_2}) and increased partial pressure of carbon dioxide (P_{CO_2}), increased levels of K^+ and adenosine.

The metabolic control of *local* blood flow undoubtedly assists in maintaining the vascular supply equal to the needs of the tissues. This mechanism also will be discussed in the section on autoregulation. It is sufficient here to point out that when blood flow to a local area becomes inadequate, the P_{O_2} of both capillary blood and interstitial fluid will fall due to the lack of supply, whereas P_{CO_2} and the concentration of other metabolites will increase because of a lack of removal. The increased concentration of these substances then produces vasodilation of the resistance vessels by their local action on the vascular smooth muscle, and blood flow increases. The increased flow then acts to close the loop of the feedback control circuit by both increasing the oxygen supply to the tissues and washing the vasoactive metabolites out of the vascular bed.

The vascular effect of alterations in local levels of these metabolic factors can be illustrated by observing the marked vasodilation that occurs in most organs if their blood supply is momentarily interrupted (Fig 11–2). This phenomenon *(reactive hyperemia)* results from the acute hypoxia and increase in extracellular concentration of vasoactive metabolites. On release of the vascular occlusion, tissue blood flow is increased above the resting level and remains elevated until metabolic conditions have returned to normal. During this interval, the blood flow "debt" is usually more than paid back.

Myogenic Action.—The terminal arterioles and the muscular layer in at least some of the venules are composed of *single-unit* smooth muscle.

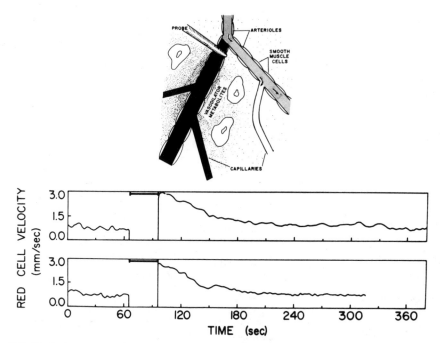

FIG 11–2.

Top, diagram showing effect of arteriolar occlusion. Depletion of oxygen and an increase in tissue metabolites cause relaxation of vascular smooth muscle along the occluded arteriole. *Bottom,* red cell velocity profiles in two arterioles before and after occlusion. Occlusion is indicated by *horizontal bar.* The reactive hyperemia response is indicated by the increased flow after release. (Modified from Gentry RM, Johnson PC: *Circ Res* 1972; 31:953. Used by permission of the American Heart Association.)

These muscle cells have an unstable resting electric membrane potential that undergoes wave-like changes similar to the fluctuation that occurs in the polarization of visceral smooth muscle. This electric instability can act as a local pacemaker and periodically triggers the development of "spike" potentials (Fig 11–3). These spike depolarizations can then spread to adjacent cells and cause the entire muscle mass to contract.

The discharge rate of these vascular pacemakers is increased by passive stretch. It is postulated that the stimulus for this response is the level of microvascular wall tension. (See Chapter 8 for discussion of the Laplace relationship and the development of wall tension.) Thus, augmentation of microvascular flow and the concomitant increase in arteriolar diameter due to an elevation in perfusion pressure will, for example, be countered by increased vascular tone, vasoconstriction, and an increase in vascular resis-

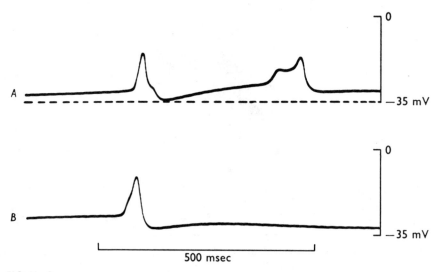

FIG 11–3.
Action potentials recorded intracellularly from the wall of a mesenteric arteriole, 120 μ in diameter, in the rat. **A,** two spikes arising from a slow wave of amplitude greater than 30% of maximum membrane polarization. **B,** single spike on the succeeding wave, which had an amplitude 20% of maximum polarization. (From Steedman WH: *J Physiol* 1966; 186:382. Used by permission of Cambridge University Press.)

tance. This *myogenic* or *Bayliss* mechanism appears to operate to maintain a constant microcirculatory flow in organs and organ systems such as the kidneys, the gastrointestinal tract, and the arterial supply to the liver.

Vasomotion.—Periodic closure of individual arterioles with interruption of flow to the capillary units they supply is a common feature of many capillary beds. Two mechanisms for this vasomotion have been suggested: (1) Interruption in capillary flow will result in local accumulation of vasodilatory metabolites in the area supplied by that vessel. These substances, as discussed above, then exert a direct effect on the sphincter, causing it to relax. Opening of the vessel, however, causes capillary flow in that area to increase. This washes out the vasoactive metabolites and removes the stimulus for vasodilation. The vessel then constricts, and the cycle starts over. (2) Shortening of the vascular smooth muscle fibers during contraction removes the length stimulus for electric activity, and pacemaker activity in the sphincter area stops. This lack of electric stimulation permits the vascular muscle to relax. However, opening of the vessels permits the internal pressure to restretch the vascular muscle cells and stimulates them to resume their pacemaker activity. Time delays in both these feedback mechanisms make the contraction-relaxation cycle oscillatory. These mechanisms will be discussed in more detail in the section on autoregulation.

In the larger collections of vascular smooth muscle, such as occur in arterioles, the electric activity of several pacemakers may operate independently. This will cause at least some of the fiber to be contracted at all times and produce a degree of muscular tension. The magnitude of this basal arteriolar tone is a function of the discharge rate of the individual pacemaker cells and thus can then be modulated by factors that affect their rhythmic activity. This is accomplished by vasomotor nerve fibers, circulating vasoactive chemicals and hormones, and local feedback systems (Fig 11–4).

Regulation of capillary flow to organs that require a high rate of blood flow during peak activity, such as the myocardium and skeletal muscles, is facilitated by the presence of considerable resting arteriolar tone. For example, blood flow to these organs can be quickly and substantially increased by reducing the resting level of arteriolar vascular muscle tension. This drop in wall tension permits the blood pressure to rapidly dilate the vessels. In contrast, the vascular bed in organs such as the kidney, which have a constant need for blood and consequently are not called on to undergo rapid vasodilation, do not have or need a high degree of basal tone.

The resting level of arteriolar tone in a vascular bed can be estimated, as discussed earlier, from the blood flow changes that occur when the vas-

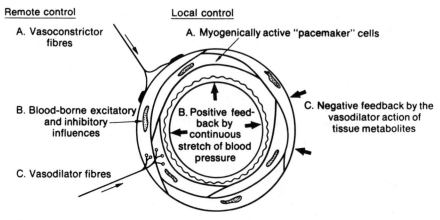

FIG 11–4.

Basic mechanisms for control of local blood flow. Myogenically active pacemaker cells in vascular sphincters are stimulated by blood pressure to produce a basal level of vascular tone. This tone is modulated by the negative feedback effect of tissue metabolites and by effects of nervous and blood-borne factors. (From Folkow B, Neil E: *Circulation.* New York, Oxford University Press, 1971. Used by permission.)

cular bed is rapidly dilated. The results of such measurements (see Table 11–1) show that the normal resistance of skeletal muscle vessels is approximately 24 times the minimal resistance obtained when the resistance vessels are fully dilated. In contrast, the kidneys, under the same conditions, show a resting resistance only 1.2 times their minimal value.

It is significant that the venous capacitance vessels do not contain single-unit smooth muscle but rather have the multiunit type that usually does not exhibit tonic pacemaker activity. As a result, the circular smooth muscle of veins does not have a significant degree of basal tone, and the vasomotor activity of these vessels is largely determined by extrinsic factors such as the vasoconstrictor impulses from sympathetic nerves. This mechanism appears to be consistent with the role of these vessels as storage reservoirs and the fact that they are not involved to any great extent in regulation of tissue blood flow (see below).

Neural Factors.—The basal level of arteriolar tone can be modulated by neural input from the "cardiovascular center" in the medulla (see Chapter 10). Sympathetic vasoconstrictor fibers innervate resistance vessels throughout the body, but there are quantitative differences in their distribution. Precapillary vessels of skeletal muscle and the mesenteric area have a much richer supply of these vasoconstrictor fibers than do the cerebral or coronary vessels. The response of a vascular bed to sympathetic stimulation is dependent on other factors besides the magnitude of the sympathetic supply. However, in general terms, the maximum vasoconstrictor tone generated by the sympathetic outflow is greatest in skin vessels; somewhat less in arterioles of the liver, gastrointestinal tract, and skeletal muscles; and least (as expected from the anatomical findings listed before) in the brain and myocardium.

The neurotransmitter liberated at the neuroeffector junction of the vasoconstrictor fibers is *norepinephrine*. This catecholamine reacts with specific sites on the vascular smooth muscle membranes that have been designated α-*receptors*. Recent studies have suggested that these receptors occur on nerve terminals (α_2-receptors) as well as on the postsynaptic muscle membrane (α_1-receptors). α_2-Receptors may respond to stimulation by decreasing the release of norepinephrine at the nerve ending, while activation of α_1-receptors, probably acting via an increase in the cell membrane conduction of sodium and perhaps other ions, typically leads to an increased discharge frequency of spike potentials and an increase in vascular tone. The sensitivity of these receptors to agonists and blocking agents differs so that α_1- and α_2-receptors can be differentiated pharmacologically. This factor may be important in the action of some antihypertensive drugs. (The dilator action of β$_2$-receptor stimulation will be discussed later with the endocrine factors.)

The cholinergic vasodilatory fibers that travel with the cranial nerves to the precapillary vessels in the tongue and salivary glands and with the sacral nerves to the genital area and the bladder have been described in Chapter 10. The mechanism for their parasympathetic vasodilatory action is still unclear. However, as discussed later, it appears, at least for the salivary glands, to be involved with formation of the vasodilatory substance *bradykinin*. In other tissues, the neurotransmitter *acetylcholine* has been postulated to activate endothelial cholinergic receptor sites. These receptors, in turn, appear to inhibit formation of spike potentials by the vascular muscle cells. This reduction in pacemaker activity results from hyperpolarization of the cell membrane probably due to a selective increase in membrane permeability to potassium.

Acetylcholine has a vasodilatory effect on all vascular beds, even though most of them do not have a cholinergic nerve supply. (See Chapter 10 for a discussion of cholinergic sympathetic fibers to skeletal muscle.) It is interesting that the vasodilator effect of pelvic parasympathetic fiber stimulation is, however, only partially blocked by atropine. This suggests that other, so far unidentified, vasoactive substances also may be involved in the response of these vessels. Recent studies indicate that vascular endothelial cells play an important role. Removal of the endothelial lining of the dog femoral or pulmonary artery, for example, prevents the vasodilation response of that vascular bed to acetylcholine. Recent studies suggest that acetylcholine binds to endothelial muscarinic binding sites and results in the liberation of the so-called *endothelium–derived relaxing factor (EDRF)*. The composition of this factor is currently under intense study. It may be the nitric oxide radical released by some intermediary compound.

Chemical and Endocrine Factors.—Many endocrine substances have vasomotor activity (Table 11–2). With perhaps the exception of bradykinin, mentioned earlier as being important in regulation of blood flow in some glands, the role of these substances in normal control of tissue blood flow is not clearly defined.

The relative role of adrenal catecholamines in the control of peripheral vascular function has been a controversial subject for years. Much of the confusion stems from the fact that, when stimulated, the adrenal medulla produces both *epinephrine* and *norepinephrine*. Epinephrine may have a dual effect on the control of vascular resistance because of its ability to bind to both the α-receptor sites found on all vascular muscle membranes and to the β-receptor sites of the vascular muscle membranes of coronary and skel-

TABLE 11–2.

Humoral and Chemical Substances Implicated in Regulation of Microcirculation*

Endocrine (Blood Borne)		Locally Produced (Chemicals)	
Substance	Role†	Substance	Role†
Catecholamines		Adenosine and adenine	C,D
Epinephrine	C,D	nucleotides	
Norepinephrine	C	Hypoxemia	D
Dopamine	C,D	H$^+$	D
Amines		K$^+$	D
Serotonin	C,D	Inorganic phosphate	D
Histamine	D	Hypercapnia	D
Acetylcholine	D	Krebs cycle intermediates	D
Polypeptides		Gastrointestinal polypeptides	
Angiotensin	C	Glucagon	D
Kinins	D	Cholecystokinin	
Vasopressin	C	Secretin	D
Oxytocin	C,D		
Vasoactive intestinal	D		
peptide			
Glucocorticoids	Modifiers	Prostaglandins	C,D modifiers
Estrogens	Modifiers	Hyperosmolarity	D
Plasma factors	Modifiers		
Substance P	D		
Thromboxanes	C		
Leukotrienes	C		

*Modified with additions from Altura BM: *Microvasc Res* 1971; 33:361.
†C = constrictor; D = dilator. Modifiers modify blood flow by potentiating or inhibiting action of other humoral vasoactive agents.

etal muscle blood vessels and the vascular bed of the liver. These latter receptors have a different dose-response reaction to various pharmacologic agonists and blocking drugs than myocardial β-receptors. For this reason, β-receptors have been divided into cardiac β$_1$-*receptors* and vascular bronchial β$_2$-*receptors*. The binding of epinephrine to α$_1$-receptors produces the same effect in the vascular smooth muscle as does norepinephrine (i.e., vasoconstriction). However, activation of the β$_2$-receptors by epinephrine produces vasodilation. The result of this action (i.e., vasodilation) is apparently the same as that produced by acetylcholine (Fig 11–5).

The β$_2$-receptor sites have sufficient affinity for epinephrine that at blood levels of this substance, usually produced by stimulation of the adrenal medulla (i.e., 0.02 μg/kg/minute or less), the vascular response is vasodilation. With higher epinephrine levels, in addition to vasodilation, va-

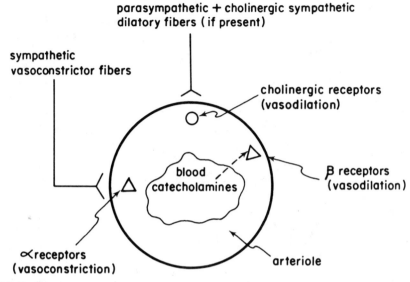

FIG 11–5.
Simplified schematic diagram of vasoactive receptor sites used in neural control of arteriolar resistance.

soconstriction is also produced via activation of the α-receptors (Fig 11–6). The concentration of norepinephrine produced at the vascular sympathetic neuromuscular junction by sympathetic stimulation is, however, likely to reach a much higher local concentration (1 to 2 μg/ml of junctional space) than will the circulating epinephrine from the adrenal medulla. The result is that the stimulation effect of norepinephrine predominates, and sympathetic stimulation causes arterioles throughout the body to constrict. The dilating effect of circulating epinephrine will, however, produce a lower net level of constriction in these vascular beds with β₂-receptors. Moreover, because of the proportionally greater reduction in flow to the vascular beds without β-receptors, blood flow will be shunted to organs with both α- and β-receptors, i.e., the myocardium, skeletal muscle, and liver.

The octopeptide *angiotensin II*, which is produced in the bloodstream through a series of steps after release of the kidney enzyme *renin* (see Chapter 7), is one of the most potent biologic vasoconstrictors so far identified. Although this substance may be important in intrarenal regulation of arteriolar resistance and in the acute stages of renal hypertension, it appears that its primary function is regulation of aldosterone production, and it probably does not play a major role in local regulation of blood flow.

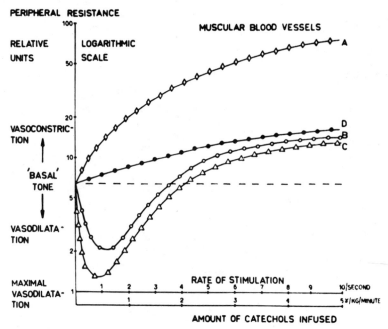

FIG 11–6.
Effect of adrenergic stimulation of skeletal muscle vascular resistance. Curve *A,* stimulation of sympathetic vasoconstrictor fibers; *B,* stimulation of adrenal medulla; *C,* epinephrine infusion; *D,* norepinephrine infusion. (From Celander O: *Acta Physiol Scand* 1954; 32[suppl 116]:1. Used by permission.)

Blood flow to the salivary and sweat glands and the exocrine pancreas is rapidly increased when the resting tone of the resistance vessels is inhibited. This is accomplished during glandular activity by direct action of cholinergic vasodilatory fibers on the larger resistance vessels and indirectly (as discussed earlier) by liberation of the vasodilatory substance bradykinin. This substance (or perhaps a similar decapeptide, kallidin) also is involved in the cutaneous vasodilation that often accompanies activation of the sweat glands (see Fig 11–5).

Some vasoactive substances, such as *histamine, serotonin* (5-hydroxy-tryptamine), and *prostaglandins,* are present in tissues and may be involved in the regulation of vascular resistance. Histamine probably causes the vasodilation that accompanies inflammation, and serotonin may be important in constriction of small vessels following vascular injury. The role of the ubiquitous prostaglandins, some of which have either potent vasoconstrictive or vasodilatory properties, remains to be clarified.

SUMMARY

The pivotal factor in local control of peripheral resistance appears to be the resting level of arteriolar muscle tension. This state of partial contraction is produced by the pacemaker activity of the single-unit smooth muscle cells and is indirectly related to the level of precapillary blood pressure. Inhibition of this basal tone by neurotransmitters (acetylcholine), hormones (e.g., epinephrine, bradykinin), or metabolic end products (e.g., low P_{O_2}, high P_{CO_2}, adenosine) permits resistance vessels to rapidly dilate and increase tissue perfusion. Augmentation in the degree of vascular muscle contraction by the action of neurotransmitters (norepinephrine) or hormones (angiotensin) increases peripheral resistance and reduces local tissue flow. No one single factor appears to play a major regulatory role in all tissues, and it is reasonable to assume that several may operate together. These mechanisms provide a feedback system for local regulation of blood flow so that each tissue receives its share of the cardiac output based on its individual need.

AUTOREGULATION OF PERIPHERAL BLOOD FLOW

It has been pointed out that blood flow to local areas appears to be internally regulated so that vasodilator substances do not accumulate, and substrate concentrations are maintained at adequate levels for cellular needs. These control mechanisms also operate to minimize the effect of alterations in perfusion pressure on tissue flow. This independence between pressure and flow over a wide range of pressure values is frequently referred to as *autoregulation* (Fig 11–7). The ability to maintain a constant flow rate despite changes in arterial pressure has obvious advantages for tissues such as the kidney that depend on a relatively fixed blood flow. The mechanism responsible for this self-regulation is still open to discussion. Considerable evidence suggests that it is a function of either or both the local length-dependent myogenic activity of vascular smooth muscle or the vasodilatory effect of local metabolites discussed earlier.

The interaction of these factors can be shown by considering the events that follow a sudden increase in arterial pressure to an individual organ. As discussed previously, the higher pressure in the precapillary vessels stimulates myogenic activity of the vascular smooth muscle. At the same time, the increased blood flow, produced by the elevated pressure, acts to wash out local tissue metabolites. The combined effect of these mechanical and chemical events is a local increase in vascular resistance and a reduction in

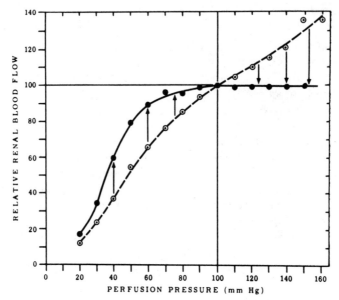

FIG 11–7.
Autoregulation of blood flow to the kidney. Initial effect *(open circles)* on blood flow of changing perfusion pressure and steady-state effect *(closed circles)*. (From Rothe CF, Nash FD, Thompson DE: *Am J Physiol* 1971; 220:1624. Used by permission.)

blood flow. On the other hand, a fall in arterial blood pressure, with its accompanying reduction in flow, results in the opposite series of events; that is, myogenic tone is decreased, and vasodilator metabolites accumulate in the interstitial fluid. These events combine to cause relaxation of resistance vessels and increase in blood flow. The negative feedback effects of these two mechanisms operate together to maintain tissue flow relatively constant over a wide range of perfusion pressures.

DISTRIBUTION OF BLOOD FLOW WITHIN THE BODY

Arterial Perfusion

Control of the circulation has so far been considered in terms of mechanisms that regulate tissue perfusion, either, as discussed earlier, through control of arterial pressure or by adjusting the caliber of the individual resistance vessels through local feedback systems. These mechanisms can be basically antagonistic and, if applied equally throughout the body, would tend to counteract each other. For example, the compensatory vasoconstriction that reflexly follows a drop in arterial pressure returns the blood pressure to normal by reducing peripheral runoff. However, the reduction in capillary flow that results from this action can lead to the local vasodilatory response of autoregulation. Fortunately, this direct confrontation usually is avoided by the competitive interaction between the two control systems. In the example used above, the major constriction takes place in organ systems such as the skin that can best withstand reduced flow. It is interesting that these organs also show the least tendency for autoregulation. At the same time, adequate perfusion of vital tissues such as the myocardium and brain is maintained because of their less profound vasoconstrictor mechanism and active tissue feedback control.

The basic pattern for the integration between central and local regulation of blood flow is determined by the anatomical distribution of vasomotor fibers to the various organs and tissues. As discussed earlier, these nerve fibers are sparsely distributed to the arterioles of the myocardium and brain. The vasculature of the skin, the viscera, and the kidneys have a rich sympathetic innervation. In addition to the density of their innervation, these vascular beds also vary in their ability to respond to sympathetic stimulation. For example, the degree of vasoconstriction produced in skeletal muscle by sympathetic stimulation is moderated by the vasodilatory effect of the circulating catecholamines from the adrenal medulla binding to β_2-receptors. The effect of sympathetic stimulation to the coronary vessels is vasodilation. This is probably a secondary effect of the increased level of metabolites produced as a result of the changes in myocardial contractility (see Chapter 14).

The net effect of these structural and functional differences among vascular beds is that blood flow to the heart and brain is protected during general sympathetic stimulation. Skeletal muscle flow is moderately reduced, and depending on degree of stimulation, blood flow to the skin, kidneys, and viscera can be markedly reduced. Under normal conditions of muscular activity and changes in body position, the differential effects of sympathetic stimulation and autoregulatory activity on vascular resistance provide that each tissue receives a share of the cardiac output according to its metabolic needs, while at the same time arterial perfusion pressure is maintained.

Vascular Capacitance

Shifts of blood within the vascular system also can be produced by changes in the capacity of the venous system. The blood volume normally stored in the capacitance vessels can be quickly mobilized, for example, by constriction of the circular multiunit vascular muscle in their walls to maintain venous return during periods of vascular adjustment. This mechanism can be illustrated by considering the effect of suddenly changing from a recumbent to an upright position. Under these circumstances, pooling of blood in the dependent venous circulation would be sufficient to reduce cardiac output if reflex venoconstriction did not take place. Under normal conditions, the change in carotid blood pressure associated with assuming the upright position is sufficient to stimulate the baroreceptor reflex; however, if this reflex fails to operate promptly, which may happen in patients with debilitated conditions, momentary dizziness or fainting may occur due to a fall in arterial blood pressure and cerebral ischemia.

In addition to its role in maintaining the return of blood to the heart, the venous system is able to take up relatively large volumes of fluid without a major change in pressure because of the distensible volume-pressure relationship of the veins (see Chapter 2). Thus, the venous capacitance vessels are able to serve as storage reservoirs that can take up or lose relatively large volumes of blood. This feature provides ballast for the maintenance of normal venous return but requires close coordination of the action of the cardiac pump, tone of the venous vascular muscles, and venous pressure by the central cardiovascular regulatory centers.

SUMMARY

Blood flow to individual vascular beds is controlled by the diameter of the resistance vessels. Myogenically active vascular muscle pacemakers are stimulated by stretch to produce a basal level of constriction. This muscular tone is modulated by the negative feedback effect of local tissue metabolites, the effect of nervous system stimulation, and by blood-borne factors. Organ perfusion is independent of a wide range of pressure values (autoregulation) due to the local metabolic regulation of tissue blood flow. Blood is preferentially shunted to specific organs due to the integrating action of both the central nervous system and local metabolic factors so that each tissue receives its share of the cardiac output according to its metabolic need.

BIBLIOGRAPHY

Ahlquist RP: A study of the adrenotropic receptors. *Am J Physiol* 1948; 153:586.
Bevan JA, Bevan RD, et al: Adrenergic regulation of vascular smooth muscle, in Bohr DF, Somlyo AP, Sparks HV Jr (eds). *Handbook of Physiology*, Section 2: *The Cardiovascular System*, vol 2. Bethesda, American Physiological Society, 1980.

Bohr DF: Vascular smooth muscle updated. *Circ Res* 1973; 32:665.

Brady MJ, Kadowitz PJ: Prostaglandins as modulators of the autonomic nervous system. *Fed Proc* 1974; 33:48.

Duling BR: Local control of microvascular function: Role of tissue oxygen supply. *Annu Rev Physiol* 1980; 42:372.

Folkow B: Description of the myogenic hypothesis. *Circ Res* 1964; 15(suppl 1):279.

Folkow B, Neil E: *Circulation.* New York, Oxford University Press, 1971.

Granger HJ, Goodman AH, Cook BH: Metabolic models of microcirculatory regulation. *Fed Proc* 1975; 34:2025.

Hermsmeyer K: Multiple pacemaker sites in spontaneously active vascular muscle. *Circ Res* 1973; 33:244.

Ignarro LJ, Byrns RE, et al: Endothelium-derived relaxing factor from pulmonary artery and vein possesses pharmacological and chemical properties identical to those of nitric oxide radical. *Circ Res* 1987; 61:866.

Johansson B, Mellander S: Static and dynamic components in the vascular myogenic response to passive change in length as revealed by electrical and mechanical recording from the rat portal vein. *Circ Res* 1975; 36:76.

Johnson PC: Autoregulation of blood flow. *Circ Res* 1964; 15(suppl 1):1.

Johnson PC: Local regulatory mechanism in the microcirculation. *Fed Proc* 1975; 34:2005.

Johnson PC: Renaissance in the microcirculation. *Circ Res* 1972; 31:817.

Johnson PC, Henrick HA: Metabolic and myogenic factors in local regulation of the microcirculation. *Fed Proc* 1975; 34:2020.

Kaiser L, Sparks HV Jr: Endothelial cells. Not just a cellophane wrapper. *Arch Intern Med* 1987; 147:569.

Mellander S, Johansson B: Control of resistance, exchange and capacitance function in the peripheral circulation. *Pharmacol Rev* 1968; 20:117.

Mellander S, et al: The effect of hyperosmolarity on intact and isolated vascular smooth muscle: Possible role in exercise hyperemia. *Angiologica* 1967; 4:310.

Murphy RA, Mras S: Control of tone in vascular smooth muscle. *Arch Intern Med* 1983; 143:1001.

Renkin EM: Control of microcirculation and blood tissue exchange, in Bohr DF, Somlyo AP, Sparks HV Jr (eds): *Handbook of Physiology, Section 2: The Cardiovascular System*, vol 2. Bethesda, American Physiological Society, 1980.

Rodbard S: Local regulation of blood flow. *Circ Res* 1971; 28(suppl. 1):1.

Rosell S: Neuronal control of microvessels. *Annu Rev Physiol* 1980; 42:359.

Rothe CF: Physiology of venous return. An unappreciated boost to the circulation. *Arch Intern Med* 1986; 146:977.

Somlyo AP, Somlyo AV: Vascular smooth muscle. I. Normal structure, pathology, biochemistry, and biophysics. *Pharmacol Rev* 1968; 20:197.

Chapter 12 _____

Tissue Perfusion and the Microcirculation

The general physical characteristics of the arterioles, capillary vessels, and venules that make up the microcirculation were discussed in Chapter 2, and the regulation of arteriolar blood flow was covered in the preceding chapter. In this section, the physiologic significance of alterations in capillary perfusion will be covered and related to the microvascular exchange between blood and interstitial fluid.

CAPILLARY FUNCTION

The capillary vessels are ideally designed for the exchange of fluids, dissolved gases, and small solute molecules between blood and interstitial fluid. The small size of these vessels gives them a maximal diffusing surface for their total volume. Because of the Laplace relationship between wall tension, internal pressure, and radius, discussed earlier in regard to the heart (see Chapter 8), the narrow diameter of the capillary vessels allows them to have a higher internal pressure than do the larger veins and still have a thin wall because it must only sustain a small amount of wall tension. The large number of vessels that share the capillary flow permits the velocity of flow in each individual vessel to be very slow (see Chapter 9). This ensures adequate time for interchange to take place across the vessel wall.

Capillary Circulation

The movement of water and dissolved solute through the clefts in the wall of the exchange vessels takes place both by diffusion and bulk flow. It is important to distinguish between these types of flow because each serves a different physiologic function.

Diffusional Flow.—Diffusion results from the random motion of particles due to their thermal energy. While this movement leads, as described in Chapter 1, to a net flux of diffusing particles from areas of high concentration to areas of lower concentration, movement also takes place, albeit at a lower rate, in the opposite direction. As a result, water and metabolic materials flow back and forth through the fluid-filled pores of the exchange vessels. This bidirectional exchange represents a high flux rate. J. R. Pappenheimer, for example, calculated that in the human forearm there is a bidirectional water flux of nearly 300 ml/minute for each 100 gm of tissue. The enormity of this exchange becomes apparent when it is realized that the plasma flow to such a sample of tissue is only about 3 ml/minute. In a similar manner, the plasma concentrations of sodium chloride, urea, and glucose exchange 120, 100, and 40 times a minute, respectively, with an equal volume of extracellular fluid. These rapid bidirectional flux rates result from the highly permeable nature of the capillary wall and the fact that most, if not all, metabolically active cells are less than a 20-μm diffusion distance from a capillary vessel. This large bidirectional exchange is important for the rapid, efficient transfer of metabolic material between capillary blood and interstitial fluid; however, as discussed below, it does not result in a significant net movement of water.

Bulk Flow.—Bulk flow, in contrast to diffusional flow, occurs under the influence of a pressure gradient; fluid and solute move as a unit. This flow can be simply expressed as

$$\dot{Q} = K_B(P_1 - P_2) \tag{12–1}$$

where $\dot{Q}$ is the flow rate; K_B, the bulk flow constant; and the difference between P_1 and P_2, is the pressure gradient. This relationship governs the flow of blood in the vascular system because of the pressure generated by the cardiac pump. This aspect is expanded and discussed in more detail in Chapter 9. There is a transcapillary pressure gradient in most exchange vessels that favors the bulk flow of fluid in or out of the vessel. This flow, as described below, depends on the energy supplied either by the heart in the form of blood pressure or by the osmotic force represented by the plasma oncotic pressure.

Bulk capillary filtration-absorption flow is important in the regulation of the circulating blood volume and is a factor in a number of conditions in which there are changes in the interstitial fluid volume; however, the amount of fluid moved by this mechanism is not large. It is estimated, for example, that only about 40 ml/24 hours/100 gm of tissue leave the capillary by bulk flow.

Solute moves with the bulk flow of fluid into and out of the exchange vessels. The magnitude of this solute drag is limited to the concentration of material in the plasma or interstitial fluid that is filtered or absorbed. This is only a small fraction of the potential diffusional movement of the same material. Thus, bulk flow is not a major factor in the interchange of fluid and solute at the capillary bed.

Filtration-Absorption Relationships.—As indicated in the previous section, there is bulk flow of an ultrafiltrate of plasma that moves from the circulation to the interstitial space and back to the vascular system. The forces responsible for this capillary circulation were first formulated in 1896 by Ernest Starling in what is now called *Starling's hypothesis*. This should not be confused with Starling's "law of the heart" discussed in Chapter 7. The mechanism proposed by Starling can be best described for an "average" capillary vessel (Fig 12–1). It should be clear to the reader that this is a model system and that the situation in individual capillaries may be quite different.

The flux of material across the wall of a capillary results from an interaction between two forces: the *effective hydrostatic pressure* and the *effective colloid osmotic* (oncotic) *pressure*. Each of these, in turn, represents the difference between the hydrostatic pressure or osmotic force operating on each side of the capillary wall. The effective hydrostatic pressure is the difference between the capillary blood pressure and the pressure exerted by the fluid in the interstitial space. The latter pressure is difficult to measure. Recent evidence has now convincingly shown that the true interstitial fluid pressure in most tissues is slightly subatmospheric. The magnitude of this negative pressure has not been settled. Most current investigators report it to vary from -1 to -10 mm Hg. The mechanism responsible for the negative tissue pressure remains uncertain, though it appears to be due to the efficient removal of protein by the lymph vessels and to the physical-chemical characteristics of the interstitial gel.

The concept of an effective oncotic pressure is somewhat more complicated and requires a brief explanation. Oncotic, a word that literally means swelling, is used to describe the osmotic effect of the plasma proteins. The

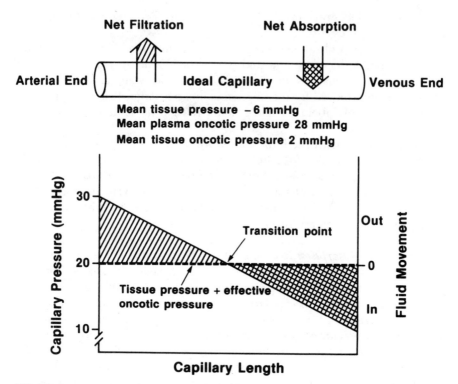

FIG 12–1.
Top, the Starling forces for filtration and reabsorption of fluid by an idealized capillary. *Bottom,* the relative amount of fluid moving out of the capillary is shown by the single *cross-hatched area,* the relative amount entering the capillary is shown by the *double cross-hatched area.* Effective oncotic pressure is the plasma oncotic pressure minus the tissue oncotic pressure. (From Little RC, Ginsburg JM: *Arch Intern Med* 1984; 144:1661. Used by permission of the American Heart Association.)

sieving action of the narrow fluid-filled pores in the capillary endothelium restricts passage of protein out of the vascular system, and only a small amount enters the tissue space. As discussed below, most of this filtered protein is promptly returned to the vascular compartment by the lymphatic system with the result that interstitial protein concentration remains quite low. Plasma, because of its high protein content, has less space for water per unit volume than interstitial fluid. As a result, the transcapillary protein concentration in large measure determines the gradient for the diffusional flow of water in the exchange vessels. Dissolved electrolytes and other freely diffusible solutes are entrained in this osmotic flow, and the fluid transfer becomes nearly equivalent to the bulk flow of an ultrafiltrate of plasma driven by a pressure equal to the effective oncotic pressure.

TABLE 12–1.

Comparison of the Contribution of Plasma Proteins to Osmotic Pressure of Plasma

Protein	Molecular Weight	Normal Conc. in Plasma (gm/100 ml	Oncotic pressure (mm Hg)	% of Total Pressure
Albumin	69,000	4.0	18.4	68.0
Globulin	100,000–450,000	1.2	1.7	6.0
Fibrogen	333,000	0.3	0.2	0.7
Others		1.5	6.7	25.3
Total		7.0	27.0	100.0

The osmotic pressure produced by a solute is defined by van't Hoff's rule as a function of the number of particles in solution. Therefore, albumin (the smallest and most concentrated of the proteins in plasma) provides the major oncotic activity (Table 12–1). The magnitude of the osmotic pressure produced by the plasma proteins is greater than that predicted by van't Hoff's rule (Fig 12–2). The precise mechanism for this anomalous behavior has not been explained, although it is thought to result from protein-protein interactions. This increased osmotic activity becomes of physiologic significance because it permits the normal level of plasma proteins to supply an oncotic pressure equivalent to nearly twice the amount that the normal protein concentration would produce if it were an ideal solution. This has the practical effect of maintaining a high plasma oncotic pressure while minimizing the effect of plasma protein concentration on blood viscosity and on flow resistance (see Chapter 9).

The electrolyte content of plasma passes easily through the wall of the exchange vessels. As a result, its osmotic effect is distributed* between the intravascular and interstitial space, and it does not exert a significant effect on the diffusional movement of water. The concentration of protein in the extracellular space varies depending on the integrity of the microvascular endothelium. In the liver, for example, capillary endothelium is discontinuous, and the only physical barrier between blood and interstitial fluid is the basement membrane. As a result, the protein content of liver interstitial fluid may be as high as 25% of the plasma concentration. In muscle, the endothelium is nearly continuous with only occasional intercellular junctions, and interstitial protein averages about 10% of the plasma concentra-

---

*The concentration of electrolytes on each side of the capillary wall is slightly different. This is due to the requirements of the Gibbs-Donnan equilibrium established by the different protein concentration between intravascular and interstitial fluid (see Chapter 1).

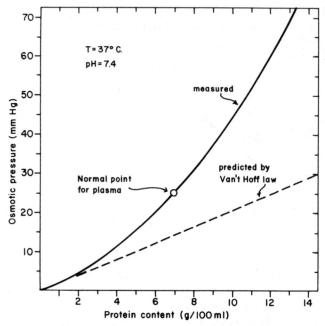

FIG 12–2.
Graph showing the relationship between protein content of plasma and osmotic pressure, as measured and predicted by van't Hoff's law. (Data calculated from Pappenheimer JR: *Physiol Rev* 1953; 33:387.)

tions. The most impermeable endothelium occurs in the brain and peripheral nerves where interstitial protein is nearly absent.

The effective plasma oncotic pressure is the difference between the osmotic pressure generated by the protein content of plasma and the protein content of interstitial fluid. The magnitude of this pressure difference will vary in different tissues because, as listed above, the protein content of interstitial fluid is not the same in all organs; however, this force (plasma oncotic pressure) tends to draw fluid into the capillary and has a usual range of 20 to 26 mm Hg. Although this pressure represents only a small part of the osmotic force exerted by the dissolved crystalloids, it represents a gradient across the capillary wall and, therefore, plays an important role in the movement of fluid in the microcirculation.

The factors responsible for the movement of fluid in and out of a typical capillary vessel are diagrammatically illustrated in Figure 12–1. The hydrostatic pressure at the arterial end is arbitrarily set in this example at 30 mm Hg. This is opposed by an effective oncotic pressure of 26 mm Hg and a tissue pressure of −6 mm Hg. These representative values have been selected to illustrate the filtration-absorption mechanism; the actual values may vary in various tissues. In this example, a force of 10 mm Hg (i.e., 30 mm Hg minus −6 mm Hg minus 26 mm Hg) is available to move fluid out of the arterial end of the capillary and produce an ultrafiltrate of plasma. Energy is lost as blood is driven through the capillary vessel. At the venous end, blood pressure is reduced, reaching, in this example, a value of 10 mm Hg. The effective oncotic pressure and the tissue pressure remain essentially the same; thus the algebraic sum of these pressures provide an inward absorbing force of 10 mm Hg at the venous end of the capillary.

This simplified example demonstrates how a balanced system of filtration-reabsorption is produced. There is flow of fluid out of the arterial end of the capillary vessel, while fluid returns to the vascular system at the venous end. It should be clear that in the body this mechanism is more complicated than is shown by this model. A balance between filtration and reabsorption is probably rarely achieved in any one vascular bed. Depending on the status of the precapillary and postcapillary resistance vessels, the level of tissue and plasma oncotic pressure and tissue pressure, individual capillary networks may act as filtering or reabsorbing surfaces. In fact, the normal vasomotion activity of arterioles (see Chapter 11) results in intermittent capillary flow in many vascular beds. As a result, filtration probably occurs throughout that capillary network when the arteriole is relaxed and capillary pressure is high. However, only absorption of fluid into the capillary bed takes place when the arteriole constricts and capillary pressure is low. If a balance between filtration and absorption is achieved, it probably occurs only over a period of time. As indicated in the next section, the lymphatic system is available to remove any excess fluid.

CIRCULATORY FUNCTION OF LYMPHATICS

The major circulatory function of the lymphatic system is to remove fluid and large-diameter molecules from the interstitial space. The endothelium of the exchange vessels is relatively impermeable to the plasma protein. Nevertheless, during a 24-hour period, between 100 and 200 gm of protein is estimated to move from the vascular system into the interstitial space. During this same period, approximately 2 L more fluid is filtered than is reabsorbed. This fluid, along with the protein and any other substances that may be present in the interstitial space (bacteria, blood cells, other small particles), enters the lymphatic capillaries through their open end or by diffusing through gaps in their walls. The sac-like terminal lymphatic vessels are suspended in the interstitium by connective tissue filaments. Expansion of the extracellular space by an increase in interstitial fluid causes these filaments to pull the lymphatic sacs open, and the hydrostatic pressure in the interstitium propels the tissue fluid into the vessel. This fluid and its dissolved material are then returned to the circulation in the form of lymph, while the particulate matter is removed by the lymph nodes.

The contents of individual lymphatic capillaries are swept into the larger impermeable lymphatic vessels by the milking action of transmitted pulsations from neighboring small arteries and muscle groups. Reflux is prevented by the lymphatic valves. Lymph flow in the thoracic duct averages about 1.3 ml/kg of body weight per hour. This slow rate is materially increased by bodily activity and factors that increase capillary filtration. However, the ability to increase lymph flow is not infinite, and for most organs, flow rate plateaus at approximately 20 times normal. Thus, the capacity for lymph drainage to increase is limited, and it can be overloaded at high filtration rates.

The smaller albumin molecules are able to penetrate the interstitial space more readily than are the larger globulin molecules. As a result, the albumin/globulin (A/G) ratio of interstitial fluid is greater than that of plasma. However, because of variations in the capillary membrane, the protein composition of lymph from different organs shows considerable variation.

The recycling of plasma proteins that enter the interstitial space is essential for maintenance of normal osmotic gradients between plasma and interstitial fluid. For this reason, injury or blockage of the thoracic duct or other main lymphatic channels may be life threatening. Localized blockage of lymph flow from a small area will lead to an accumulation of protein and a smaller amount of water in the affected tissue. This localized area of swelling *(lymphedema)* differs from an accumulation of extracellular fluid *(edema)* because of its high protein content.

CAPILLARY CIRCULATIONS

In the previous section, four different types of capillary circulations have been discussed. These can be summarized as follows:

1. Blood flow.—In a normal adult at rest, approximately 8,400 L of blood or 4,620 L of plasma (blood contains about 45% formed elements) travels through the total capillary system every 24 hours.

2. Capillary diffusional circulation.—Plasma water exchanges with interstitial fluid by diffusion through the capillary wall 120 times per minute.

This can give a total diffusional circulation of as much as 85,000 L per day.

3. Interstitial fluid circulation.—About 0.25% of the blood volume is filtered per minute throughout the capillary bed into the interstitial space (exclusive of glomerular filtration in the kidney). During a 24-hour period, this amounts to almost 20 L of fluid. Of this volume, 80% to 90%, or about 18 L, is reabsorbed into the capillary bed at its venous end.

4. Lymph flow.—The approximately 2 L of fluid that is filtered but not absorbed by the capillary bed is returned to the circulation via the lymphatic circulation per 24 hours.

EDEMA

The term "edema"comes from a Greek word meaning tumor or swelling and is used to describe a collection of interstitial fluid that distends the tissues. If the edema fluid collects in the peritoneal cavity, it is called *ascites;* a collection of serous fluid in the pleural cavity is referred to as *hydrothorax* or *pleural effusion*. Edema develops when the capillary filtration-reabsorption relationship, described in the previous section, is disturbed (see Fig 12–1) and interstitial fluid is formed at a rate faster than it is removed by capillary absorption or lymph drainage. This relationship is not as delicately balanced as the previous statement might suggest. For reasons that are discussed below, a deviation of 5 to 10 mm Hg is required from the normal venous pressure or plasma oncotic pressure before there is a significant redistribution of fluid between intravascular and extravascular compartments.

Edema occurs in a number of diseases and it is a valuable diagnostic sign for the physician. The following brief summary of the circulatory mechanisms involved in the production of edema will serve to illustrate how capillary function can be modified by alterations in Starling forces, capillary surface area, and capillary permeability. Important causes of edema are (1) a fall in oncotic pressure of the plasma as a result of starvation, liver disease, or other conditions that reduce the plasma protein level; (2) increased capillary hydrostatic pressure that may result from local obstruction of veins or postural changes such as prolonged standing; (3) increase in the extracellular fluid volume as a result of conditions associated with fluid retention; and (4) increase in capillary permeability due to local toxins, hypoxia, or inflammation.

Pulmonary edema due to transudation of fluid from the pulmonary capillaries into the alveolae is a potentially serious complication of congestive heart failure or other conditions where pulmonary capillary pressure is increased (see Chapter 13).

Interstitial Compartment Compliance

The interstitial compartment is quite stiff under normal conditions, and a small change in volume will result in a large change in tissue pressure. This relationship is usually described in terms of compliance, i.e., the ratio of change in volume to change in pressure (Fig 12–3). This low interstitial compliance at normal tissue pressure is important to the regulation of interstitial compartment size. The relatively large increase in interstitial pressure that accompanies even a small increase in interstitial volume due to an increase in capillary filtration will, for example, have a negative effect on interstitial fluid formation by opposing further movement of fluid out of the vascular compartment. At the same time, the increase in tissue pressure will increase lymph flow. These mechanisms thereby limit the increase in interstitial volume. Conversely, a small decrease in interstitial fluid forma-

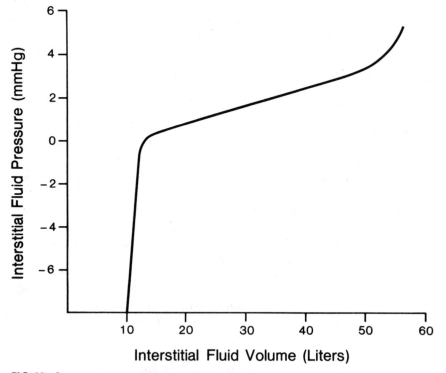

FIG 12–3.
Idealized pressure-volume relationship of the human interstitial space based on experimental animal data. Data from Guyton AC: *Textbook of Medical Physiology*, ed 7. Philadelphia, WB Saunders Co, 1986.

tion will act to decrease lymph flow and facilitate filtration. Thus, the low interstitial compliance normally serves to maintain interstitial volume in the normal range.

However, the low interstitial compliance just described changes abruptly as tissue pressure moves into the positive range. When this occurs, the interstitial compartment becomes quite distensible. Accordingly, a significant increase in interstitial fluid volume, such as occurs with sodium retention due to heart or kidney failure, leads to loss of the safety factor provided by the normally stiff tissue compartment. Under these conditions, interstitial volume can expand easily, and massive edema can result.

Low Plasma Proteins

Reduction of the oncotic pressure of blood due to a drop in plasma protein concentration will increase net filtration pressure and reduce net reabsorption forces. This change also will shift the transition point in the capillary bed at which filtration and reabsorption of fluid are equal toward the venous end of the capillary network (Fig 12–4, bottom). A larger than normal capillary surface then becomes available for filtration and, as a result, there will be a corresponding reduction in the absorptive surface. The end effect of these shifts is an increase in the net volume of fluid that enters the interstitial space. If this influx overloads the ability of the lymphatic vessels to remove the extra fluid, edema will develop. This tendency will be greatest in the dependent parts of the body due to the additive effect of the higher venous pressure in those areas (see below).

The protein albumin, as discussed earlier, provides the major osmotic activity of the plasma proteins. When its concentration falls below 2.5 to 3 gm/100 ml of plasma, edema usually becomes clinically evident. Massive generalized edema *(anasarca)* may occur with lower albumin levels.

Increased Capillary Pressure

The resistance to capillary drainage produced by elevated venous pressure causes both capillary pressure and volume to increase. This change is accompanied by increased transudation of fluid into the interstitial space due to the higher filtration pressure and larger exchanging surface. The change in venous pressure and the edema it produces may be localized or generalized depending on the cause. For example, thrombophlebitis of a deep vein in the calf will produce localized swelling of the lower leg, whereas generalized edema may occur with an elevation in systemic venous pressure in conditions such as congestive heart failure or renal disease

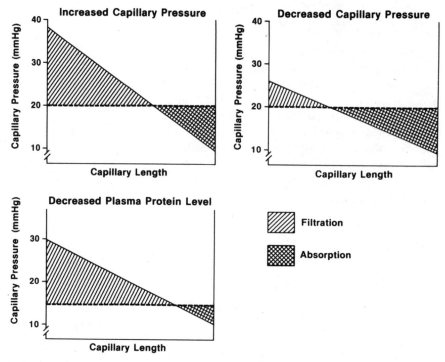

FIG 12–4.
Effect of abnormalities in capillary pressure or plasma protein level on fluid movement in and out of an ideal capillary and on capillary filtration and absorption surface. (From Little RC, Ginsburg JM: *Arch Intern Med* 1984; 144:1661. Used by permission.)

where there is an increase in volume of the extracellular fluid compartment. In both cases, the equilibrium point between filtration and reabsorption is shifted toward the venous side of the affected capillary bed (see Fig 12–4, top, left). In this situation, just as described above for hypoproteinemia, there is an increase in both net filtration pressure and filtration surface and a reduction in the absorbing area.

Edema produced by a localized elevation in capillary pressure frequently is minimal in amount and, provided the basic cause does not change, usually remains more or less stationary. This occurs because the tissue pressure in the affected area is increased sufficiently to bring filtration and reabsorption back into equilibrium. Such an equilibrium is most easily obtained when the edema is limited to a tight anatomical compartment such as the dorsum of the foot or the ankle so that the marked increase in interstitial compartment compliance that normally occurs with elevation of the tissue pressure (see above) is prevented. This mechanism may explain why the edema that accompanies prolonged standing (see Chapter 13) is usually mild. However, severe edema may accompany congestive heart failure or renal disease due to the extensive enlargement of extracellular fluid volume in those conditions in addition to the elevated venous pressure.

Increased Capillary Permeability

A number of toxins and other substances involved with the inflammatory reaction act on the capillary endothelium (see Chapter 2) to increase capillary permeability. As a result, fluid and protein leave the capillary vessels, and swelling becomes one of the first clinical signs of inflammation. Histamine, serotonin, and various kinins also increase vascular permeability and undoubtedly play a role in the production of allergic edema. In a rather rare disease, *hereditary angioneurotic edema,* the periodic attacks of swelling, which can obstruct the airway and be life threatening, apparently occur because of the congenital lack of a serum, α_2-globulin, which normally inhibits the kinin-forming enzymes.

Other Causes of Edema

Obstruction of lymphatic vessels will interfere with the removal of excess extracellular fluid and may result in edema. This mechanism may, for example, explain the localized swelling that frequently occurs for some weeks following a fracture of one of the long bones. It also underlies the edema associated with tropical parasitic infection in which the organism invades and blocks the lymphatic vessels. However, as mentioned above, chronic lymphatic obstruction produces a type of edema (lymphedema) that is quite different from that of ordinary swelling. A number of other conditions such as allergic reactions, insect bites, and food poisons also may cause localized areas of edema. The mechanism responsible for these events is not always clear and frequently no satisfactory explanation is available.

SUMMARY

The arterial system receives the pulsatile flow from the left ventricle and delivers nearly steady flow to the capillaries. Here, the interaction of the circulatory pressure, oncotic pressure, tissue pressures, and capillary surfaces provide for the efficient exchange with the tissue.

Movement of fluid and dissolved material through the exchange vessels takes place by diffusion and by bulk flow due to the transcapillary pressure gradient (Starling's hypothesis). The capillary circulation includes (1) blood flow, (2) diffusional circulation with interstitial fluid, and (3) filtration-absorption (Starling forces). Disturbances of the filtration-absorption mechanism may lead to excess production of interstitial fluid (edema).

BIBLIOGRAPHY

Airkland K, Nicoloysen G: Interstitial fluid volume: Local regulatory mechanisms. *Physiol Rev* 1981; 61:556.

Brace RA: Progress toward resolving the controversy of positive vs negative interstitial fluid pressure. *Circ Res* 1981; 49:281.

Burton AC: Physical principles of circulatory phenomena: The physical equilibria of the heart and blood vessels, in Hamilton WF (ed): *Handbook of Physiology, Section 2: Circulation*, vol 2. Washington DC, the American Physiological Society, 1963.

Burton AC: Relation of structure to function of the tissue of the wall of blood vessels. *Physiol Rev* 1954; 34:619.

Grega GJ (ed): Symposium. Role of the endothelial cell in the regulation of microvascular permeability to molecules. *Fed Proc* 1985; 45:75.

Guyton AC, Granger HJ, Taylor AE: Interstitial fluid pressure. *Physiol Rev* 1971; 51:527.

Landis EM, Pappenheimer JR: Exchange of substances through the capillary walls, in Hamilton WF (ed): *Handbook of Physiology, Section 2: Circulation*, vol 2. Washington DC, The American Physiological Society, 1963.

Little RC, Ginsburg JM: The physiological basis for clinical edema. *Arch Intern Med* 1984; 144:1661.

McDonald DA: *Blood Flow in Arteries*, ed 2. Baltimore, Williams & Wilkins Co, 1974.

Pappenheimer JR: Passage of molecules through capillary walls. *Physiol Rev* 1953; 33:387.

Sparks HV Jr (ed): Symposium. A metabolic barrier for solute transport. *Fed Proc* 1985; 44:2602.

Staub NC, Taylor AE: *Edema*. New York, Raven Press, 1984.

Taylor AE: Capillary fluid filtration; Starling forces and lymph flow. *Circ Res* 1981; 49:557.

Van Citters RL, Wagner BM, Rushmer RF: Architecture of small arteries during vasoconstriction. *Circ Res* 1962; 10:668.

Chapter 13 _____

Venous and Pulmonary Circulation

_____

The conduit function of the arterial system and details of the microcirculation have been covered in earlier sections. The activities of the venous and pulmonary circulation will be summarized in this chapter.

VENOUS CIRCULATION

General Considerations

A driving force of 7 to 8 mm Hg is normally available at the end of the capillary bed to propel blood through the venous system (see Chapter 7). This pressure *(vis a tergo)* plus a negligible kinetic component due to the velocity of flow represents the remainder of the energy imparted to the blood by cardiac contraction. This force is sufficient to return blood to the heart from the dependent parts of the body because of the unique construction of the venous circulation.

Venous Distensibility

As pointed out earlier, most peripheral veins act as collapsible structures and become elastic vessels only when distended (see Fig 2–7). This has led to confusion regarding the distensibility characteristics of veins and the venous system. For example, at low pressure (P) levels (0 to 6 mm Hg), the venous system can accommodate a considerable change in volume (V) with very little alteration in pressure, making $\Delta V/\Delta P$ (the compliance) large. This occurs because the cross-sectional area of the elliptic veins will increase as these structures approach a circular shape. However, some physiologists have erroneously concluded from this ability of the venous system to store fluid at low pressures that the vein wall is very elastic. In fact, the contrary is correct. The true distensibility of the veins becomes apparent when the internal volume is increased sufficiently for the vein to operate as an elastic structure (Fig 13–1). Under these conditions, which may be achieved in the veins of the lower legs during quiet standing (see below), the slope of the venous volume-pressure plot is greater than comparable values for the arterial system (see Fig 10–11). At greater filling volumes the distensibility characteristics of veins change as the inelastic collagen of the outer wall begins to be stretched and the vessel becomes very stiff. This latter ability to withstand high internal pressures without dilating has permitted the use of vein segments as arterial grafts during vascular surgery.

Effect of Hydrostatic Level

When an individual is supine, the major arteries and veins assume a horizontal orientation that places them in essentially the same plane as the heart. As a result, differences in hydrostatic level between the heart and veins will be quite small, and its effect on vascular pressure usually can be ignored. Because of this, the difference between the pressure at the heart and the periphery in a recumbent subject (if kinetic factors are discounted) will represent the energy expended in overcoming vascular resistance as

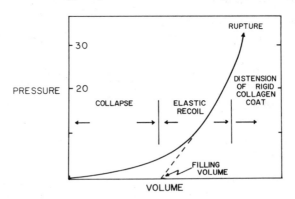

FIG 13–1.
Schematic plot of volume of a segment of vein vs. the transmural pressure, showing response to a change in volume during its phase as a collapsible structure, as an elastic structure, and when it is fully distended. See text for further discussion. (Modified from Folkow B, Neil E: *Circulation.* New York, Oxford University Press, 1971.)

blood flows to or from the heart. This value, as shown in Fig 13–2, is usually about 5 mm Hg for both the arterial and the venous systems.

The large circulatory vessels change from the horizontal plane when one assumes an upright position, and they become vertically oriented columns. In this position, these fluid-filled tubes exert an important hydrostatic effect on the vascular pressure in the dependent parts of the body. The increased pressure of blood in the legs on standing, for example, may cause dilation of venous channels and increase the ultrafiltration of fluid into the interstitial space. Because of the hydrostatic column of blood in an individual in the upright position, vascular pressures from different areas are normally related to a single reference point. The middle of the right atrium usually is used as the reference or *phlebostatic level*. This is the site in the cardiovascular system where there is the least change in pressure when the body is rotated into various positions. The use of this level, for example, will permit comparison of the effect of a drug on arterial pressure even though the pressure is measured in different vessels or with the body in different positions.

Under most conditions, the *transmural* blood pressure, i.e., the difference in pressure between inside and outside the vessel, is of physiologic interest. Measurement of this pressure requires that it be related to the

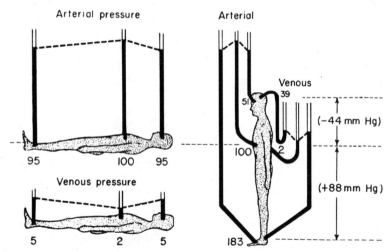

FIG 13–2.

Effect of body position on arterial and venous pressure. On the *left*, the numbers give the pressure (in millimeters of mercury) with the right atrium as the reference level. On the *right*, the numbers give the pressure (in millimeters of mercury) related to the point of measurement. See text for discussion. (From Burton AC: *Physiology and Biophysics of the Circulation*, ed 2. Chicago, Year Book Medical Publishers, 1972. Used by permission.)

point of measurement. The difference between the transmural and vascular pressure can be shown by the following illustration.

The dorsum of the foot of an upright adult can be assumed to be 120 cm below the phlebostatic level (see Fig 13–2). In this position, a mean aortic pressure of 100 mm Hg at the level of the heart will provide a transmural pressure of 183 mm Hg in the dorsalis pedis artery. This value results because the 120-cm column of blood provides a pressure of 88 mm Hg. Thus 100 mm Hg plus 88 mm Hg minus 5 mm Hg pressure lost due to resistance between the heart and the foot equals 183 mm Hg. However, when the same example is used, if the pressure in the dorsalis pedis artery is related to heart level (phlebostatic level), the hydrostatic column between the heart and the foot is subtracted and the pressure becomes 95 mm Hg. This is the same as the transmural pressure in the dorsalis pedis artery when the individual is supine.

The pressure in the veins on the dorsum of the foot in the upright position will depend on how long the individual has been standing. During a period of standing without muscular movement, the venous channels will fill from below upward as blood pools in the dependent vessels; the venous valves will be forced open and blood flow will be continuous from the periphery to the heart. Under these circumstances transmural venous pressure in the foot will be approximately 93 mm Hg (computed as 88 mm Hg hydrostatic pressure plus 5 mm Hg venous pressure). This would be 5 mm Hg if the foot were elevated to heart level. Under these conditions, the total energy used in both the arterial and venous systems to overcome vascular resistance between the periphery and the heart is the difference between the central and peripheral pressure after correction for hydrostatic pressure differences.

The practical significance of this relationship between central and peripheral vascular pressure stems from the siphon qualities of the circulation. Additional energy is not required to maintain the flow of blood through the dependent parts of the body even though the capillary pressure may be markedly elevated in those regions.

In the upright position, the pressure in the cerebral blood vessels will be lower than the corresponding pressure at heart level. In this case, the pressure exerted by the fluid column above the heart will be subtracted from the pressure at heart level. Again, the difference between central and peripheral pressure provides the energy necessary to maintain flow. These relationships stem from the fact that vascular resistance and driving force are not affected by the path taken by the blood vessels. As shown in Figure 13–3, flow is related to the pressure head (i.e., the difference in pressure between the ends of the vessel), characteristics of the fluid, and size of the tube but is independent of the path taken by the vessel.

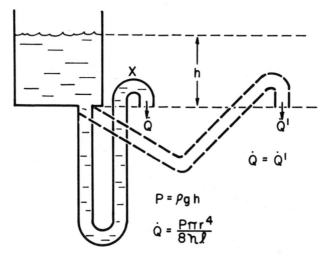

FIG 13–3.

Diagram showing a flexible tube and reservoir arranged as a reverse siphon. Flow *(Q)* through tube is a function of pressure head *(P)*, type of fluid, and dimensions of tube and is independent of the height of the bend in the tube. ρ = density of the fluid; g = gravitational constant; h = height of the hydrostatic column; r = radius of tube; η = viscosity of fluid; l = length of tube.

Muscular Activity and Venous Pressure in the Legs

The high venous pressure that develops in the lower extremities as a result of motionless standing can have serious consequences if it persists for an extended period. Fortunately, the muscular contractions associated with postural movements and activities such as walking effectively lower venous pressure in the legs and feet (Fig 13–4). This reduction occurs as a consequence of the compression applied to the leg veins as they travel through the fascial compartments that surround the active muscle groups. This *muscle pump*, aided by the venous valves, squeezes the contents toward the heart (Fig 13–5). When the muscles relax, the valves prevent backflow and each deep venous segment fills from the superficial veins and lower deep veins. In the process, the venous fluid column between the periphery and the heart is interrupted (Fig 13–6). As a result, the hydrostatic force exerted on the lower venous segment is reduced, and the venous pressure in the foot is correspondingly lower. Even a single step (see Fig 13–4) can be very effective in reducing the high venous pressure produced by standing quietly.

As discussed above, inadequate rhythmic contraction of the leg veins results in a high venous pressure, which, in turn, will cause increased

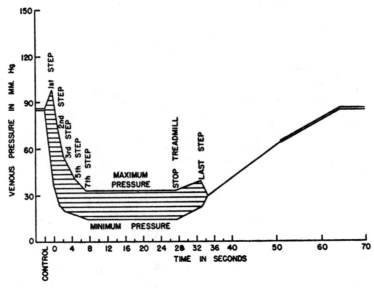

FIG 13–4.
With quiet standing, venous pressure in the dorsal vein of the foot is 85 mm Hg. Walking quickly lowers the pressure to 30 mm Hg. When walking stops, venous pressure gradually increases back to 85 mm Hg. (From Pollock AA, Wood EH: *J Appl Physiol* 1949; 1:649. Used by permission.)

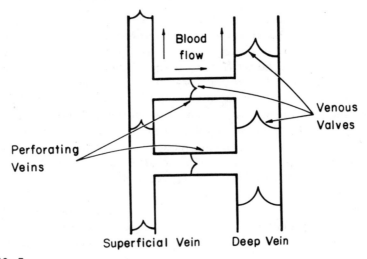

FIG 13–5.
Schematic diagram of superficial and deep venous circulation of the leg showing venous valves. The normal direction of venous flow is shown by the *short arrows.* Retrograde flow is prevented by closure of valve cusps.

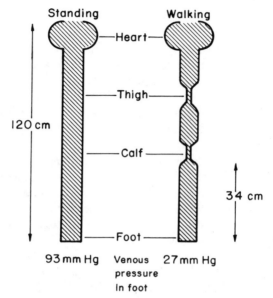

FIG 13-6.
Schematic diagram showing effect of standing and walking on the hydrostatic column of blood in veins of the leg. Compression of veins by muscular action interrupts the blood column and reduces hydrostatic pressure in lower leg and foot. (Only two of the venous values in the leg are shown.)

capillary filtration and a tendency for edema formation. Engorgement of the dependent veins also may trap a sizable amount of blood estimated to be as much as 500 ml. Prolonged standing or conditions such as venous obstruction or pregnancy that lead to chronic overstretching of the veins can cause destruction or incompetence of the venous valves. When this occurs, the muscle pump becomes ineffective and results in the superficial veins of the leg being subjected to the full hydrostatic pressure of the venous column. As these veins frequently lack supporting tissues, the increased pressure may in time lead to bulbous dilations of the veins with further destruction of the venous valves and to stasis of blood. This condition is referred to as *varicose veins*.

Some people appear to have a familial tendency to development of varicosities in the leg veins (see above), in the hemorrhoidal veins (hemorrhoids), and in other segments of the venous system (varicocele, esophageal varices). These difficulties are part of the physiologic price of an upright position. It is interesting that in four-footed animals approximately 70% of the blood volume is at or above the level of the heart, whereas in the upright human nearly the same percentage is below the phlebostatic axis.

Subatmospheric Venous Pressure

Venous Pressure Above the Heart.—If the veins were rigid tubes, the pressure at any point above the heart would be equal to right atrial pressure minus the force produced by a vertical hydrostatic column of blood between the phlebostatic axis and the point of measurement. As a result, the pressure in the neck veins of an upright normal individual becomes subatmospheric a few centimeters above heart level. Below this area, the veins act as proper conduits; however, they are not rigid and the difference between inside and outside pressure (the *transmural pressure*) above this area will cause them to collapse (Fig 13–7). It should be pointed out that the veins while collapsed are not occluded, and flow continues through tunnels formed where the walls are not in total opposition.

The collapse of the neck veins breaks the hydrostatic column so that venous pressure remains essentially zero above the point of collapse to the entrance of the vessel into the skull. This phenomenon can be used as a noninvasive method for bedside measurement of central venous pressure. The vertical distance between the heart and the point at which venous distention disappears gives the central pressure in centimeters of blood (see Fig 13–7). This is normally 3.4 to 4 cm.

For reasons that the following discussion should make clear, venous pressure inside the skull in the erect position is subatmospheric. However,

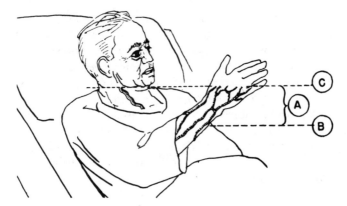

FIG 13–7.
Diagram showing how neck veins and veins in back of the hand collapse when their internal pressure becomes subatmospheric. B = heart level; C = level at which veins collapse; A = vertical height of fluid column in the veins. (From Burton AC: *Physiology and Biophysics of the Circulation,* ed 2. Chicago, Year Book Medical Publishers, 1972. Used by permission.)

because the skull forms a rigid box and cerebrospinal fluid (CSF) pressure also is subatmospheric, transmural pressure across the wall of the cerebral veins is essentially zero. As a result, the cerebral veins are neither collapsed nor distended and can again act as a hydrostatic column. The force exerted by this column must be subtracted from the essentially zero venous pressure at the entrance of the veins into the skull to give the pressure at any point within the brain (see Chapter 14).

Thoracic Venous Pressure.—The veins within the thoracic cavity are subjected to the negative intrapleural pressure. The resulting increase in venous transmural pressure causes the thoracic veins to dilate, and central venous pressure is reduced. The pressure gradient between the extrathoracic veins and the heart is increased and venous return is facilitated. During inspiration the increased negative intrapleural pressure tends to increase venous return, with the result that venous pressure just outside the chest may be reduced. If this occurs, it has the negative feedback effect of producing partial (or complete) collapse of the veins just before they enter the chest. The increase in flow resistance produced by this reduction in the lumen of the veins then acts to limit venous return. Thus, the effect of this *respiratory venous pump* is limited in its ability to increase venous return.

The action of the respiratory pump on venous return, although limited, does result in some increase in right ventricular output during inspiration via the Frank-Starling mechanism. This increase is, however, largely absorbed by the concomitant enlargement of the pulmonary vascular volume due to inflation of the lungs so that left ventricular output remains constant or may even fall during inspiration. With expiration, the extra blood that has been trapped in the lungs during inspiration is returned to the left side of the heart. The Frank-Starling mechanism now results in an increase in left ventricular output. The outcome is that cardiac output and, indirectly, arterial blood pressure increase slightly with expiration and fall with inspiration. These variations may be increased in the presence of pericardial effusions or other conditions that limit the expansion of the heart (see Chapter 2). These changes may occur slightly out of phase, particularly if there is a larger than normal pulmonary blood volume.

Right Atrial Pressure.—During the early part of ventricular systole, tension from the contracting myocardium pulls the atrioventricular (AV) valve anulus toward the apex and elongates the atria (descent of the cardiac base; see Chapter 4). This results in a sharp drop in atrial pressure (the X descent), and as a result, the venoatrial filling gradient increases. This increase in the filling gradient is particularly marked on the right side of the heart where it produces a significant spurt in venous return. A second increase in atrial filling occurs during the Y descent of the atrial pressure pulse early in diastole.

The Venous Blood Reservoir.—The venous system acts as a storage reservoir from which blood is removed to fill the heart. As indicated in Chapter 2, the venous capacitance vessels may contain up to 77% of the blood circulating in the systemic circulation. The actual amount will depend on (1) total blood volume, (2) level of cardiac output, (3) level of constriction of the smooth muscle in the wall of the veins, and (4) venous pressure. As discussed above, venous pressure, particularly in individual vessels, can be altered by hydrostatic factors. In addition, the magnitude of capillary blood flow may cause local variations in venous volume and pressure. The inotropic state of the myocardium may also affect the size of the venous reservoir. During an episode of acute heart failure, for example, the inability of the heart to maintain cardiac output may result in venous engorgement. Similarly, a loss of blood volume due to a sudden hemorrhage will lead to sympathetic stimulation and contraction of the venous reservoir (see Chapter 15). This will act to maintain venous return and cause blood to be transferred from the veins to the high-pressure arterial circulation by cardiac action.

Reflex changes in venomotor tone due to afferent input from arterial and venous baroreceptors appear to play an important role in the maintenance of a normal central venous pressure and cardiac preload. Recent studies indicate that active venoconstriction or dilation can provide rapid compensation to maintain cardiovascular hemostasis that is equivalent to a sizable change in blood volume. This is an area of intense current research; however, the details of this control remain unclear.

PULMONARY CIRCULATION

Pulmonary vs. Bronchial Circulation

The pulmonary circulation transports venous blood from the right ventricle to the alveolar capillaries and then returns the oxygenated blood to the left atrium. This vascular system should be distinguished from the bronchial circulation, which also supplies blood to the lungs. The alveoli and alveolar ducts receive their nutrients largely from the pulmonary circulation. The bronchial circulation receives arterial blood from the bronchial arteries and supplies (1) the bronchi, bronchioles, and supporting tissues of the lung; (2) vasa vasorum of the pulmonary arteries; and (3) pulmonary nerves and sensory endings (Fig 13–8).

The bronchial circulation can be of physiologic importance because (1)

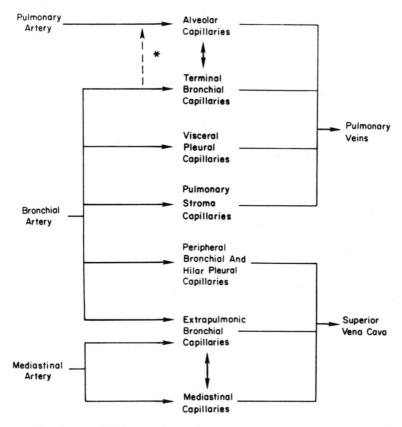

* Vasa Vasorum Of Pulmonary Artery

FIG 13–8.
Schematic diagram of vascular connections of bronchial, pulmonary, and mediastinal arteries.

there are direct anastomotic connections between the bronchial and pulmonary capillaries and (2) 75% to 80% of the bronchial venous outflow is discharged into the pulmonary veins. Bronchial blood flow is normally about 1% of the total cardiac output. At this level, the shunt of venous blood into the pulmonary veins is too small to be of practical importance. However, with long-standing bronchial infection or with conditions such as congenital cardiac malformations where pulmonary flow is reduced to one or both lungs, bronchial flow may be significantly increased. When this occurs, the venous shunt from the bronchial circulation may lead to some arterial desaturation. (The coronary venous blood that enters the left side of the heart via the thebesian veins also adds to this venous shunt.)

Pulmonary blood vessels are characteristically shorter and wider and have thinner walls than corresponding vessels in the systemic circulation. The pulmonary arterioles have less contractile tissue than systemic arterioles; however, because of their lower internal pressure, it appears to be adequate to regulate their diameter. In addition, many of the smaller arteries in the 30-50 μ range have a layer of vascular muscle that is innervated by sympathetic vasoconstrictor fibers. Selective constriction of these vessels can be used to regulate the distribution of pulmonary blood flow to various segments of the lung; however, present indications are that, at least in adults, this mechanism is not used.

The pulmonary capillaries form a sheet-like network that surrounds the alveolar sacs. This capillary space has a surface area that has been estimated to be 60 sq m at rest, and it can increase to as much as 90 sq m during exercise due to recruitment of previously collapsed vessels in the lungs. The thin endothelial capillary membrane is distinct from the equally thin lining of the alveolus (Fig 13–9). These membranes usually are very close together, and the diffusing distance between the respiratory gas and pulmonary blood is normally only 0.20 to 0.60 μ. However, under pathologic

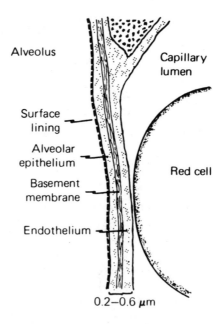

FIG 13–9.
Diagram of alveolar-capillary junction showing structures that separate alveolar gas from plasma. (From Ganong WF: *Review of Medical Physiology*, ed 7. Los Altos, Calif, Lange Medical Publications, 1975. Used by permission.)

conditions the potential space between the two membranes can become filled with edema fluid, exudate, or fibrous tissue. Any of these substances will present a barrier to the free diffusion between blood and alveolar gas and will lead to diffusion difficulties at the alveolar-capillary membrane.

Effect of Transmural Pressure

The pulmonary microcirculation differs from its systemic counterpart in that pulmonary capillaries are largely surrounded by gas and lack a firm supporting structure. As a result, these delicate vessels will expand or collapse depending on the balance between the distending capillary blood pressure and surrounding alveolar pressure. During normal breathing, alveolar pressure varies between a slightly negative value during inspiration and a slightly positive value during expiration. However, as alveoli are connected via the bronchi to the outside air, alveolar pressure usually is close to atmospheric. In addition to transmural pressure, the caliber of the pulmonary arteries and veins is also affected by traction from the surrounding lung as it expands and contracts.

Mean pulmonary arterial pressure under normal conditions is approximately 15 mm Hg, and mean pulmonary capillary pressure is 10 mm Hg (Fig 13–10). As pulmonary capillary pressure is considerably below the oncotic pressure of plasma proteins, filtration does not normally occur in the alveolar-capillary bed and the net inward-directed force aids absorption of fluid. The mechanism operates to keep the alveoli dry. If capillary pressure rises above plasma oncotic pressure, this protective mechanism will be lost and pulmonary edema can result. This is a serious matter as any appreciable layer of fluid in the alveoli will interfere with diffusion between alveolar gas and pulmonary blood. Active absorption of alveolar fluid is important, as the lymphatic vessels of the lungs do not extend below the level of the alveolar ducts. As a result, this mechanism is not available to remove fluid from the alveolar sacs.

Hydrostatic Relationships and Pulmonary Blood Flow

Because of the low level of pulmonary blood pressure compared to systemic arterial pressure, changes produced by hydrostatic differences within the lung may become important. For example, in the upright position (Fig 13–11), a mean capillary pressure of 10 mm Hg at heart level could become as low as − 2 or − 3 mm Hg at the apex of the lung and as high as 24 or 25 mm Hg at the base. The exact value in each case will depend on the distance between the top and bottom of the lung. As the gravitational effect on gas in the respiratory system is negligible, the atmospheric alveolar pres-

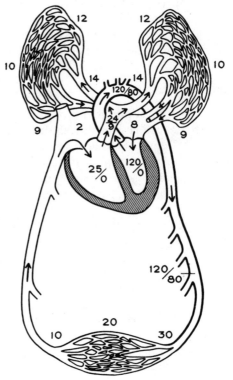

FIG 13–10.
Schematic diagram of pulmonary and systemic circulation. Average pressure values are shown. (From Comroe JH Jr: *Physiology of Respiration,* ed 2. Chicago, Year Book Medical Publishers, 1974. Used by permission.)

sure at the apex of the lung may exceed capillary pressure, and the entire capillary bed at the apex may be occluded (Fig 13–12). In the middle zone of the lung (sometimes referred to as zone 2), arterial pressure will exceed alveolar pressure; however, alveolar pressure may be higher than venous pressure. Therefore, the venous end of the capillary bed will be compressed but not necessarily occluded. In the lower part of the lung (zone 3), blood pressure in the capillary microcirculation will exceed alveolar pressure, and the vascular bed in this area will be dilated.

The illustrative relationships described above may not be precisely duplicated in vivo because of individual variations in lung size and pulmonary pressure. For example, when the body is in the upright position, pulmonary flow may not be completely prevented at the apex of the lungs in short individuals or in children, due to the lower hydrostatic pressure at that

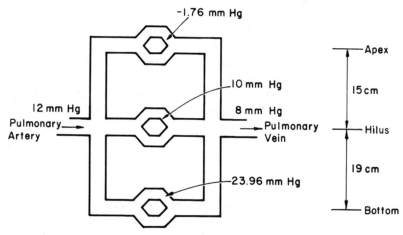

FIG 13–11.
Schematic diagram of the lung in the upright position. Capillary pressure at heart level (hilus of the lung) is 10 mm Hg. This pressure becomes −1.76 mm Hg at the apex of the lung if it is 15 cm above the hilus and 23.96 mm Hg at the bottom of the lung if it is 19 cm below the hilus.

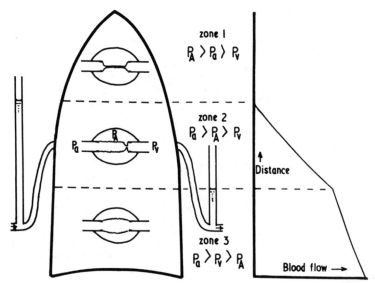

FIG 13–12.
Model of circulation illustrating the effect of hydrostatic pressure changes when the body is in the upright position on behavior of small pulmonary vessels and the resulting regional differences in blood flow. P_A = alveolar pressure; P_a = arterial pressure; P_v = venous pressure. (From West JB, Dollery CT, Naimark A: *J Appl Physiol* 1964; 19:713. Used by permission.)

point because of the smaller lungs in these individuals. In addition, because of the pulsatile nature of pulmonary capillary pressure, the capillaries at the apex of the lung in large individuals may open only during systole. In any case, these mechanisms will cause pulmonary blood flow in the upright position to vary from being small or absent at the apex to becoming maximal at the base of the lungs (Fig 13–13). In the supine position, the hydrostatic forces are reduced, and the entire lung responds much like the middle zone of the upright lung.

Pulmonary Resistance

Pulmonary vascular resistance under normal conditions is approximately one tenth that of the resistance of the systemic circulation. This value is predictable from the fact that pulmonary pressure is one tenth of the systemic value. (A cardiac output that is 5.5 L/minute at a mean systemic pressure of 100 mm Hg gives a systemic resistance of 18.1 mm Hg/L/minute, whereas the same flow at a pulmonary pressure of 10 mm Hg gives a resistance of 1.81 mm Hg/L/minute.)

The lung is unique in that an increase in either pulmonary arterial or venous pressure will result in a drop in its vascular resistance (Fig 13–14).

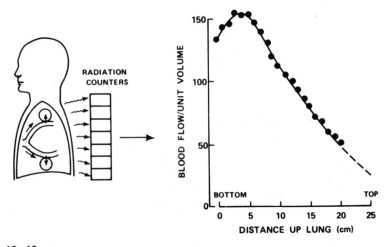

FIG 13–13.
Right, blood flow distribution in the lung in the upright position by radioactive xenon. The dissolved xenon is evolved into alveolar gas through the pulmonary capillaries. The units of blood flow are such that if flow were uniform, all values would be 100. *Left,* note the small flow *(dots)* at the apex. (Modified from Hughes JMB, et al: *Respir Physiol* 1968; 4:58 from West JB: *Respiratory Physiology: The Essentials.* Baltimore, Williams & Wilkins Co, 1974. Used by permission.)

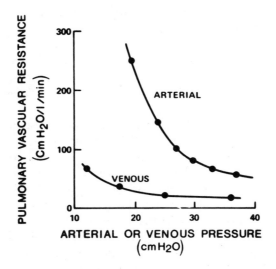

FIG 13–14.
Change in pulmonary vascular resistance in the excised dog lung as the pulmonary arterial or venous pressure is raised. During changes in arterial pressure, venous pressure was held constant at 12 cm H_2O, and when venous pressure was changed, arterial pressure was held at 37 cm H_2O. (From West JB: *Respiratory Physiology: The Essentials.* Baltimore, Williams & Wilkins Co, 1974. Used by permission.)

This decrease can result from either or both of the following mechanisms: (1) increase in the radius of the pulmonary microvasculature due to the increase in distending pressure, and (2) opening of collapsed vessels. Under most circumstances an increase in lung volume will reduce pulmonary vascular resistance. However, at very high lung volumes, the caliber of some vessels may be reduced by excessive stretch, and as a result, vascular resistance may then be increased.

Control of Pulmonary Resistance

As described above, the pulmonary circulation has a meager supply of vascular muscle in its wall. Large and medium arterioles have both a sympathetic and parasympathetic nerve supply. These vessels are capable of responding to α-stimulation by vasoconstriction and to β- and cholinergic stimulation by vasodilation. However, the mechanism responsible for these actions is not fully understood. The intrapulmonary veins and venules apparently do not have autonomic innervation. A potent stimulus for an increase in pulmonary resistance is hypoxia. A local fall in alveolar partial pressure of oxygen (P_{O_2}) will cause vasoconstriction of the pulmonary ves-

sels in that area, whereas systemic hypoxemia will produce peripheral vasodilation and only a minor degree of generalized pulmonary vasoconstriction. The mechanism for hypoxic constriction of the pulmonary vessels is
not known. In experimental animals this process is unaffected by either
vagotomy or sympathectomy. Histamine, catecholamines, some prostaglandins, and other locally active substances such as angiotensin II are also
vasoconstrictor agents.

The change in the ventilation perfusion ratio in response to a low alveolar P_{O_2} due to pulmonary vasoconstriction may have a protective function. Ventilation of a single lung with a low oxygen mixture, for example,
will shift pulmonary blood flow to the normally oxygenated lung. As a
consequence, arterial deoxygenation is minimized, and tissue oxygenation
is maintained at a higher level than if this mechanism was not present.

Despite the ability to change the vascular resistance of the lung, pulmonary blood pressure remains relatively uanffected by factors that vary
systemic blood pressure, and control of this parameter does not appear to
be an important factor in cardiovascular regulation.

Pulmonary Compliance

The pulmonary venous system is relatively elastic and able to alter its
internal volume without a major change in pulmonary blood pressure. In
this respect, its behavior is similar to that of the systemic veins. As a result, the pulmonary system serves as an important blood reservoir. Pulmonary blood volume in an adult is approximately 400 ml in the upright
position, but is increased to 600 to 700 ml when the individual lies down.
This shift of fluid may produce mechanical difficulties with respiration (or-
thopnea) if the pulmonary circulation is already engorged because of obstruction to flow by a stenotic mitral valve or by enlargement of the circulating blood volume, as may occur with congestive heart failure.

SUMMARY

Venous System.—Vascular pressure is usually related to the phlebostatic level of the heart to avoid the hydrostatic effect of different reference
levels. Transmural pressure is related to the point of measurement. Due to
the siphon qualities of the circulation, additional energy is not required to
maintain flow through the dependent parts of the body. High venous pressure in the legs due to the upright posture is avoided by venous values and
the pumping action of muscular contraction. Venous pressure in the head
is subatmospheric, but transmural pressure of cerebral veins is essentially

zero. During respiration, venous return to the heart is assisted by the respiratory pump. Most veins act as collapsible structures and can accommodate a large change in volume with only a small change in pressure. Veins can contain up to 77% of the circulating blood volume, and they serve as important blood reservoirs.

Pulmonary Circulation.—The pulmonary circulation transports venous blood to the alveolar capillaries and arterial blood to the left atrium. The bronchial circulation supplies the supporting structure of the lungs. The pulmonary capillary bed has a large surface area and a thin endothelial-alveolus membrane. Pulmonary vascular resistance and mean pulmonary blood pressure are about one tenth that of the systemic circulation. Blood flow is different in the apex and base of the lungs due to the low pulmonary pressure and the hydrostatic effect of the upright position.

BIBLIOGRAPHY

Alexander RS: The peripheral venous system, in Hamilton WF (ed): *Handbook of Physiology, Section 2: Circulation*, vol 2. Washington DC, American Physiological Society, 1963.

Brecher GO: *Venous Return.* New York, Grune & Stratton, 1956.

Burton AC: *Physiology and Biophysics of the Circulation*, ed 2. Chicago, Year Book Medical Publishers, 1972.

Comroe JH: *Physiology of Respiration*, ed 2. Chicago, Year Book Medical Publishers, 1974.

Dowling SE, Lee JC: Nervous control of the pulmonary circulation. *Annu Rev Physiol* 1980; 42:199.

Fishman AP: Vasomotor regulation of the pulmonary circulation. *Annu Rev Physiol* 1980; 42:211.

Friedman JJ: The systemic circulation, in Selkurt EE (ed): *Physiology*, ed 4. Boston, Little, Brown & Co, 1976.

Greenway CV: Role of splanchnic venous system in overall cardiovascular hemostasis. *Fed Proc* 1983; 42:1678.

Hainsworth R, Linden RS: Reflex Control of Vascular Capacitance. *Int Rev Physiol* 1979; 18:67.

Jacquez JA: *Respiratory Physiology.* Washington, DC, Hemisphere Publishing Corp, 1979.

Rothe CF: Reflex control of the veins in cardiovascular function. *Physiologist* 1979; 22:28.

Rothe CF: Reflex control of veins and vascular capacitance. *Physiol Rev* 1983; 63:1281.

Rothe CF: Physiology of venous return. An unappreciated boost to the heart. *Arch Intern Med* 1986; 146:977.

Shepherd JT, Vanhoutte PM: *Veins and Their Control.* Philadelphia, WB Saunders Co, 1975.

West JB: *Respiratory Physiology: The Essentials.* Baltimore, Williams & Wilkins Co, 1974.

West JB, Dollery CT: Distribution of blood flow and the pressure-flow relationship of the whole lung. *J Appl Physiol* 1965; 20:175.

Wiederhielm CA: The capillaries, veins and lymphatics, in Ruch TC, Patten HD (eds): *Physiology and Biophysics, II: Circulation, Respiration and Fluid Balance.* Philadelphia, WB Saunders Co, 1974.

Chapter 14 _____

Circulation to Special Areas

_____

The peripheral circulation has thus far been considered in a general way, and the special features of each vascular bed have not been singled out for discussion. This has been done because (1) space limitation prevents a systematic treatment of the vascular organization and function of even the major organ systems and (2) these special circulations are individually covered in specific monographs and texts devoted to the function of a single body system. Nevertheless, summaries of several representative organ circulations are presented in this chapter to illustrate the vascular principles discussed in earlier sections.

CEREBRAL CIRCULATION

General Considerations

Because the cerebral circulation is surrounded by essentially incompressible brain tissue within the rigid calvaria, early physiologists suggested that a lack of expansion room would prevent changes in vascular diameter, and as a result, its vasculature must contain a fixed volume *(Monro-Kellie doctrine)*. This view proved to be incorrect when observations made through a glass window placed in the skull showed active cerebral vasomotion. These studies also showed that space was provided inside the skull for changes in capillary volume by compression or dilation of the extensive cerebral venous network. As a result of these and other observations, it is now recognized that cerebral circulation adjusts its own blood flow to meet local needs; that this control is largely intrinsic to the brain, and that it is essentially independent of arterial blood pressure over the range of pressures normally encountered.

The brain, like the myocardium, must receive a continuous flow of blood. Cerebral metabolism requires a ready supply of substrate energy, largely derived from glucose and oxygen. The brain contains meager stores of both these substances so that under the best of conditions a lack of blood flow can be tolerated for only a few seconds before loss of consciousness and for only 3 or 4 minutes without permanent brain damage. This interval may be somewhat prolonged with hypothermia. Normal cerebral blood flow (CBF) in man averages between 52 and 65 ml/minute/100 gm of brain tissue or about 775 ml/minute for the entire 1,400-gm brain. The high level of this perfusion is indicated by the fact that the brain, which contains less than 2% of the body weight, receives approximately 15% of the resting cardiac output. When CBF falls below about 40 ml/minute/100 gm, clinical symptoms usually appear and syncope may occur when blood flow is reduced to 28 ml/minute/100 gm.

Anatomical Relationships.—In humans, the major cerebral blood supply is via the internal carotid arteries, and in contrast to most animals, only a small fraction of total CBF comes from the vertebral arteries. This arrangement is of physiologic importance because it permits cerebral perfusion pressure to be the variable used in the control of arterial pressure via the carotid sinus reflex (see Chapter 10), and it ensures that an adequate pressure head is available to maintain CBF.

The basilar artery formed by the union of the two vertebral arteries joins with the internal carotid arteries to form the *circle of Willis*. Branches of the basilar artery also go to the medulla, pons, occipital lobe of the cortex, and cerebellum. The circle of Willis supplies the cerebral cortex and upper brain stem. Blood from each carotid artery is distributed largely to the same side of the brain, and very little mixing occurs between the two circulations despite their connection through the circle of Willis. This separation takes place because (1) the blood pressure is approximately equal in each carotid artery so that a pressure gradient is normally not present between them and (2) the connecting vessels are too small to permit significant flow even if such a gradient is produced by sudden occlusion of one carotid artery. This has clinical importance because compression or occlusion of an internal carotid artery by any means, particularly in an individual with significant arteriosclerotic disease, may result in ipsilateral cerebral ischemia and brain damage.

The large arterial trunks from the circle of Willis curve around the cerebral hemispheres and branch extensively as they form progressively smaller vessels in a complicated geometric arrangement. The small cerebral vessels either lie on the cerebral surface *(pial vessels)* or penetrate the substance of the brain *(parenchymal vessels)*. Both the pial and parenchymal arteries terminate in arterioles. Neither the cerebral capillaries nor venules have smooth muscle in their wall. As a result, active regulation of blood flow can only be accomplished by the single layer of vascular smooth muscle in the wall of the arterioles.

Cerebral capillaries are similar to those in other organs except that the lining endothelium does not have fenestrations or clefts and the basement membrane is more prominent than in other tissues. The capillary vessels also are separated from the neural cells of the brain by a layer of astrocytes and glia cells. This intact capillary endothelium and thick basement membrane may explain the slow diffusion of large molecular weight substances such as dyes, antibiotics, and many water-soluble substances into the brain (so-called *blood-brain barrier*). The cerebral endothelium, however, contains specific transport mechanisms for ions and some metabolic substrates. Lymphatic vessels are not present.

A complex and extensive network of small cerebral veins receives blood from superficial and deep cerebral capillaries. These vessels empty into the dural sinuses or make connections with the paravertebral veins or other cranial veins. Blood from the cerebral sinuses leaves the skull on each side via the internal jugular vein. Approximately two thirds of the carotid artery flow normally drains via the ipsilateral internal jugular vein and most of the remainder by the contralateral jugular. This anatomical feature may become important, as discussed below, in determination of CBF to each hemisphere.

Innervation of Cerebral Vessels

Both adrenergic and cholinergic nerve fibers accompany the cerebral arteries. The larger arteries have a rich sympathetic supply; innervation of the pial vessels is somewhat less; and few, if any, adrenergic fibers accompany the penetrating parenchymal arteries. The role of this innervation is obscure (see below). Local application of catecholamines or acetylcholine to pial vessels will alter their diameter; however, it is generally agreed that the sensitivity of these vessels and the magnitude of their response to neural transmitters are considerably less than for similar arteries elsewhere in the body.

The cerebral vasculature receives a number of myelinated sensory fibers. These nerves are probably involved in the classic migraine headache associated with cerebral vasodilation and the painful sensations produced by traction on cerebral vessels.

Measurement of Cerebral Blood Flow

Quantitation of brain blood flow presents a number of specific problems, and only in the last few years have continuous measurements been possible. Blood enters and leaves the brain through a number of vascular channels. In addition, the regulatory mechanisms for cerebral blood flow, as discussed below, are different than for other tissues of the head. As a result, the arterial supply to the brain must be separated from noncerebral blood flow.

A fundamental step in the study of cerebral circulatory dynamics occurred in the 1940s when the indicator-dilution principle discussed in Chapter 7 was adapted to the measurement of CBF.* However, this technique in which subanesthetic amounts of nitrous oxide are used as the indicator was only able to measure CBF over a period of several minutes. In addition, the calculation depended on a number of questionable assumptions. These included the following: (1) blood flow is constant during the measurement period; (2) jugular blood is representative of mixed cerebral venous return; and (3) significant arterial venous shunts are not present. As a result, highly accurate measurements were difficult, if not impossible to accomplish.

More recently, radioactive substances such as ^{85}Kr and ^{133}Xe have been used as tracer substances. This is accomplished by breathing the radioactive gas and counting the radioactivity of the tracer compounds through the skull. Studies of this type have shown blood flow variations from a high of 180 ml/minute/100 gm for the midbrain (inferior colliculus) to 130 ml/minute/100 gm for the sensorimotor cortex and a low of 14 ml/minute/100 gm for the spinal cord.

Simultaneous measurement of the blood flow to each cerebral hemisphere by collecting the venous drainage separately from each jugular bulb shows a right-to-left-side variation of only about 15%; however, the flow is not consistently higher on either side. Magnetic resonance imaging and ultrasound measurement of blood flow velocity are currently under investigation for use in the measurement of CBF.

Regulation of CBF

The cerebral circulation is normally so closely regulated that total CBF is maintained nearly constant even though local variations may occur in the flow to individual areas of the brain. The major factors in this regulation can be divided into extracranial and intracranial groups. The first group

*See Kety SS, Schmidt CF: *J Clin Invest* 1948; 24:476.

contains (1) arterial perfusion pressure, (2) cardiovascular reflexes, and (3) blood viscosity. The second group includes (1) cerebrospinal fluid pressure (intracranial pressure), (2) the metabolic activity of the brain, and (3) intraluminal pressure within the cerebral vessels.

Extracranial Factors.—The driving force for cerebral perfusion is arterial blood pressure at the level of the head minus the pressure in the internal jugular veins. When the body is in the upright position, this latter pressure is subatmospheric, and in the recumbent position, it becomes at most a few millimeters of mercury (see Chapter 13). As a result, venous pressure usually is ignored in calculations of cerebral perfusion pressure. Because of the marked autoregularity activity of the cerebral circulation (see below), the ability of the perfusion pressure to influence CBF is limited, and it becomes a factor only when the blood pressure falls below about 60 mm Hg or increases to above 150 mm Hg.

The role of vascular reflexes and the neurogenic control of the cerebral circulation is not settled. As indicated earlier, the blood vessels of the brain receive both adrenergic and cholinergic nerves and can respond to local application of sympathetic and parasympathetic neurotransmitters. Nevertheless, present evidence suggests (1) that neurogenic influences are limited at most to the larger blood vessels on the surface of the brain and perhaps to some of the extraparenchymal pial vessels and (2) that intraparenchymal vessels, at least in man, are largely unresponsive to autonomic influences. In the human, bilateral stellate ganglion blockade or sympathectomy does not alter CBF, and intra-arterial injection of small doses of norepinephrine has been reported to cause only minimal changes. Thus, it appears that extrinsic neurogenic influences do not play a major role in the regulation of cerebral circulation in man. A different situation occurs in animals. In the dog, monkey, baboon, and other species, cervical sympathectomy results in an increase of CBF, whereas stimulation of the stellate ganglion caused this flow to be reduced.

Reflex alterations in CBF have been described in various clinical conditions such as orthostatic hypotension and vasovagal syncope. There is no evidence, however, that the cerebral circulation is involved in these conditions other than as a secondary result of a marked drop in arterial pressure. Localized areas of vascular constriction or venospasm occasionally occur, particularly in association with a hemorrhage into the subarachnoid space. The cause of this spasm is obscure. It is, however, apparently not due directly to the release of local vasoconstrictive substances, although they may play a role in combination with other, so far unknown, factors.

As in other tissues, cerebrovascular resistance is affected by the viscosity of the blood (see Chapter 9). For this reason, anemia is accompanied by an increase in CBF, whereas in conditions in which blood viscosity is increased, such as polycythemia and macroglobulinemia, it may be decreased as much as 30%.

Intracranial Factors.—The pressure of the *cerebrospinal fluid* (CSF) in the subarachnoid space that surrounds the brain is normally only slightly higher than venous pressure and thus too low to materially affect blood flow to the brain. However, if intracranial pressure is acutely elevated as a result, for example, of a blow to the head or an expanding brain tumor, it may compress cranial blood vessels and significantly interfere with CBF unless arterial pressure also is elevated. Fortunately, the medullary cardiovascular pressor centers discussed earlier that are involved in the regulation of systemic arterial pressure are stimulated when their blood flow is reduced. Under these conditions, generalized peripheral vasoconstriction with concomitant reflex bradycardia results. The increased arterial blood pressure that follows this change in systemic resistance is then usually sufficient to maintain CBF despite elevated cerebrospinal fluid (CSF) pressure. This mechanism, sometimes called the *Cushing reflex*, is quite effective over a considerable range of CSF pressures in maintaining minimal cerebral perfusion. However, the increased cardiac afterload produced by this reflex often leads to such high left atrial and pulmonary arterial pressures that massive pulmonary edema may result.

Intense peripheral vasoconstriction and elevation of the arterial blood pressure as a result of the Cushing reflex is not only a compensatory reaction to an elevated CSF pressure, but the same mechanism also operates a final compensatory response in severe hypotension and circulatory shock (see Chapter 15). In this situation the reduction in blood flow to the brain stem because of a fall in arterial pressure below the autoregulatory level leads to a marked peripheral sympathetic discharge and increase in vascular resistance.

The cerebral arterioles appear to be sensitive to changes in the partial pressure of carbon dioxide (P_{CO_2}) and pH. An increase in P_{CO_2} is particularly potent in producing cerebral vasodilation and an increase in CBF. This response undoubtedly results from the action of the CO_2, which easily penetrates the blood-brain barrier of the cerebral capillaries and is not the result of associated changes in blood H^+ concentration as cerebral vascular resistance is unaffected by acute changes in blood pH (at least within the physiologic range) unaccompanied by changes in P_{CO_2}. However, the increased level of CO_2 in the cerebral spinal fluid in this situation causes a drop in CSF pH which, in turn, leads to cerebral vascular vasodilation.

Cerebral vessels respond to a drop in P_{CO_2} with vasoconstriction. It is not clear, however, if this is in direct response to the hypocapnia or if it is a secondary response as a result of the lack of the normal CO_2-mediated vasodilation. The CBF may be reduced as much as 35% by voluntary hyperventilation. This reduction is more than sufficient to cause cerebral ischemia and to explain the symptoms of dizziness and tingling that often accompany a maneuver of this type.

A number of vasoactive substances associated with tissue metabolism such as acetylcholine and adenosine have been suggested as being important in the chemical regulation of the cerebral circulation. Adenosine is a potent dilator of pial vessels, and its level increases in the brain following ischemia, hypoxemia, or hypotension. However, its role in the autoregulation of CBF is still unclear.

Autoregulation of Cerebral Blood Flow

Cerebral circulation has a marked tendency to undergo autoregulation (see Chapter 11) and is able to maintain a normal flow despite large variations in arterial pressure (Fig 14–1). This ability to alter its vascular resistance appears to depend on a combination of (1) the local metabolic environment and (2) the level of arterial perfusion pressure. Although various metabolic vasoactive compounds have been suggested, the main regulating

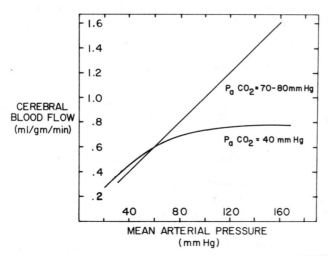

FIG 14–1.
Schematic pressure-flow relationships of cerebral circulations of the dog at two levels of P_{CO_2}. The normal autoregulation shown in the *lower curve* at a P_{CO_2} of 40 mm Hg is lost *(upper curve)* during hypercapnia (P_{CO_2} 70 to 80 mm Hg). (Modified from data of Harper AM, in Lassen NA: *Circ Res* 1964; 15:I–201.)

substance appears to be CO_2. The responsiveness of cerebral arterioles is indicated by the local vasodilation that occurs in the involved areas of the brain during nervous activity. This reaction presumably results from the increased metabolic activity associated with the electric activity of the nerve cells.

Cerebral precapillary vascular smooth muscle also is quite sensitive to stretch and responds to an increase in arteriolar pressure with an increase in tone (see Chapter 11). This vasoconstriction acts to counter the elevation in perfusion pressure by increasing vascular resistance and thus limits blood flow (see Fig 14–1). The importance of CO_2 to this mechanism, as suggested above, is indicated by the absence of any autoregulation due to changes in pressure in the presence of a high P_{CO_2}.

CORONARY CIRCULATION

General Considerations

The anatomical arrangement of the coronary vessels was summarized in Chapter 2. Blood flow to the heart, just as to any organ, is determined by the driving pressure and resistance of the vascular bed (see Chapter 9). As the coronary vessels originate directly from the aorta, the reflex mechanisms that control arterial pressure maintain a relatively constant driving pressure for myocardial perfusion. As a result, cardiac blood flow is largely regulated by alterations in coronary resistance. It is helpful in considering coronary resistance to separate the *intrinsic* and *extrinsic* components. Intrinsic resistance is determined largely by the tone of the circular vascular muscle of the coronary arterioles, whereas the extrinsic component results from the mechanical effect of cardiac contraction on the coronary vessels that travel through the myocardium.

Mechanical Obstruction to Coronary Flow

During the early part of cardiac ejection, left ventricular pressure exceeds aortic pressure. As a result, subendocardial pressure in the left ventricle will be higher during systole than the distending pressure in the coronary arteries, and the vessels will collapse (Fig 14–2). This systolic obstruction to blood flow provides a rational explanation for the greater susceptibility of this area to ischemic injury and necrosis.

Intramyocardial force during systole is greatest near the inner border of the left ventricular wall, and it becomes progressively less toward the epicardial surface. This force is also considerably lower throughout the right ventricular myocardium because of the smaller right ventricular con-

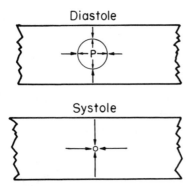

FIG 14–2.
Schematic diagram of intramyocardial blood vessel. During diastole the vessel is held open by its internal blood pressure. During systole the intramyocardial force due to cardiac contraction is greater than the internal pressure, and the vessel is squeezed closed.

tractile tension, although the same gradient exists as in the left ventricle. As a result of this difference in intramyocardial compressive force, the coronary vessels are not all restricted to the same degree. Overall coronary flow is reduced during systole (Fig 14–3). Some studies, in fact, have suggested that left ventricular subendocardial flow may occur only during diastole. This same constricting effect may also increase coronary sinus outflow during systole because of its stripping action on the cardiac venous system.

The magnitude of the reduction in coronary flow produced by myocardial contraction can be estimated by perfusing the coronary circulation of an experimental animal at a constant pressure. When the heart in such an experiment was suddenly stopped, as shown in Figure 14–4, flow in the right coronary artery increased 22% and left coronary artery flow increased 44%. As the extrinsic resistance to coronary flow was presumably removed in this heart by the production of asystole, the larger flow reflected only the effect of the intrinsic resistance of the coronary system.

During the interval between heartbeats, the mechanical effect of cardiac contraction on coronary flow is removed, and the situation is similar to the period of asystole described above. As a consequence, the heart receives most of its nutrient blood flow between beats. Under normal circumstances, the total flow over the cardiac cycle is sufficient to maintain myocardial metabolism. However, in individuals with occlusive disease of the coronary arteries and a restricted coronary blood flow, a significant increase in heart rate may lead to difficulties. This follows because there are (1) increased metabolic requirements of the heart because of the faster rate and (2) decreased diastolic time available for myocardial perfusion. The latter

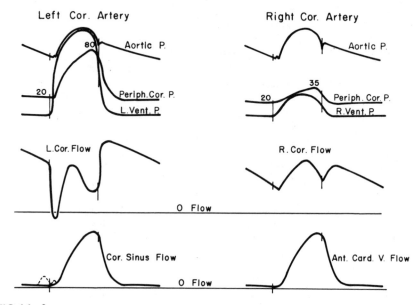

FIG 14–3.
Series of curves showing the variation in left and right coronary inflow and coronary sinus and anterior cardiac vein flow compared to aortic, ventricular, and peripheral coronary artery pressure. (Modified from Gregg DE, in Luisado AA [ed]: *An Encyclopedia of the Cardiovascular System.* New York, McGraw-Hill Book Co, 1959. Used by permission.)

event occurs because the duration of systole is relatively fixed and an increase in heart rate is accomplished largely by reducing the interval between beats. For example, at a heart rate of 70 beats per minute, the time available for maximum coronary perfusion is approximately 34 seconds out of each minute. At a heart rate of 150 beats per minute, the same diastolic interval becomes approximately 23 seconds. Thus, an increase in cardiac rate from 70 to 150 beats per minute leads to a 35% reduction in the time available for maximal coronary flow. This observation explains the frequent association between a rapid heart rate and anginal attacks in patients with coronary insufficiency.

Myocardial Oxygen Requirements and Coronary Flow

The normal metabolic activity of the heart in a person resting quietly requires approximately 10 ml of oxygen per minute per 100 gm of myocardium. To meet the high basal demand for oxygen and not exceed the normal resting coronary flow of 70 to 80 ml of blood per minute per 100 gm

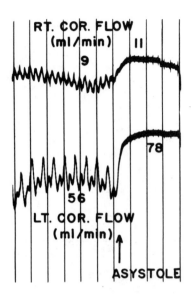

FIG 14–4.
Record of coronary flow in right and left coronary arteries with perfusing pressure maintained at a constant level. With onset of cardiac asystole, flow increased in both vessels. (From Sabiston DC Jr, Gregg DE: *Circulation* 1957; 15:14. Used by permission of the American Heart Association.)

of heart, the myocardium must extract 65% to 70% of the oxygen carried by the coronary blood supply (Fig 14–5). This extraction equals the maximum achieved by skeletal muscles under conditions of severe metabolic stress. As this extraction rate cannot be materially improved, the only way the delivery of oxygen to the myocardium can be increased is to increase coronary blood flow. It is, therefore, not surprising that coronary blood flow and myocardial oxygen consumption have a fixed relationship to each other and go up and down together. During maximal exertion the myocardium requires as much as 50 ml of oxygen per minute per 100 gm of heart. To deliver this amount of oxygen, coronary flow must become as high as 350 ml/minute/100 gm of tissue.

Myocardial hypoxia is one of the most potent stimuli known to reduce intrinsic coronary resistance. This vasodilatory response appears to be activated when the oxygen content of venous coronary blood falls below the critical level of 5.5 ml of oxygen per 100 ml of blood. The association between hypoxia and vasodilation suggests that a reduction in the oxygen content of the myocardium may permit metabolic end products to build up in the tissue. These metabolites, in turn, lead to dilation of the precapillary coronary resistance vessels. A number of metabolites have been suggested (see Chapter 11); however, recent evidence points to the formation of aden-

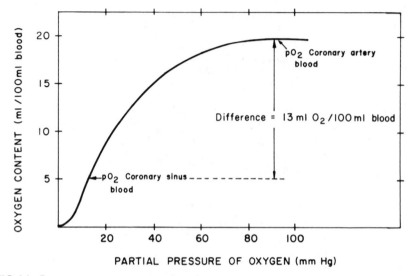

FIG 14–5.
Oxygen saturation curve for hemoglobin showing typical values for coronary arterial and coronary sinus blood. The myocardium extracts approximately 13 ml of the oxygen carried by each 100 ml of blood as it travels through the coronary circulation.

osine from adenine nucleotides as a likely candidate. An increase in P_{CO_2} or a decrease in blood pH has a similar, but considerably less effective, dilatory action than that of hypoxia. Recent evidence has suggested that the prostaglandin, prostacyclin (PGI_2), which is synthesized from arachidonic acid by vascular endothelial cells, may play an important role in the regulation of coronary flow. This compound is a potent coronary vasodilator, and it appears in increased amounts in coronary venous blood following myocardial hypoxemia.

When the myocardium becomes hypoxic, the balance between the breakdown and synthesis of ATP is disturbed and adenylic acid (AMP) and inorganic phosphate accumulate within the cardiac cell. Enzymes associated with the cell membrane dephosphorylate the AMP to form adenosine, which is then able to diffuse through the cell wall. The formation, distribution, and metabolism of adenosine are summarized in Figure 14–6. This substance has a powerful vasodilatory effect on coronary resistance vessels. Presumably the reduction in intrinsic coronary resistance produced by the interstitial adenosine increases coronary flow sufficiently to return myocardial oxygen to normal. The increased flow also completes the negative feedback loop by washing the extra adenosine out of the heart.

Autoregulatory mechanisms maintain myocardial blood flow ade-

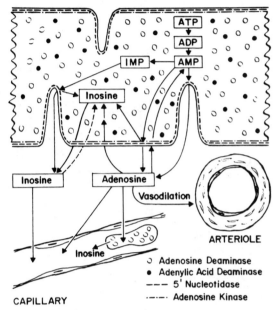

FIG 14–6.
Schematic diagram of part of a myocardial cell illustrating the formation, rate, and site of action of adenosine arising from intracellular adenosine triphosphate *(ATP)*. AMP = adenosine monophosphate; ADP = adenosine diphosphate; *IMP* = inosine monophosphate. (From Berne RM, Rubio R: *Am J Cardiol* 1969; 24:776. Used by permission.)

quately for the needs of the heart over a wide range of conditions. This can be illustrated by plotting the coronary blood flow recorded from an experimental animal at various pressure levels against the perfusion pressure. As shown in Figure 14–7, a 50% variation in perfusion pressure above and below the control value of 120 mm Hg will produce a maximum variation of only about 20% in the steady-state coronary flow. Animal studies suggest, however, that a reduction in coronary perfusion pressure below the point of maximal autoregulatory vasodilation will cause inadequate subendocardial perfusion and local myocardial ischemia. In addition to the low perfusion pressure, this may also be due to a higher diastolic extravascular pressure in that layer.

Hormonal and Neurogenic Regulation

Stimulation of the sympathetic nerves to the heart produces a marked increase in coronary flow (Table 14–1). This observation suggested to ear-

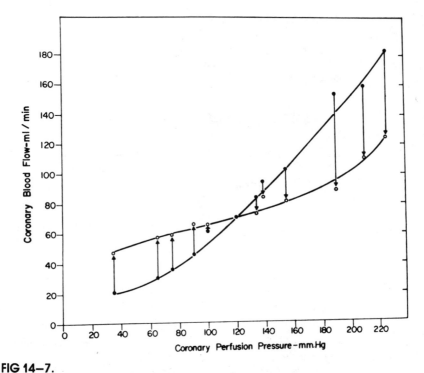

FIG 14–7.
Pressure-flow relationship in coronary vascular bed. Aortic pressure, cardiac output, and heart rate remained constant. Perfusion pressure was abruptly increased or decreased from control (indicated by point where the two lines cross). *Closed circles* show coronary flow immediately after the intervention. *Open circles* show the steady-state flow. Over the range of 60 to 180 mm Hg perfusion pressure, flow returned to a relatively constant level (autoregulation). (From Berne RM, Levy MN: *Cardiovascular Physiology,* ed 2. St Louis, CV Mosby Co, 1972. Used by permission.)

lier workers that the coronary resistance vessels responded to sympathetic stimulation by vasodilation. However, recent studies using pharmacologic blocking agents have shown that the coronary vessels, like the blood vessels of skeletal muscle, contain both vasoconstrictive α-receptors and vasodilator β-receptors. Cardiac arterioles do not, however, have cholinergic sympathetic vasodilator fibers. As a result, a more complex mechanism than direct dilation is required to explain the increased flow that accompanies adrenergic stimulation.

The vasoconstrictor action of the coronary α-receptors is relatively weak and at least in the dog after β-receptor blockade, maximum sympathetic stimulation produces only a moderate increase in coronary artery re-

TABLE 14–1.

Effect of 3 μg Epinephrine (Administered Intravenously) on Main Left
Coronary Artery Flow in the Conscious Dog*

Factor	Control	12 Sec After Drug	% Change
Heart rate (beats/min)	83.0	88.0	+6
Mean aortic pressure (mm Hg)	117.0	115.0	−2
Left coronary flow			
Mean (ml/min)	79.0	204.0	+158
Systolic flow/beat (ml)	0.10	0.42	+320
Diastolic flow/beat (ml)	0.85	1.90	+123

*Data from Rayford CR, Khouri EM, Gregg DE: *Am J Physiol* 1965; 209:680.

sistance compared to the fivefold or sixfold increase obtained under the
same circumstances in skeletal muscle. However, sympathetic stimulation,
in addition to its weak vasoconstrictor effect, leads to a sizable increase in
the metabolic activity of the myocardium. Current evidence suggests that
the increased demand for oxygen, produced by this enhanced metabolic
activity, probably working through the adenosine mechanism described
above, overrides the direct sympathetic vasoconstriction and causes coronary resistance to fall.

RENAL CIRCULATION

General Considerations

The kidneys are designed to maintain the volume and composition of
the aqueous phase of the blood by selectively excreting water and dissolved
materials. In carrying out this task, the kidneys process nearly 400 ml of
blood per minute per 100 gm of renal tissue for a total organ blood flow of
approximately 1,200 ml/minute. Although this level of perfusion is just
behind that of the carotid body and the thyroid gland in volume flow per
100 gm, in terms of total organ flow the kidney outranks all other organs.

Kidney function is so closely tied to the structure of its vascular system
that it is not possible to discuss renal circulatory dynamics without at least
briefly considering other aspects of kidney physiology. However, as the
emphasis in this section is on the vascular system, no attempt will be made
to provide a balanced treatment of renal activity, and the interested reader
is referred to specific texts for such information.

Structural Aspects of Kidney Circulation

Functional Anatomy.—Blood enters the kidney from the abdominal aorta via the *renal artery*. This vessel promptly divides after entering the hilus to form the *interlobar arteries*, which radiate outward toward the cortex (Fig 14–8). At the margin between the cortex and medulla, the interlobar arteries again divide and turn at right angles to form the *arcuate arteries*. *Interlobular arteries* then branch off and travel toward the surface of the kidney. Small lateral branches, the *afferent arterioles*, arise at right angles from the interlobular arteries and supply blood to individual *glomerular capillary tufts*. From the glomeruli, blood enters the *efferent arterioles* and is distributed to the network of small *peritubular capillaries* that surrounds the renal tubules and in some nephrons (see below) to the *vasa recta*. Blood then returns to the vena cava by way of the renal venous system and renal vein.

Renal Nephron.—The renal nephron is the functional unit of the kidney. It consists of *Bowman's capsule*, the *proximal* and *distal convoluted tubules*

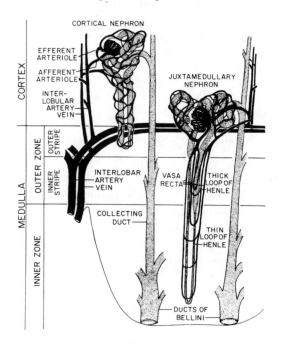

FIG 14–8.
Diagram of a cortical and a juxtamedullary nephron showing their blood supply. (From Pitts RF: *Physiology of the Kidney and Body Fluids,* ed 3. Chicago, Year Book Medical Publishers, 1974. Used by permission.)

with an intervening *loop of Henle*, and the *collecting duct*. The glomerular tufts, along with their basement membrane, serve as a semipermeable membrane for production of an ultrafiltrate of plasma. This fluid collects in Bowman's capsule and is then converted into urine as it travels through the remainder of the nephron toward the renal pelvis.

Peritubular Capillaries.—There are important differences in arrangement of the peritubular capillaries in individual nephrons depending on their location within the kidney. Nearly 85% of the nephrons in man originate from glomeruli in the renal cortex. These *cortical nephrons* have a short loop of Henle, which extends toward the hilus only as far as the outer layer of the medulla. The remaining nephrons originate near the margin between the cortex and the medulla. These *juxtamedullary nephrons* have a long loop of Henle that penetrates deep into the medulla and may even reach the tip of the renal papillae.

The efferent arteriole from cortical glomeruli subdivides rapidly into a rich network of peritubular capillaries that surrounds the entire nephron. These vessels anastomose freely with peritubular capillary vessels from adjoining nephrons so that this peritubular network receives blood from several efferent arterioles. These capillaries function as an absorptive surface and pick up from the renal interstitium the large volume of fluid, electrolytes, and other substances that are removed from the tubular urine as it progresses through the nephron.

Juxtamedullary nephrons have a peritubular circulation quite different from that just described for cortical nephrons. The efferent arterioles from these glomeruli provide several side branches, which supply a network of capillaries that surround their proximal and distal convoluted tubules. These vessels serve the same function as the peritubular capillaries described above. In addition, the efferent arterioles form a series of wide, straight vessels, the vasa recta, which follow the descending loop of Henle to its tip and then return to the upper medulla. Fine capillary vessels arise at various levels from the vasa recta. Each of these capillaries surrounds the loop of Henle for a short distance.

Arteriocapillary vessels (Treueta shunts), which bypass the glomeruli and permit blood to pass directly from small branches of the renal artery to capillaries in the medulla as well as other arterioarterial and venovenous shunts, have been described. However, these vessels occur infrequently, and their functional significance is not clear.

Renal Nerves.—The kidney has a rich supply of both afferent and efferent nerves. It receives sympathetic vasoconstrictor fibers from the thoracic and lumbar sympathetic chain. Recent evidence suggests that cholinergic vasodilator fibers also may travel with these nerves. The adrenergic constrictor nerve fibers travel with the blood vessels and innervate primarily the afferent arterioles and, to some extent, the descending vasa recta. The vasodilator fibers appear to supply primarily the efferent arterioles, particularly of the juxtamedullary nephrons.

Afferent sensory fibers have been identified coming from the renal pelvis and the capsule as well as from various areas of the renal parenchyma. The physiologic role of these sensory fibers is speculative.

Lymphatics.—The renal cortex has an extensive lymphatic network. Lymph vessels follow the major blood vessels and leave at the renal hilus. The fact that the renal medulla is devoid of lymphatics should not be surprising in view of the countercurrent mechanism that operates in that area (see below).

Countercurrent Mechanism

The hairpin loop of the vasa recta and its parallel alignment with the renal tubules provide the configuration for a countercurrent exchanger. In such a system, opposite flow in parallel paths is arranged so that the contents of one tube affect the material flowing in the other. This same principle permits birds, for example, that stand in cold water to conserve body heat. The warm blood in the arteries of the upper leg transfers heat to the cold venous return in neighboring veins coming from the lower leg and foot. In this fashion, venous blood is warmed, and heat, which is shunted away from the feet, is retained by the body.

A similar arrangement in the renal medulla permits the loop of Henle to function as a *countercurrent multiplier* and produce an osmotic gradient between systemic blood and renal medullary interstitial fluid. Present evidence suggests that, as discussed below, the active transport of Cl^- out of the ascending limb of the loop of Henle causes an increase in the solute concentration of the medullary interstitial fluid. In addition, because the descending limb of the loop of Henle is more permeable to water than to solute (sodium), water leaves the tubules as a consequence of the hyperosmotic medullary interstitial fluid and the increased intraluminal concentration. In the thin segment of the loop, this difference in permeability is reversed and the tubule wall becomes permeable to Na^+ and urea but not water. As a result, both Na^+ and urea diffuse down their concentration gradients and move out of the thin segment, and the osmolarity of the interstitial space in the medullary pyramids is increased. Chloride is actively pumped out of the lumen of the ascending thick segment of the loop of Henle, and Na^+ follows passively. As this segment is also relatively impermeable to water, the removal of solute causes the tubular fluid left behind to become dilute so that by the time it enters the distal convoluted tubules, it is hypotonic with respect to systemic plasma.

In distinction to the countercurrent multiplier function of the loop of Henle, the countercurrent exchange activities of the vasa recta protect the medullary osmotic gradient while at the same time removing extra fluid and solute in its venous effluent. This entire passive activity takes place as follows: solute (sodium) diffuses into the descending limb of the vasa recta from the medullary interstitium, where it is present in high concentration, while water moves in the opposite direction. In the ascending limb, solute diffuses back out of the vasa recta, and water moves into the blood (Fig 14–9). As a result, the hypertonicity of the inner medulla is maintained by a recirculation of solute while water is shunted away from the renal pyramids.

The distal convoluted tubules and the collecting ducts are quite per-

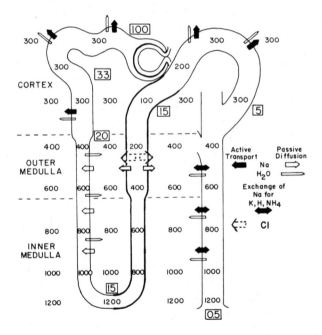

FIG 14–9.
Diagram showing exchange of water and ions across the wall of a nephron during production of hypertonic urine. Concentrations of tubular urine and peritubular fluid are given in milliosmoles per liter; *boxed numbers* are estimated percentages of glomerular filtrate remaining within the tubule at that level. (Modified from Pitts RF: *Physiology of the Kidney and Body Fluids,* ed 3. Chicago, Year Book Medical Publishers, 1974. Used by permission.)

meable to water in the presence of antidiuretic hormone (ADH); however, the upper end of the collecting duct is relatively impermeable to urea. As a result of these relationships, much more water than urea leaves the nephron, and the concentration of urea inside the tubule increases. The lower collecting duct is again quite permeable to urea. In the presence of ADH, water as well as urea diffuses out of this area, and a concentrated urine is delivered to the renal pelvis. This concentrating ability is one of the interesting complexities of renal function; unfortunately, further discussion of this mechanism and its effect on kidney function is outside the area of this book.

Regulation of Renal Circulation

Autoregulation.—The series arrangement of the two major renal capillary networks just described permits both glomerular filtration (*glomerular filtration rate*, GFR) and *renal blood flow* (RBF) to be controlled by regulating the diameter of either or both the afferent or efferent arterioles. For example, elevation of mean arterial pressure is prevented from significantly increasing either glomerular capillary pressure or RBF by an increase in renal vascular resistance due to constriction of afferent arterioles. As capillary pressure is the major determinant of filtration (see Chapter 12), regulation of that parameter will also prevent changes in GFR. In a similar manner, a moderate reduction in mean perfusion pressure is prevented from unduly influencing either GFR or RBF by relaxation of the afferent arterioles. With more marked reduction in mean arterial pressure (down to 70 to 80 mm Hg), GFR is still maintained reasonably constant by constriction of the efferent arterioles and limitation of the outflow from the glomerular capillary network. Under these circumstances control of GFR is attained at the expense of RBF, and blood flow to the kidney is markedly reduced. At lower perfusion pressures, neither GFR nor RBF is regulated, and both decrease to low levels as arterial pressure falls.

The vascular reactions just described occur in the denervated kidney and thus appear to be due to an intrinsic mechanism. It should, however, be pointed out that this autoregulation is limited to the cortex of the kidney and that the smaller medullary blood flow via the vasa recta varies more directly with perfusion pressure.

The mechanism for intrinsic regulation of renal circulation has not been completely settled. Current evidence points to a myogenic (Bayliss) mechanism triggered by intra-arterial pressure similar to that discussed in Chapter 11. Support for this hypothesis is given by the loss of autoregulation that follows poisoning of the vascular smooth muscle by drugs such as procaine or papaverine and the observation that a sudden increase in vascular pressure requires 5 to 10 seconds before any vasoconstrictive adjustment occurs. This latter delay is approximately the latent period of vascular muscle. Other theories include the following: (1) Changes in blood viscosity occur within the kidney due to axial streaming (see Chapter 9) so that vascular resistance increases with flow velocity. Most physiologists now believe this mechanism has little if any effect on regulation of RBF; (2) Changes in intrarenal pressure with changes in arterial blood pressure affect transcapillary pressure and cause vascular resistance to vary with capillary pressure; (3) The renin-angiotensin system of the juxtaglomerular cells (see Chapter 7) relates the release of renin from the juxtaglomerular cells (probably the polkissen) to a reduction in mean intraluminal pressure and subsequent production of the vasoconstrictor agent, angiotensin. The role of these systems in the autoregulation of renal blood flow has not been precisely determined; however, recent evidence suggests that the juxtaglomerular cells may play a more important role in renal autoregulation than previously suspected.

It has recently been shown that the kidney is a major site of prostacyclin and prostaglandin E_2 and $F_{2\alpha}$ synthesis. These ubiquitous compounds appear to play a role in the regulation of salt and water excretion via their vasodilatory action, particularly of medullary blood vessels, and through their direct effect in inhibiting sodium and chloride absorption by the nephron.

Renal blood flow also correlates well with oxygen consumption by the kidney. In distinction to other tissues such as muscles, the arterial-venous oxygen extraction by the kidney is relatively constant (14 ml of O_2 per liter). Thus, any increase in renal oxygen consumption must be accompanied by an increase in RBF. The mechanism for this regulation has not been clearly defined, although some vasoactive metabolites have been suggested, including renin and prostaglandins. It is interesting that renal oxygen consumption correlates best with the rate of active sodium transport by the kidney tubules.

Neural Control.—Stimulation of the sympathetic vasoconstrictor fibers to the renal vasculature or injection of catecholamines such as epinephrine or norepinephrine causes a marked reduction in RBF due to constriction of the renal vasculature. This action is superimposed on the autoregulatory activity described above. The increased vascular resistance produced by stimulations of this type results from constriction of both the afferent and efferent arterioles so that GFR usually does not decrease as much as RBF.

The role of the cholinergic vasodilatory fibers, which supply the efferent arterioles and vasa recta, remains to be completely defined. They appear to be anatomically located to assist in control of medullary flow. Renal vasodilation is produced in addition by bacterial pyrogens and by some drugs such as hydralazine that are used in treatment of hypertension.

Neural regulation of renal blood flow is of primary importance in the circulatory adjustments that accompany stress or emergency situations. Changes in body position or moderate exercise, for example, are accompanied by vasoconstrictor impulses to the renal vasculature. The increase in vascular resistance that results from this stimulation reduces RBF slightly, but GFR is maintained by the autoregulatory mechanisms. However, with severe stress such as hemorrhage, maximal exercise, or inadequate cardiac output, the level of vasoconstrictor stimulation is increased, and both RBF and GFR may be profoundly reduced.

Distribution of Renal Blood Flow.—The excretory function of the kidney, and particularly the countercurrent mechanism described earlier, requires that the blood flow to the cortex and medulla be regulated separately. Cortical blood flow in the dog is about 4 to 5 ml/gm/minute, whereas medullary flow averages only 0.7 to 1 ml/gm/minute. The regulatory mechanisms that control medullary blood flow are not as well understood as those involved with cortical vasomotor activity. However, as discussed above, the presence of both sympathetic and parasympathetic innervation to the vasa recta and other vessels in the medulla suggests that control is available.

CUTANEOUS CIRCULATION

General Considerations

The skin comprises 4% of the normal adult body mass and, depending on the skin and body temperature, receives from 150 to 500 ml of blood per minute. In addition to meeting the circulatory needs of the skin, the cutaneous circulation plays an important role in the regulation of body temperature. Because of their large capacity, subcutaneous venous plexuses serve, in addition, as an important blood depot. Vasomotor activity of these capacitance vessels can shift as much as 1,000 ml of blood into and out of the active circulation as needed to maintain homeostasis.

Skin and mucous membrane color results in large measure from the amount and color of the hemoglobin in the cutaneous capillaries. There is usually sufficient oxyhemoglobin with its red color to provide for the normal skin color. However, if the concentration of reduced hemoglobin is increased to 5 gm/ml or more due either to reduced availability of oxygen, increased extraction of oxygen by the tissues, or other causes, the skin and mucous membranes will turn a blue-purple color. This condition is called *cyanosis.* A reduction in skin blood flow may lead to increased extraction of oxygen in the skin capillaries, and the skin will turn a pale gray color. However, in a very cold environment dissociation of oxyhemoglobin is inhibited by the low skin temperature, and cyanosis does not usually appear.

Control of the Skin Microcirculation

The skin has two types of circulations: a superficial arteriolar-capillary-venous network and a series of arteriovenous anastomotic vessels. The first type is similar to the microcirculation of other tissues except that it also has a prominent collection of subcutaneous venous plexuses. The arteriovenous anastomotic vessels are large-diameter, muscular structures in the skin of the fingers, toes, palms of the hand, and the face that can shunt blood from the arterioles directly to the venules. These thick-walled coiled structures do not serve to exchange fluids, solute, or gas but instead are efficient heat exchangers between the warm blood coming from the body core and the cooler body surface.

Skin arterioles are under the dual control of local metabolic factors and the sympathetic nervous system. These vessels normally have a high level of resting tone due to tonic sympathetic stimulation. Vasodilation is produced by decreasing this sympathetic stimulation since skin vessels do not receive vasodilatory parasympathetic fibers. However, parasympathetic stimulation to sweat glands results in the liberation of *bradykinin*, a polypeptide with vasodilator properties (see Chapter 12). It is thought that diffusion of this material into the perivascular space aids in the dilation of local vessels as part of the response to an increase in body temperature.

Local application of cold to the skin results in vasoconstriction and may reduce blood flow to the affected area to a very low level. In a cold environment, this may lead to tissue damage due to freezing. It is interesting that the application of cold for a prolonged period of time may, however, produce vasodilation and lead to localized areas of skin redness. It has been suggested that this rosy color, particularly in the face and nose, probably results more from the reduced oxygen extraction by the cold skin than from an increase in tissue blood flow. However, the precise mechanism for this reaction is not known. The local application of heat, in contrast, leads to vasodilation and an increase in skin blood flow. This reaction is initiated by temperature receptors in the skin and at first may be localized to the area of increased temperature. However, as warmed venous blood returns to the brain, general reflex vasodilation occurs.

The sympathetic supply to the cutaneous blood vessels of the face, neck, and upper thorax are especially sensitive to modulation by the higher brain centers. Embarrassment may lead to vasodilation and blushing, while anger, fear, or anxiety may be accompanied by vasoconstriction and loss of the normal skin coloration.

SKIN MICROCIRCULATION AND HEAT TRANSFER

Under conditions of normothermia, skin blood flow is predominantly controlled by tissue metabolic factors. However, under conditions of heat stress, sympathetic input to both the resistance vessels and the large arteriovenous anastomotic vessels is reduced, the vessels dilate, and skin blood flow is markedly increased.

The anastomotic blood vessels are not involved in the local metabolic control of blood flow, and they do not show autoregulation. However, opening of these vessels in response to reflexes from heat sensitive receptors both in the skin and in hypothalamic centers permits a large proportion of the warm arterial blood to bypass the capillary network. The high heat conductivity of the tissues then permits the effective transfer of this heat to the skin as the blood travels directly to the venous system.

FUNCTIONAL ASPECT OF THE SKIN CIRCULATION

While β-adrenergic receptors have been reported for cutaneous vascular smooth muscles of the nutrient arterioles, all skin resistance vessels act as though they have only α-adrenergic receptors. Vasoconstriction is produced by both epinephrine and norepinephrine, and maximal blood flow results after sympathetic blockage. In addition, sympathetic stimulation causes constriction of both large and small veins. These vessels apparently have their own nervous supply as they can constrict independently of the arteriolar vessels.

Blood vessels in the skin may become overly sensitive to nervous vasoconstrictive influences. In *Raynaud's phenomenon*, for example, there may be severe vasospasm of the skin vessels that leads to pain, skin changes (especially of the hands), and even tissue necrosis. Following exposure to cold or frostbite, the skin vessels may become sensitized to recurring exposure to low temperatures and respond by localized constriction of surface vessels and production of burning and itching sensations. This condition, sometimes called *chilblains*, may become chronic and cause considerable discomfort.

SUMMARY

Blood flow to the brain, heart, kidneys, and skin are summarized in this chapter as illustrative of the special features needed to meet the vascular requirements of different vascular beds. In the discussion of each organ system, emphasis has been given to the principles of cardiovascular function and regulation of the circulation presented in earlier chapters.

BIBLIOGRAPHY

Abboud FM, Heistad DD (eds): Regulation of the cerebral circulation. *Fed Proc* 1981; 40:2296.

Berne RM, Rubio R: Acute coronary occlusion: Early changes that induce coronary dilation and the development of collateral circulation. *Am J Cardiol* 1969; 24:776.

Chapman WH, Bulger RE, et al: *The Urinary System: An Integrated Approach.* Philadelphia, WB Saunders Co, 1973.

Feigl EO: Parasympathetic control of coronary blood flow in dogs. *Circ Res* 1969; 25:509.

Feigl EO: Sympathetic control of coronary circulation. *Circ Res* 1967; 20:262.

Folkow B, Neil R: *Circulation.* New York, Oxford University Press, 1971.

Gregg DE: The coronary circulation, in Best CH, Taylor NW (eds): *The Physiological Basis of Medical Practice*, ed 8. Philadelphia, Williams & Wilkins Co, 1966.

Helvig EB, Mostofi FK (eds): *The Skin.* New York, RE Krieger Co, 1980.

Kontos HA: Regulation of the Cerebral Circulation. *Annu Rev Physiol* 1981; 43:397.

Kontos HA: Mechanism of regulation of the cerebral microcirculation. *Curr Concepts Cerebrovasc Dis* 1975; 10:7.

McHenry LS Jr: Cerebral blood flow measurements and regulation in man. *Curr Concepts Cerebrovasc Dis* 1976; 11:1.

Needleman P: The synthesis and function of prostaglandins in the heart. *Fed Proc* 1976; 35:2376.

Rayford CR, Khouri EM, Gregg DE: Effects of excitement on coronary and systemic energetics in unanesthetized dogs. *Am J Physiol* 1965; 209:680.

Renkin EM, Robinson RR: Glomerular filtration. *N Engl J Med* 1974; 290:785.

Rosenblum EI: Neurogenic control of cerebral circulation. *Stroke* 1971; 2:429.

Rouleau J, Boerboom LE, et al: The role of autoregulation and tissue diastolic pressure in the transmural distribution of left ventricular blood flow in anesthetized dogs. *Circ Res* 1979; 45:804.

Scheinberg PS, et al: Cerebral circulation and metabolism in stroke. *Stroke* 1976; 7:213.

Stein PM, MacAnespie CL, et al: Total body vascular capacitance changes during high intracranial pressure in dogs. *Am J Physiol* 1983; 245:H947.

Vander AJ: *Renal Physiology.* New York, McGraw-Hill Book Co, 1975.

Wilken DEL: Local factors controlling coronary circulation. *Am J Cardiol* 1983; 52:8A–14A.

Chapter 15 _____

Response of the Heart and Circulation to Stress

_____

An efficient method for studying circulatory regulation is to apply a specific stress and observe the compensatory mechanisms that operate to maintain blood flow equal to the needs of the body. A summary of the dynamic events that follow such a maneuver will serve both as a review of the compensatory mechanisms discussed individually in earlier chapters and perhaps more important, as an illustration of the close coordination that is required for these mechanisms to maintain circulatory integrity. In this chapter, two types of disturbances will be discussed: (1) the normal stress placed on the circulation by muscular exercise and (2) the abnormal stress of a sudden blood loss such as occurs with a major hemorrhage.

MUSCULAR EXERCISE

The response of the body to muscular exercise involves most, if not all, of the organ systems. Active muscles, for example, must receive sufficient oxygen and energy-rich substrate to meet their metabolic needs, while the by-products of that activity must be removed. These wastes include carbon dioxide, a variety of breakdown products of cellular metabolism such as lactic acid and polypeptide metabolites, electrolytes such as potassium, and a significant amount of heat. To meet these requirements for oxygen and energy substrate, the rate and depth of respiration must be closely regulated, the absorption and intermediary metabolism of food must be controlled, and the removal of waste products becomes of prime importance. At the same time, body temperature and pH must be maintained within physiologic limits. Finally, a fine degree of neuromuscular control is required to coordinate the mechanical results of muscle actions. These activities must all be accomplished without disruption of the organism's vital activities. Such multiorgan system adjustments are complicated and in some cases not entirely understood. Our attention is directed here to the circulatory system. Information on the activities of other organ systems is included only as it relates directly to cardiovascular function.

Oxygen Consumption

While working muscles are able to anaerobically utilize the energy of adenosine triphosphate (ATP) and creatine phosphate, intramuscular stores of these materials are limited, and their resynthesis requires oxidative metabolism. Thus, the performance of muscular work ultimately depends on the transport of oxygen to the muscle mitochondria. For this reason, oxygen consumption, usually expressed as liters of oxygen per minute ($\dot{V}_{O_2}$), becomes a reliable measure of muscular activity (Table 15–1). Early studies showed that when an individual was subjected to increasing work levels, $\dot{V}_{O_2}$ increased with the severity of the work until it finally plateaued at a

TABLE 15–1.

Average Energy Cost of Muscular Exercise (Sedentary Adult)

Type of Activity	MRER*	Energy Utilized	
		Oxygen Consumption (ml/min)	Calories/Min†
Supine, at rest	1.0	250	1.21
Slow walking (1.0 mile/hr)	1.7	438	2.11
Walking (3.0 mile/hr)	3.5	875	4.22
Tennis—doubles	4.5	1,125	5.42
Walking (4.0 mile/hr)	5.5	1,375	6.62
Tennis—singles	6.5	1,625	7.83
Jogging (5.0 mile/hr)	7.5	1,875	9.03
Running (5.5 mile/hr)	8.5	2,125	10.24
Competitive handball	10.0	2,500	12.05

*Multiple of resting energy requirement; i.e., 2 MRER indicates twice the rest energy is utilized.
†One liter O_2 = 4.82 calories.
Data, in part, from Zohman LR: *Beyond Diet: Exercise Your Way to Fitness and Heart Health.* Coventry, Conn, CPC International Inc, 1974, and Judy WV: Physiology of exercise in Selkurt EE: *Physiology,* ed 4. Boston, Little, Brown & Co, 1976.

maximal value. This maximal oxygen consumption ($m\dot{V}_{O_2}$), while subject to improvement with physical conditioning, is a rather constant and reproducible measurement for a given person.

Average sedentary adults performing muscular work on a treadmill are able to increase their $\dot{V}_{O_2}$ to about 10 times their rest level and obtain $m\dot{V}_{O_2}$ of approximately 2.5 L/minute (Table 15–2). Outstanding athletes, however, are able to do much better and can increase their $\dot{V}_{O_2}$ as much as 24 or 25 times. In fact, values of 6 or 7 L/minute are often obtained. For this reason, $m\dot{V}_{O_2}$ is used as a functional index of the ability to do muscular work. In normal individuals, the limiting factor for $m\dot{V}_{O_2}$ does not appear to be either the ability of the pulmonary system to supply oxygen or the capacity of the muscles to use it; rather, $m\dot{V}_{O_2}$ is determined by the ability of the circulation to deliver oxygen to the working muscles.

Delivery of Oxygen

Transport of oxygen from the pulmonary capillaries to active muscular tissues depend on (1) oxygen-carrying capacity of blood, (2) magnitude of blood flow, and (3) ability of the tissues to extract oxygen from capillary blood. The ability of blood to transport oxygen is primarily a function of the oxygen-carrying capacity of hemoglobin and the amount of that substance present in the blood, while tissue blood flow depends on the interaction among vascular resistance, arterial pressure, and cardiac output. The output of the heart per minute is, in turn, a function of heart rate and

TABLE 15–2.

Effect of Work Load on Cardiovascular Parameters (Average Steady-State Values)*

	Level of Work (kg/min)		
	600	900	1,400
$\dot{V}_{O_2}$ (L/min)	1.50	2.17	3.46
% $m\dot{V}_{O_2}$	44	63	100
Heart rate (beats/min)	115	154	186
Stroke volume (ml)	112	125	127
Cardiac output (L/min)	12.9	19.2	23.7
Arterial pressure (mm Hg) (mean)	150/68 (95)	169/66 (99)	187/75 (113)
Total peripheral resistance	0.0052	0.0051	0.0043
Lactic acid (mEq/L)	2.78	5.28	12.55
Arteriovenous O_2 difference (vol %)	10.8	11.4	14.6

*Data from Stenberg J, Ekblom B, Messin R: *J Appl Physiol* 1966; 21:1589.

stroke volume. Unloading of oxygen from hemoglobin in the microcirculation and its diffusion to tissues depend on physical factors present in the
capillary vessels. Each of these factors will be discussed individually.

Oxygen Carriage in Blood.—Each liter of arterial blood normally contains about 2.9 ml of dissolved oxygen and 195 ml of oxygen loosely bound
to the hemoglobin contained in the red blood cells. The chemistry of oxygen carriage by hemoglobin is beyond the scope of this chapter; however,
the following will serve as a brief summary. Oxygen is loosely bound to
the hemoglobin molecule. The major factors that affect this binding are the
partial pressure of oxygen (P_{O_2}) temperature, pH, and the presence of 2,3-
diphosphoglycerate (2,3-DPG), a by-product of glucose metabolism, that
decreases the affinity of hemoglobin for oxygen. In the lungs, hemoglobin
readily accepts oxygen due to the high level of alveolar P_{O_2} and the biochemical events associated with the movement of carbon dioxide into the
pulmonary system. In the microcirculation of active muscles, the normal
unloading of oxygen is facilitated by (1) a low tissue P_{O_2}, (2) increased
temperature (it may reach 40°C in exercising muscles), (3) decreased pH
due to the liberation of acid metabolites and carbon dioxide by the tissue,
and (4) an increased level of 2,3-DPG.

Muscle Blood Flow.—During intense exercise, oxygen consumption by
skeletal muscles may increase to as much as 50 or 60 times rest level. The
amount of oxygen that can be supplied by deoxygenation of capillary
blood, however, is limited so that supplemental oxygen must be provided
by increasing muscle blood flow. In this way, the extraction of oxygen per
unit of blood as described above and the number of such units per minute
are both increased.

The mechanism responsible for the increased blood flow to active muscles has been the subject of intense study. The weight of current evidence
suggests that, at least at the onset of exercise, the increased flow occurs as
a result of central nervous system action. For example, anticipation or
preparation for exercise will usually result in (1) activation of cholinergic
sympathetic vasodilator fibers with relaxation of arterioles in the muscles to
be used and (2) stimulation of medullary sympathetic centers and inhibition
of parasympathetic cardiac inhibitory centers. This will result in a modest
increase in the heart rate and augmentation of cardiac output.

Shortly after the onset of muscular work, there may be a further increase in heart rate, cardiac output, and blood pressure, perhaps as a result
of local reflexes from active muscles and joints. Moreover, because of the
liberation of vasoactive metabolites by the contracting muscles and autoregulation of their vascular bed, sympathetic vasoconstrictor input to these

active tissues is overcome and the resistance vessels dilate. The result is that the centrally mediated vasoconstriction in other vascular beds is counterbalanced, and there is a net fall in total peripheral vascular resistance (Fig 15–1). This causes blood to be diverted to the active muscles where flow may reach as much as 20 times that of normal.

Relaxation of precapillary arterioles in the active muscles permits previously underperfused capillaries to fill. This leads to a marked increase in the surface area available for interchange between blood and extracellular fluid. At the same time, postcapillary resistance undergoes only minor changes so that capillary pressure in the active muscles remains high and filtration is facilitated. At moderate or greater levels of work, this results in a significant increase in muscular interstitial fluid and lymph flow. Movement of fluid out of the vascular system under these conditions may be sufficient to reduce the circulating plasma volume as much as 10% to 12%. The hemoconcentration produced by this movement of fluid may help in the carriage of oxygen to active muscles, but this is probably offset by the coincident increase in vascular resistance produced by the greater viscosity of the blood. The reduction in plasma volume with muscle work may be

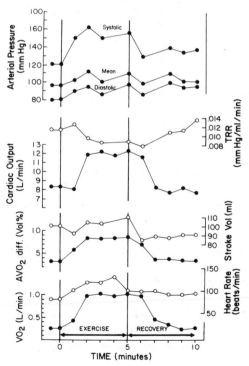

FIG 15–1.
Average cardiovascular parameters before, during, and after light exercise in four human subjects. (Data from Donald KW, Bishop JM, Cumming G, et al: *Clin Sci* 1955; 14:37.)

exacerbated by excess sweating (see below), particularly when exercise is carried out in a warm, humid environment.

Tissue Extraction of Oxygen.—The factors discussed above that facilitate the unloading of oxygen from hemoglobin are increased during exercise. As a result, the extraction of oxygen from the circulation by working muscles can be increased to more than three times basal levels. This means that the arteriovenous oxygen difference across active skeletal muscles may increase to as much as 13.8 ml of oxygen per 100 ml of blood. The myocardium is an exception to this mechanism. As discussed in Chapter 14, cardiac extraction of oxygen is always at or near maximal. As a result, the heart must depend on increased coronary blood flow to augment its oxygen supply.

Muscle Blood Volume.—The volume of blood required to fill the muscle capillaries and small veins in active skeletal muscles that are perfused as a consequence of vasodilation may equal 1 to 1.5 ml/100 gm of tissue. As a normal adult may have 35 to 45 kg of muscle, the extra volume contained in the active muscles may equal several hundred milliliters of fluid. The rapid removal of this blood from active circulation at the onset of muscular activity, as a result of storage in muscle capillaries, could result in a serious loss of venous return if a compensatory constriction of the venous reservoir did not occur. The mechanism for this reduction in venous volume is probably a vascular reflex triggered from the venous pressor receptors in the vena cava, right heart, and pulmonary artery (see Chapter 10).

Nonmuscle Blood Flow.—To maintain sufficient blood flow during exercise for physiologic function in essential nonmuscular vascular beds, local autoregulation quickly acts to counter the generalized increase in vasoconstrictive sympathetic tone. As a result, cerebral blood flow remains essentially normal during even heavy exercise. However, the combination of vasoconstriction of nonessential vascular beds and vasodilation of arterioles in active muscles shunts the unused flow plus the increased cardiac output to the active tissues. Coronary blood flow increases in proportion to the increase in myocardial work and with heavy exercise may increase from three to five times.

Kidney blood flow is markedly reduced during exercise. In recent animal studies, for example, renal blood flow was reduced from a total of 9% of the cardiac output at rest to 2% with light work and 0.5% with heavy exercise. This reduction in renal perfusion is at least a partial explanation for the reduction in urine formation that accompanies heavy work.

Venous Return, Stroke Volume, and Cardiac Output.—The increase in muscle blood flow and massaging action of muscular contractions during exercise leads, particularly when the body is in the upright posture, to a marked increase in venous return to the heart. The greater cardiac filling, in turn, leads to increased ventricular end-diastolic volume and augmentation of cardiac stroke volume via the Frank-Starling "heterometric" mechanism. At the same time, the increased sympathetic discharge provides inotropic stimulation to the myocardium to increase cardiac contractility. This "homeometric" mechanism produces an increase in both stroke volume and ejection fraction so that heart size may actually be reduced. The comparative roles of venous return, the inotropic effect of sympathetic stimulation, and the Frank-Starling mechanism (the chronotropic effect is discussed below) in producing the increased cardiac output of muscular exercise are not settled (see Chapter 7); however, they are clearly interrelated, and all play a part.

Heart Rate.—The increase in heart rate that begins just before or simultaneously with the onset of muscular exercise reaches a peak value for that level of work within 15 to 20 seconds. This initial tachycardia results primarily from a reduction in vagal impulses to the sinoatrial (SA) node (see above). During the next 10 to 15 seconds, the heart rate frequently slows slightly (i.e., 10 to 15 beats per minute) before undergoing a secondary increase to its steady-state level, which is reached after 1 or 2 minutes.

The tachycardia of exercise occurs despite the associated increase in blood pressure (see below). This suggests that the baroreceptor reflexes, which normally respond to an elevated arterial pressure by slowing the heart rate, fail to operate during muscular exercise. In fact animal studies have shown that the same steady-state heart rate is obtained with exercise before and after denervation of the carotid and aortic baroreceptors. It is interesting to speculate that the brief dip in heart rate in normal individuals shortly after the onset of exercise described above may reflect an abortive effect of the baroreceptor reflex.

With increased levels of muscular work, the heart rate increases linearly up to the maximal obtainable rate. This value is the same for normal men and women and can be approximated by subtracting the individual's age from 220. As discussed earlier, the time available for cardiac filling is progressively reduced as the heart rate increases. As a result, the effectiveness of venous return in increasing the stroke volume will be inversely related to the heart rate. It is, therefore, not surprising that with increasing levels of work, the stroke volume will soon reach a maximum value. This occurs at a level of exercise that requires a $\dot{V}_{O_2}$ of approximately 40% of the $m\dot{V}_{O_2}$. With work loads above that level, further increases in cardiac output then occur only as the result of the additional increase in heart rate.

This relationship between heart rate and level of exercise has been used in physical conditioning. It has been suggested, for example, that in a normal individual a level of exercise sufficient to promote physical fitness will result in a heart rate 70% to 80% of the maximal attainable rate. This level of work turns out to require between 60% to 80% of the $m\dot{V}_{O_2}$. Most authorities suggest that a maximum of 20 to 30 minutes of exercise at this level three times a week is needed for cardiovascular conditioning.

Cardiac Output.—The cardiac output of an average adult increases in a linear fashion with the intensity of muscular work and reaches a maximum of about four times the basal level with exhausting exercise (see Table 15–2).

As indicated above, this increase results from the combination of a larger stroke volume and an increase in heart rate. At low levels of work the increase in cardiac output comes primarily from the increase in stroke volume, while at high work levels the major factor is the increase in heart rate. For reasons that are not clear, the point at which these factors are equal, usually at 40% to 50% of maximal oxygen uptake, tends to move to high work levels with physical conditioning. Thus, the same work load will lead to a lower heart rate in a "trained" individual than in one who is not physically fit.

Arterial Blood Pressure.—The arterial blood pressure starts to increase at the beginning of muscular exercise coincident with the increased heart rate and reaches a steady-state value that parallels the level of work performed. Systolic pressure and the pulse pressure both increase (see Fig 15–1) as a result of the large cardiac output, while diastolic pressure increases only slightly or may not change because of the increased runoff through the microcirculation of the active muscles.

Core Temperature.—Continuation of active muscular work leads to the liberation of a significant amount of heat and an increase in body temperature. Elevation of the core temperature, in turn, stimulates hypothalamic centers to reflexly inhibit the normal vasoconstrictive sympathetic impulses to skin arterioles and arteriovenous shunts. As a result, these vessels dilate, cutaneous blood flow increases, and the heat content of the perfusing blood is lost by convection and radiation from the skin. If this mechanism for heat loss is insufficient and the core temperature continues to increase, sweating begins. These compensatory mechanisms that operate to maintain the normal body temperature counteract the central vasoconstriction of cutaneous blood vessels. As a result, cutaneous arterioles lose their vasoconstrictive tone and skin blood flow returns to normal or, depending on the degree of exercise, to greater than normal levels. As a result of this vasodilation, there will be some diversion of blood flow from the active muscles unless it can be prevented by further constriction of arterioles elsewhere in the body.

Cardiac Size and the Effect of Exercise

A number of studies have shown that trained athletes regularly performing endurance exercise frequently have a larger cardiac mass than matched sedentary controls. The increase in cardiac size, which in the absence of heart disease is usually not excessive, apparently develops in response to the volume load associated with the increased stroke volume. The larger myocardial mass then acts to reduce the cardiac wall tension required for cardiac ejection (see Chapter 8). This mechanism serves to at least partially compensate for the greater systolic tension required via the Laplace relationship because of the increased end-diastolic volume. The larger myocardial mass, however, does not lead to an increase in oxidative metabolism as occurs with hypertrophy of skeletal muscle, although there may be some increase in cardiac adenosine triphosphatase (ATPase) activity.

Earlier histologic studies reported that the density of myocardial capillaries decreased in hypertrophied hearts. This suggested that the blood supply available for the larger myocardial fibers would be reduced. Findings from recent animal studies have now put these observations in question and suggest that cardiac hypertrophy due to chronic exercise may increase the ratio of capillaries to myocardial cells. As a result, it now appears that the mild cardiac hypertrophy that develops as a result of training may improve the oxygen supply to the myocardium. This factor could contribute to the superior performance of world class athletes. In contrast, marked cardiac enlargement, the so-called "athletic heart," is still considered a pathologic response to exercise.

SUMMARY

The mechanisms that operate to maintain the circulation during muscular exercise and their interrelationships are summarized in the block diagram shown in Figure 15-2. The dynamic nature of these circulatory events requires close integration with the activities of the other organ systems. As a result, the effect of exercise on the heart and circulation cannot be separated from the total response of the body.

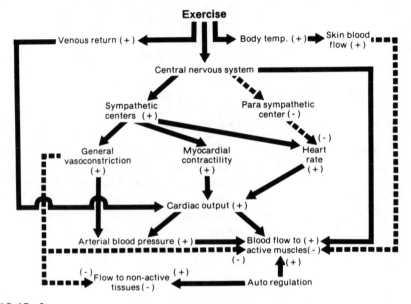

FIG 15–2.
Schematic diagram of the major factors that operate to maintain the circulation during muscular exercise. Increased activity is shown by *solid lines,* decreased activity by *dashed lines.* See text for discussion.

CIRCULATORY RESPONSE TO BLOOD LOSS

Compensatory Mechanisms

The compensatory mechanisms that operate to immediately stabilize the circulation after an acute hemorrhage are summarized in Figure 15–3. If the loss of blood is promptly stopped and the hemorrhage has not been excessive, these reactions usually are adequate to return the blood pressure to at least near-normal range and to provide for perfusion of vital tissues. In fact, the immediate adjustments that follow a donation of 250 to 500 ml of blood to a blood bank are so effective that, in most instances, arterial pressure is only momentarily disturbed, if at all, and untoward side effects are rarely encountered. These acute compensatory reactions provide time for restoration of body fluid stores over the next few hours and the somewhat slower regeneration of proteins, blood cells, and other blood constituents.

Hypovolemic Shock

If the compensatory mechanisms set in play following a loss of circulating blood volume are not adequate to maintain cardiac output and arterial

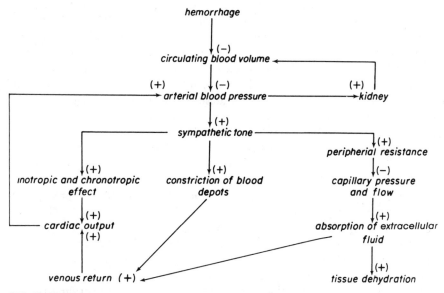

FIG 15–3.
Schematic diagram of acute compensatory reactions that operate to maintain arterial blood pressure following a hemorrhage. (+) = increased activity; (−) = decreased activity. See text for discussion.

blood pressure falls, the condition of hypovolemic shock develops. As most of the signs and symptoms of this syndrome result from the full development of the compensatory mechanisms, their circulatory responses will be summarized as part of the discussion of hypovolemic (circulatory) shock.

An acute loss of circulating blood volume leads to a reduction in baroreceptor input to the brain stem and, as a result, a corresponding increase in the activity of the sympathetic nervous system. If arterial pressure falls to low levels, this sympathetic activity is augmented by facilitatory impulses from the arterial chemoreceptors. These receptors are stimulated by the local tissue hypoxia that results from the decrease in their blood supply. Increased sympathetic discharge causes three general types of cardiovascular reactions: (1) Generalized arteriolar constriction occurs particularly in the skin and to a lesser extent in the viscera and muscles (see above). This increase in peripheral resistance limits capillary flow in these tissues and tends to raise arterial pressure by retaining blood in the arterial system. Because of the relatively minor constriction of the resistance vessels in the brain and heart (coronary arterioles actually may dilate), the outflow from the arterial system is preferentially shifted to these organs and their perfusion is maintained at the expense of the other tissues. (2) Constriction of the capacitance vessels, particularly those in the viscera and intrathoracic area, squeezes the blood normally stored in these depot areas into the active circulation. (3) The heart rate and level of myocardial contractility increase. These positive chronotropic (heart rate) and inotropic (contractility) effects serve to maintain cardiac output by increasing both the rate and vigor of myocardial contraction. The increased contractile force also tends to empty the heart more completely, and as a result, some of the blood normally stored as end-systolic ventricular volume is put in active circulation. This mobilization of stored and slowly circulating reserve blood from the capacitance vessels and other storage areas has been called *"autotransfusion."*

The drop in capillary perfusion pressure that follows the loss of blood volume and the constriction of the resistance vessels lead to a reduction in capillary filtration. This reduction is accentuated in some tissues because arterioles constrict more than do venules and the ratio between precapillary and postcapillary resistance increases. The change in normal capillary dynamics leads to a net movement of interstitial fluid into the vascular compartment. This reabsorption of fluid and electrolytes acts to restore the circulating volume without adding blood cells or osmotically active plasma proteins. For this reason, it has been called *"autoinfusion."*

The amount of fluid that can be mobilized by reabsorption from the interstitial space is limited by the dilution of plasma proteins and the corresponding reduction in oncotic pressure. Nevertheless, this volume can represent as much as 2 to 3 ml/100 gm of soft tissue. With severe hypotension and maximal vasoconstriction, this mechanism can mobilize up to 1 L of fluid per hour and reduce the level of plasma proteins as much as 27%.

The generalized reduction in capillary filtration that follows a loss of blood becomes of particular importance to the function of the kidneys. If the reduction in arterial pressure is only moderate, the intrinsic autoregulatory mechanism of the kidney tends to maintain renal blood flow. However, with a severe hemorrhage the intense vasoconstriction produced by the sympathetic stimulation to these organs may reduce glomerular filtration to the point that urine flow is severely reduced or stopped entirely. This has the compensatory effect of saving water and electrolytes to replace the depleted vascular volume. However, if the renal ischemia persists for too long a period, it may lead to permanent renal difficulties or kidney failure.

The reduction in afferent arteriolar pressure due to renal vasoconstriction also results in the saving of sodium and water via the renin-angiotensin-aldosterone mechanism described in Chapter 7. In addition, the reduction in the size of the extracellular fluid compartment stimulates the thirst mechanism and, operating perhaps through the atrial volume receptors (see Chapter 7), causes the release of antidiuretic hormone from the posterior pituitary. These mechanisms together act to restore the lost fluid volume by stimulating oral ingestion of fluid and further reducing renal loss of water and salt.

Besides producing generalized vasoconstriction, the intense sympathetic stimulation that follows a hemorrhage leads to increased blood levels of the adrenal hormones epinephrine and norepinephrine. These catecholamines reinforce the vasoconstrictive activity of sympathetic stimulation. They also produce metabolic effects such as increased breakdown of liver glycogen and an increase in blood glucose levels as well as protein catabolism to supply material for the synthesis of plasma proteins and blood cells. A marked reduction in visceral blood flow may also produce swelling and dysfunction of liver cells and sloughing of the intestinal mucosa.

The compensatory mechanisms that respond to a loss of blood volume produce as a side effect most of the signs and symptoms observed in man following severe hemorrhage (Table 15–3). For example, the pale, slightly cyanotic color and coolness of the skin reflect intense cutaneous vasoconstriction. The rapid pulse, small pulse pressure, and increased sweat gland activity result from the increased sympathetic stimulation, whereas the sunken features and lack of skin turgor are a result of tissue dehydration.

TABLE 15–3.

Signs and Symptoms Following a Severe Hemorrhage (Hypovolemic Shock) and Their Causes

Signs and Symptoms	Causes
Pale, cyanotic skin color	Vasoconstriction of skin arterioles
Decreased skin temperature	
Tachycardia	Sympathetic stimulation and increased circulating norepinephrine
Sweating	
Weak, thready pulse	Generalized vasoconstriction, reduced cardiac output
Hypotension	
Increased respiratory rate	Chemoreceptor stimulation by anemia, anoxia, and lactic acidosis; lack of inhibition of arterial baroreceptors input to respiratory center
Increased absorption of interstitial fluid and tissue dehydration	Low capillary blood pressure
Reduced urine formation	Constriction of afferent and efferent renal arterioles; increased circulatory aldosterone and vasopressin
Thirst	Loss of extracellular fluid, increased circulating angiotensin II
Dulled sensorium	Cerebral ischemia and acidosis
Collapsed peripheral veins	Reduction in venous return due to autoregulatory pooling of blood in active vascular beds

Increased respiratory activity occurs with a marked drop in arterial pressure as a consequence of chemoreceptor stimulation. The intense thirst, dry mouth, and scanty urine volume also reflect the attempt by the body to replenish its lost fluid volume.

Irreversible Circulatory Shock

Both the volume of blood that can be returned to the active circulation by constriction of the capacitance vessels and blood depots and the amount of fluid that can be mobilized from the interstitial space are limited. If these compensatory reactions are not successful in rapidly restoring the circulating blood volume, the patient will enter a critical stage. Unless external therapy such as intravenous fluids or a transfusion of blood is available at this point, the blood pressure will slowly decline and a state of irreversible circulatory shock will develop.

Recent evidence suggests the metabolic effects of a period of hypotension and cellular anoxia are largely responsible for conversion of circulatory shock into its irreversible form. During prolonged cellular asphyxia, for example, a number of products of tissue damage are released that are deleterious to the circulation. These include vasoactive polypeptides such as bradykinin and substances such as histamine and adenosine, which have vasodepressor actions. A myocardial depressant factor, perhaps working in conjunction with a plasma substance, has recently been identified in the blood of patients in shock. Following hemorrhage, hormones such as renin, vasopressin, and catecholamines are present in increased amounts. The role of prostaglandins, the production of endogenous opiates such as endorphins, and the presence of increased plasma levels of superoxide-free radicals during hypotensive shock are also under investigation. The combined effects of these events are that vascular permeability is increased, vasodilation continues, and the patient remains in shock.

It should be pointed out that the generalized vasoconstriction that follows a loss of blood is a *negative* feedback control reaction. The drop in arterial pressure results in vasoconstriction, which acts to counter (i.e., is opposite in sign) the falling blood pressure. However, if for some reason the compensatory reactions set in motion by a severe hemorrhage are unable to stabilize the circulation and this intense vasoconstriction is maintained for some time, the negative feedback aspect changes and the system becomes a *positive* feedback reaction. Under this circumstance the compensatory system then acts to lower the blood pressure even more.

The reason for the reversal in the feedback effect of vasoconstriction is as follows: The marked reduction in tissue blood flow that follows an intense constriction of the resistance vessels leads, with time, to tissue hypoxia and local accumulation of acid metabolic end products and other vasodilatory substances (see above). Depending on the metabolic activity of the tissue and severity of the reduction in flow, these vasoactive materials eventually reach a level where they override the vasoconstrictor effect of sympathetic stimulation, and both precapillary and postcapillary resistance falls. This permits the capillary bed to fill with blood at the expense of arterial volume, and peripheral runoff is increased. The result is a further fall in arterial blood pressure.

The reduction in arterial pressure due to the opening of local vascular beds acts to intensify the level of sympathetic discharge. In addition, when arterial pressure falls to the point that cerebral blood flow is impaired, a further powerful sympathetic discharge is produced. However, the additional vasoconstriction produced by these mechanisms soon leads to the same local vasodilation and an even further drop in blood pressure. As a consequence, tissue blood flow may be reduced to the point that insufficient oxygen is present to permit entry of pyruvate from the metabolism of glucose into the Krebs cycle and the level of pyruvate increases in the plasma. A severe acidosis then results from the conversion of the pyruvate to lactic acid, which is a strong organic acid. This acidosis may, in turn, depress myocardial contractility and interfere with the vasoconstrictor action of norepinephrine.

The end result of these reactions is a lack of tissue perfusion, cell damage, and ultimately death unless the vicious, positive feedback cycle just described can be promptly broken by effective treatment before tissue damage is irreparable.

Other Forms of Circulatory Shock

Circulatory failure and the symptoms of shock can result from noncirculatory causes such as trauma, infection, acute myocardial infarction, or dehydration. For example, patients with severe infections, often from gram-negative organisms, may develop shock-like symptoms due to peripheral vasodilation, pooling of blood, and a reduction in the effective circulating blood volume. A similar condition may occur with severe dehydration from vomiting, diarrhea, or other causes. Cardiogenic shock caused by a marked acute reduction in cardiac output often accompanies occlusion of one or more coronary vessels and production of an extensive myocardial infarction. While the clinical picture early in these conditions may vary, inadequate blood flow aggravated by increased sympathetic activity and the development of acidosis usually leads to the typical signs and symptoms of circulatory shock.

SUMMARY

The response to the stress of exercise or hemorrhage illustrates the integrated control that regulates the circulation. During exercise, the cardiac output increases to meet the increased skeletal muscle needs for oxygen and substrate. This is accomplished by an increase in heart rate, myocardial contractility, and venous return as well as by changes in the arterial system. During hemorrhage, the arterial pressure is protected by arterial and venous constriction as well as by sympathetically mediated inotropic and sympathetic stimulation of the heart.

BIBLIOGRAPHY

Anderson KL: The cardiovascular system in exercise, in Falls HB (ed): *Exercise Physiology*. New York, Academic Press, 1968.

Astrand PO: Quantification of exercise capability and evaluation of physical capacity in man. *Prog Cardiovasc Dis* 1976; 19:51.

Brengelmann GL: Circulatory adjustments to exercise and heart stress. *Annu Rev Physiol* 1983; 45:191.

Chapman CB (ed): *Physiology of Muscular Exercise*, monograph 15. New York, American Heart Association, 1967.

Clausen JP: Effect of physical training on cardiovascular adjustments to exercise in man. *Physiol Rev* 1977; 57:779.

Lefer AM, Saba TM, Mela LM (eds): *Advances in Shock Research*, vol 1, New York, Liss, 1979.

Miloy P (ed): *The Marathon: Physiological, Medical, Epidemiological and Psychological Studies*. New York, New York Academy of Science, 1977.

Moss GS, Saletta JD: Current concepts: Traumatic shock in man. *N Engl J Med* 1974; 290:724.

Nadel ER: Circulatory and thermal regulations during exercise. *Fed Proc* 1980; 39:1491.

Roskoll WJ, Goldman S, Cohn K: The "athletic heart": Prevalence and physiological significance of left ventricular enlargement in distance runners. *JAMA* 1976; 236:1515.

Rowell LB: Human cardiovascular adjustments to exercise and thermal stress. *Physiol Rev* 1974; 54:75.

Saunders M, Rasmussen S, Cooper D, et al: Renal and intrarenal blood flow distribution in swine during severe exercise. *J Appl Physiol* 1976; 40:932.

Slutsky R: Response of the left ventricle to stress: Effects of exercise, atrial pacing, afterload stress and drugs. *Am J Cardiol* 1981; 47:357.

Smith EE, Guyton AC, Manning RO, et al: Integrated mechanisms of cardiovascular response and control during exercise in the normal human. *Prog Cardiovasc Dis* 1976; 18:421.

Sparks HV: Mechanisms of vasodilation during and after ischemic exercise. *Fed Proc* 1980; 39:1487.

Vatner SF, Pagani M: Cardiovascular adjustments to exercise: Hemodynamics and mechanisms. *Prog Cardiovasc Dis* 1976; 19:91.

Weiner DA: Normal hemodynamic, ventilatory and metabolic response to exercise. *Arch Intern Med* 1983; 143:2173.

Zweifach BW, Fronk A: The interplay of central and peripheral factors in irreversible hemorrhagic shock. *Prog Cardiovasc Dis* 1975; 18:147.

Index

797-1466

Mon.
10:00   Dr. Jame(g) 524-8286

         Dr. Secur - 861-6533
            10:00   831